Education Centre Library
William Harvey Hospital
Kennington Road,
Ashford,
Kent TN24 0LZ

An Outline of Fractures and Dislocations

An Outline of Fractures and Dislocations

David Sutherland Muckle MB BS(Dunelm) FRCS MS MD

Consultant Orthopaedic and Accident Surgeon,
Middlesbrough General Hospital, North Tees,
Hemlington and the Cleveland Nuffield Hospitals;
Research Associate, University of Durham;
Fellow of the British Orthopaedic Association and
the British Orthopaedic Research Society;
Medical Adviser and Medical Instructor to the FIFA;
Member of the Medical Committee of the
Football Association, England; formerly Medical
Adviser and Club Surgeon to Oxford United FC,
Middlesbrough FC and Oxford University FC

WRIGHT

1985   Bristol

© **John Wright & Sons Ltd.** 1985

All Rights Reserved.
No part of this publication may be reproduced,
stored in a retrieval system, or transmitted
in any form or by any means, electronic,
mechanical, photocopying, recording or
otherwise, without the prior permission
of the Copyright owner.

Published by
John Wright & Sons Ltd
Techno House, Redcliffe Way,
Bristol BS1 6NX, England

British Library Cataloguing in Publication Data

Muckle, David Sutherland
   An outline of fractures and dislocations.
   1. Fractures   2. Dislocations
   I. Title
   617'.15   RD101

ISBN 0 7236 0805 9

Education Centre Library
William Harvey Hospital,
Kennington Road,
Ashford,
Kent TN24 0LZ

11316

Typeset by Activity Limited,
Salisbury, Wiltshire

Printed in Great Britain by
John Wright & Sons
(Printing) Ltd at
The Stonebridge Press,
Bristol BS4 5NU

To
Dr Harry Burbidge
Dr John O'Hara
Professor Denys Morgan
Professor Stewart Adams
Professor Frank O'Gorman

Outstanding by Example

Preface

Most students would agree that a textbook should be both interesting and informative, although it is often difficult to enliven the basic scientific literature. In a fresh approach this book has been designed to give a concise visual outline to a subject which relies heavily on observations of movement, posture and deformity as well as those useful albeit limited two-dimensional (black-and-white) photographic shadows called X-rays.

One of the most frequent misconceptions made about orthopaedics is that it is the study of immobility (of bed rest, splints and plasters). Nothing is further from the truth! Those rapid, powerful movements that grace the animal kingdom are the true domain of the orthopaedic practitioner and all treatment has one aim—notably to restore form and function as fully and as quickly as possible.

Remember the triad: diagnosis ... accurate
treatment ... immediate
duration ... minimum

What is the current state of the art? This book intends to sift through the plethora of facts (both old and new) while encouraging the reader to pause, think and research the literature. It has a broad design—for medical, nursing and fellowship students (as a base), as well as general practitioners, radiographers and physiotherapists.

D.S.M.

Acknowledgements

Many people have been involved with the production of this book and I would like to thank them all, with special mention of the following: Margaret Stevenson MA, who typed the manuscript; Julie McHale who gave additional typing and retrieved the many hundreds of X-rays reviewed; J. Hudson for the general support; K. Watson and staff, especially K. Lloyd, at North Tees Photographic Department; K. Goult, Middlesbrough General Hospital Photography Department; Dr Aideen Irwin, Dr William Irwin and staff, Park View, Radiology Clinic, Middlesbrough; K. Whittam and other staff, Department of Radiology, MGH; the staff of the Orthopaedic Department, MGH, Norton Nuffield Hospital and Hemlington Hospital; Louise Hetherington for the line drawings; the following consultants and medical staff who gave permission to use their material: Mr J. W. Hooley (MGH) (*Figs.* 1.8*c,d*; 5.8*h*, 6.11); Mr W. Ellis (N. Tees) (*Fig.* 2.14); Professor C. Burri (Ulm, W. Germany) (*Fig.* 2.17); Mr D. Caird (MGH) (*Figs.* 3.8*c*, 3.9, 5.18, 5.19); Dr W. Granger (MGH) (*Fig.* 4.7*b*); Mr J. Stothard (MGH) (*Fig.* 5.11); Professor R. Szyszkowitz (Graz, Austria) (*Figs.* 6.1*b*, 6.7*a,b*); Mr T. R. Vijaya (MGH) (*Fig.* 7.8*b*); Mr B. Y. Pai (MGH) and Dr R. Krishnan (MGH) (*Fig.* 7.17*b*) and Mr M. Fansa (MGH) (*Fig.* 8.1*b*). Also Mr D. K. Evans (Sheffield) and Medical Education (International) Ltd for *Figs.* 6.1*f*, 6.3*c* and 6.6 (from *Surgery* 1984); Karen Lloyd (*Fig.* 2.10); Johnson & Johnson Ltd, Slough (Orthopaedic Division) (*Fig.* 2.11); Zimmer Ltd (Swindon) (*Fig.* 3.3). The following figures were redrawn from Zimmer *Fractures and Fracture Management* Manual (*Figs.* 5.8*a,b,c*, 7.24*a*, 7.25*a*); *Fig.* 2.13 redrawn from Müller et al. *Manual of Internal Fixation*, Springer-Verlag (see references); *Fig.* 7.1*a–h* redrawn after Peltier (1965) (see references); *Figs.* 1.13, 3.10, 4.8, 7.28, 7.29, 8.1*a* were reproduced from *Injuries in Sport* (1982), Wright PSG (D. S. Muckle); and *Figs.* 3.15*a,b,c,* 7.4, 7.5, 7.6, 7.10, 7.11 from *Femoral Neck Fractures* (1977), Chapman & Hall (D. S. Muckle); *Fig.* 8.2*i* by permission of Mr J. Kenwright (Oxford).

I would like to express my gratitude to the staff of John Wright & Sons Ltd; and to my family (especially Kim) who have been so patient during the preparation of this book.

Contents

1	An introduction to fractures and dislocations	1
2	Principles of treatment	20
3	Complications: local and general	40
4	Injuries to the shoulder, arm and elbow	70
5	Fractures of the forearm, wrist and hand	93
6	Spinal injuries	122
7	Fractures of the pelvis, thigh and knee	137
8	Fractures of the leg, ankle and foot	173
	Bibliography	194
	Index	203

1

An introduction to fractures and dislocations

- **Fractures**

- *A fracture is a break in bone continuity.* It is visible on X-rays provided the correct views are taken and more than 60% of the bony tissue is destroyed.

The type of fracture depends upon:
1. The direction of the force.
2. Its magnitude.
3. The strength and elasticity of the bone.
4. The restraining action of surrounding soft tissues.

Let us consider the following X-rays (*Fig.* 1.1)
The greenstick fracture of the radius in a child (*Fig.* 1.1*a*) is due to a relatively slight force (a fall on to the outstretched hand) in malleable bones; the comminuted fracture of the tibia (*Fig.* 1.1*b*) is in a youth with strong bones subjected to a severe force (in this case a motor cycle accident). Little wonder the soft tissues are extensively damaged, although not visible radiologically; while the fractured neck of femur in the aged (*Fig.* 1.1*c*) occurs with trivial force (such as a slip or stumble) in osteoporotic bones. Thus these three X-rays represent a broad spectrum of age, force and fracture requiring a variety of orthopaedic and rehabilitation managements.

- *When planning therapy remember the patient (age, occupation and general health) as well as the fracture.*

This may seem a very obvious remark but so often the fractured area and X-rays are subjected to the closest scrutiny to the exclusion of all else.

Forces and Types of Fractures

The force can be *direct or indirect* or a combination of the two. Impact energy is dissipated through the tissues like ripples in a pond. Thus many types of bone and soft-tissue injuries occur.

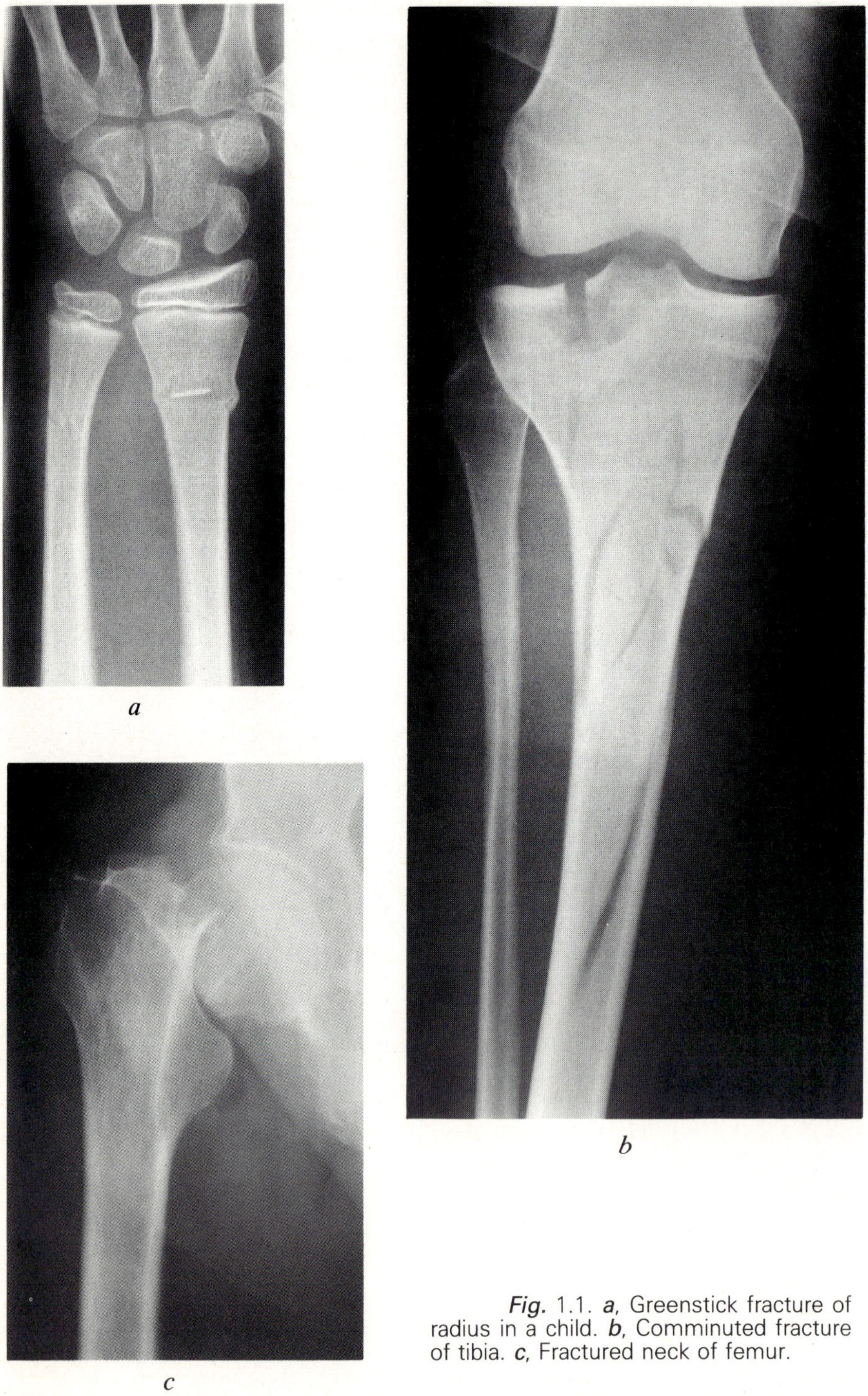

2 An outline of fractures and dislocations

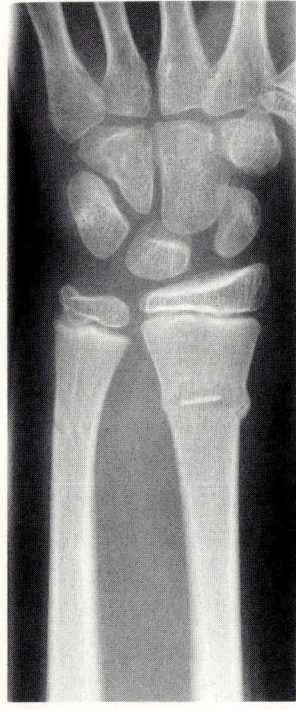

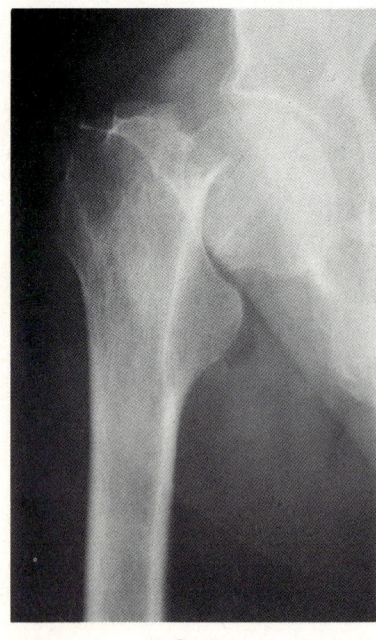

Fig. 1.1. *a*, Greenstick fracture of radius in a child. *b*, Comminuted fracture of tibia. *c*, Fractured neck of femur.

3 An introduction to fractures and dislocations

Radiological Classification

On radiological grounds alone the following classification is merited (*Fig. 1.2*):

Greenstick	Transverse	Pathological
Compression	Oblique	
Stress	Spiral	
Impacted	Comminuted	
Avulsion	Intra-articular	

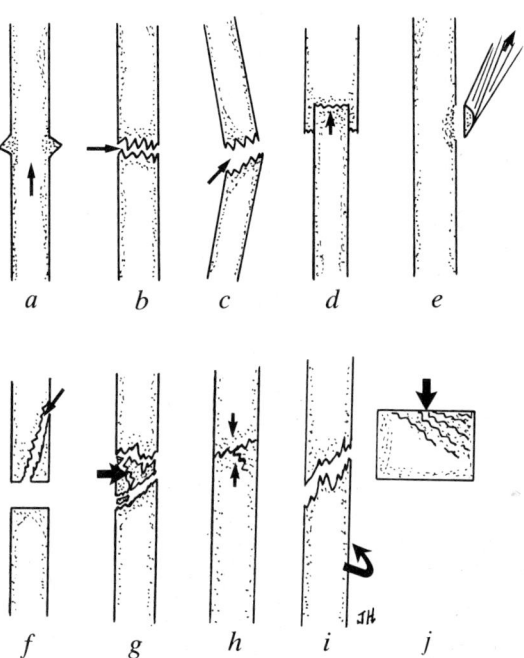

Fig. 1.2. The radiological classification of fractures. *a*, Greenstick. *b*, Transverse. *c*, Oblique. *d*, Impacted. *e*, Avulsion. *f*, Intra-articular. *g*, Comminuted. *h*, Stress. *i*, Spiral. *j*, Compression.

4 An outline of fractures and dislocations

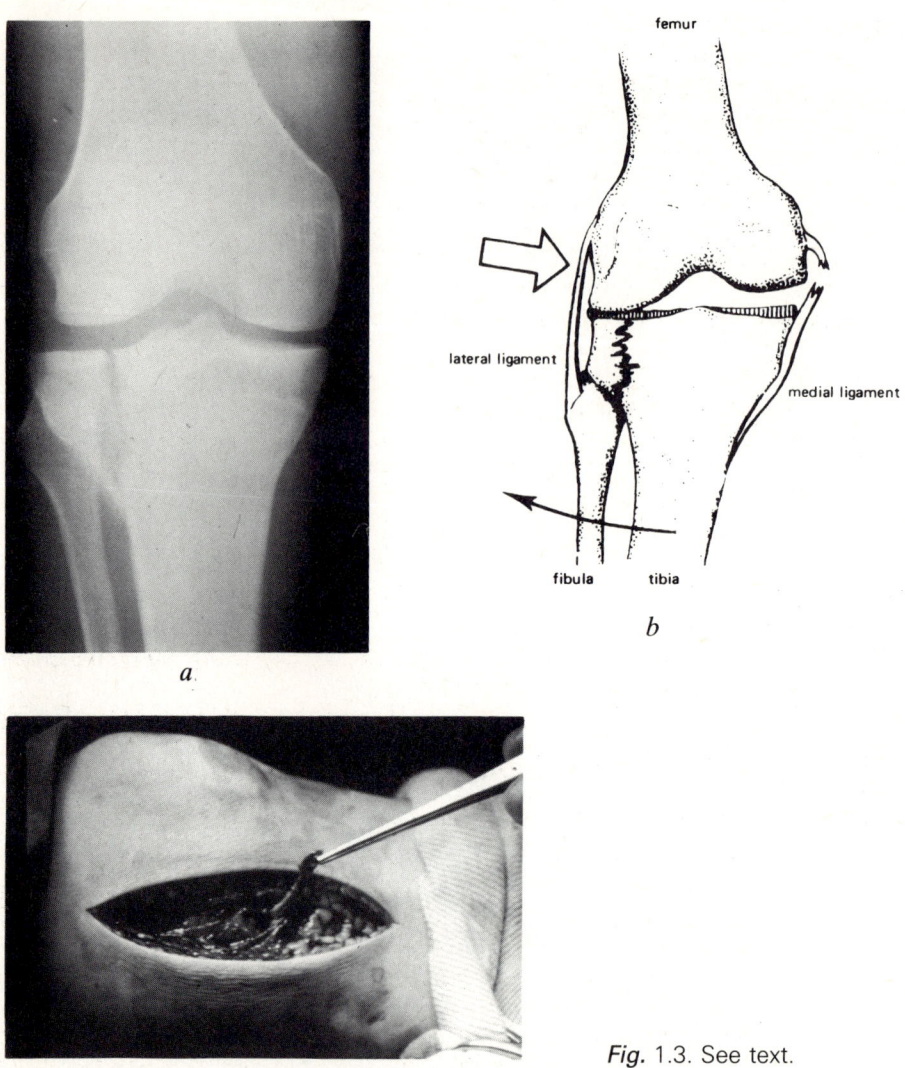

Fig. 1.3. See text.

Fracture Forces and Soft-tissue Injuries (*Fig.* 1.3)

In *Fig.* 1.3*a* the direction of the tibial plateau fracture indicates a vertical force which on consideration (*Fig.* 1.3*b*) has occurred with either stretching or tearing of the medial ligament complex (*Fig.* 1.3*c*). Other soft-tissue injuries will be described later, especially with regard to dislocations.

5 An introduction to fractures and dislocations

Diagnosis

A fracture:
1. Is generally painful.
2. Is associated with loss of function.
3. May have obvious bony deformity.
4. Commonly has associated bleeding and swelling.

- *Always confirm a fracture with an X-ray and not by eliciting movement or crepitus (a painful procedure that adds to the damage).*
- *Relate the injury to the magnitude of the forces involved and, if necessary, investigate thoroughly for pathological causes such as tumour (Fig. 1.4a), metabolic bone disease (e.g. osteomalacia), Paget's disease (Fig. 1.4b) etc. (Fig. 1.4c,d).*
- *Look for vessel and nerve injury reflected in the limb below the fracture level; while cord damage must be excluded in even minor fractures of the vertebrae.*
- *Look for evidence of shock with major long bone or pelvic fractures; as much as 2 litres or more of blood may be lost with femoral and pelvic injuries or when several fractures occur at one time (multiple injuries). Each fracture may lose half a litre into the tissues.*

X-rays

(*The rule of '2'*). X-rays are used to confirm the clinical picture. However, please note that they are only of value if:
1. At least 2 views are taken (usually anteroposterior and lateral) (*Fig. 1.5a,b*).
2. The whole of the injured area is X-rayed, including 2 joints i.e. above and below the fracture (*Figs. 1.5c,d, 5.6, 7.4*).
3. A comparison is made with the uninjured limb (i.e. 2 areas), e.g. to find out the normal epiphyseal development in a child's elbow (*Fig. 1.6*).
4. X-rays are taken at 2 different time intervals e.g. in the wrist and femoral head when avascular necrosis due to cessation of the blood supply may not be evident for several months (*Fig. 1.7*).
5. The extent of comminution is greater at surgery than appears on the X-rays (2 x the damage).
6. And remember that the soft-tissue injuries to muscles, ligaments, tendons and fasciae are not usually visible radiologically unless special films, e.g. arthrograms, are taken (*too often forgotten*).

Ancillary X-rays Investigations

Plain X-rays can be supplemented by special investigations. The most frequently used are shown on pp. 9–11 (*Figs. 1.8a–f, 1.9a–d*).

Although in its infancy and only available at a few medical centres clinical nuclear magnetic resonance imaging is clearly an important development since the study of protons (and other atomic nuclei, e.g. Na23) in a magnetic field gives pictures of better resolution than CT studies.

6 An outline of fractures and dislocations

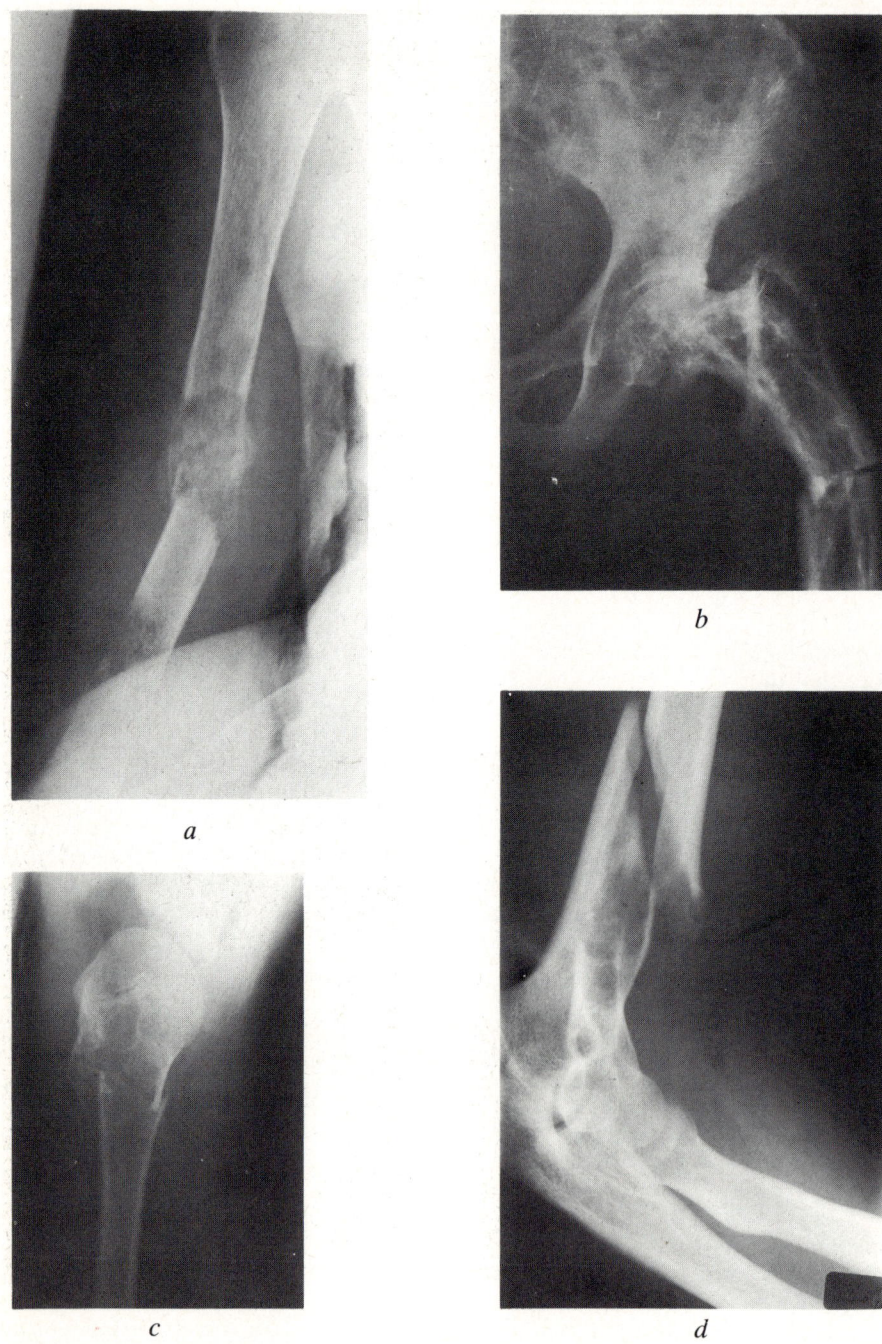

Fig. 1.4. Pathological fractures. *a*, Metastatic lesion (renal) in R humerus. *b*, Paget's disease L upper femur. *c*, Unicameral cyst, upper humerus (12-year-old girl). *d*, Fibrous dysplasia lower humerus (20-year-old man).

7 An introduction to fractures and dislocations

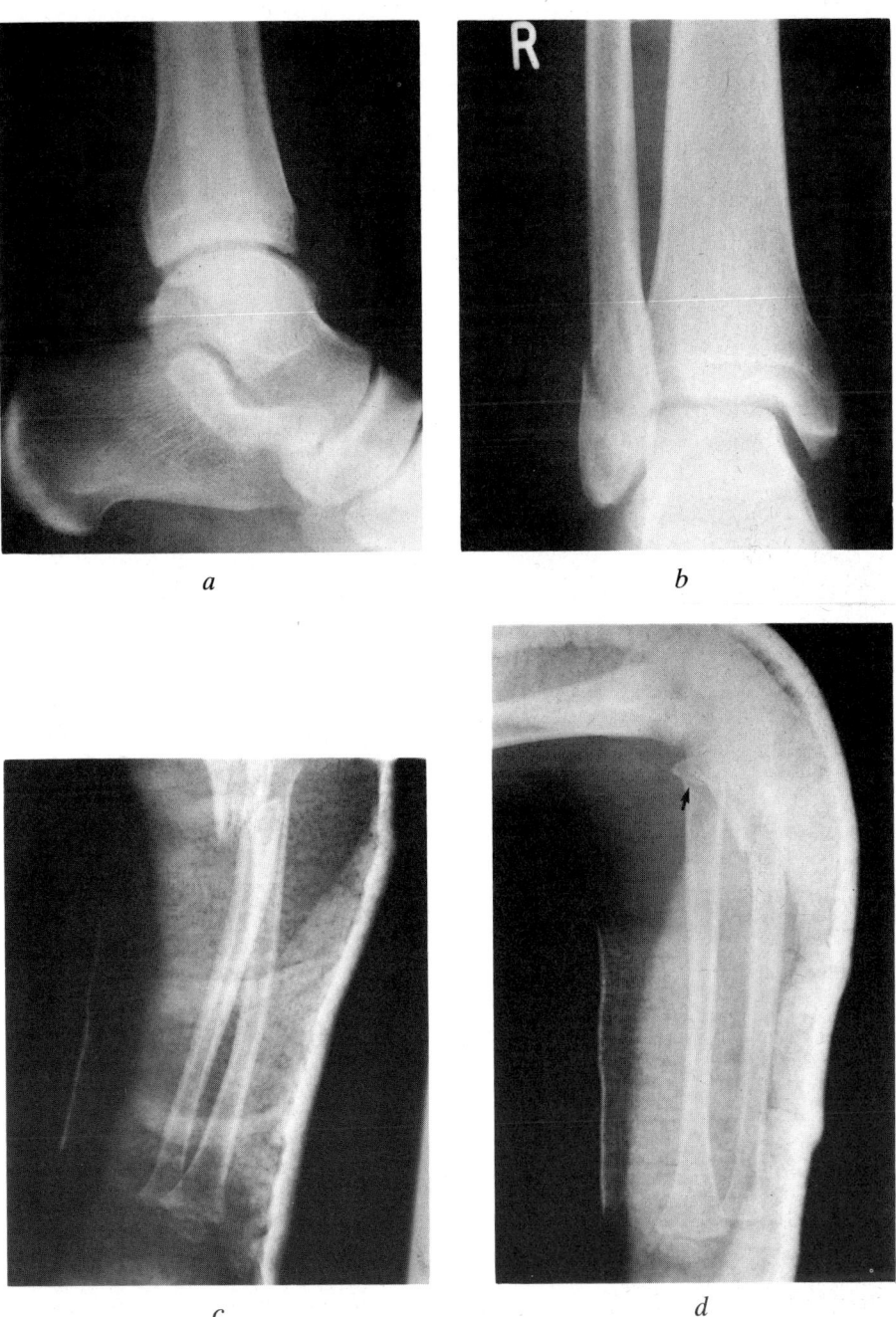

Fig. 1.5. *a*, Lateral view R ankle appears normal. *b*, AP view shows a fractured lateral malleolus. *c*, A fractured ulna in plaster with elbow not visible (5-year-old). *d*, A fractured radial head missed on the first film.

8 An outline of fractures and dislocations

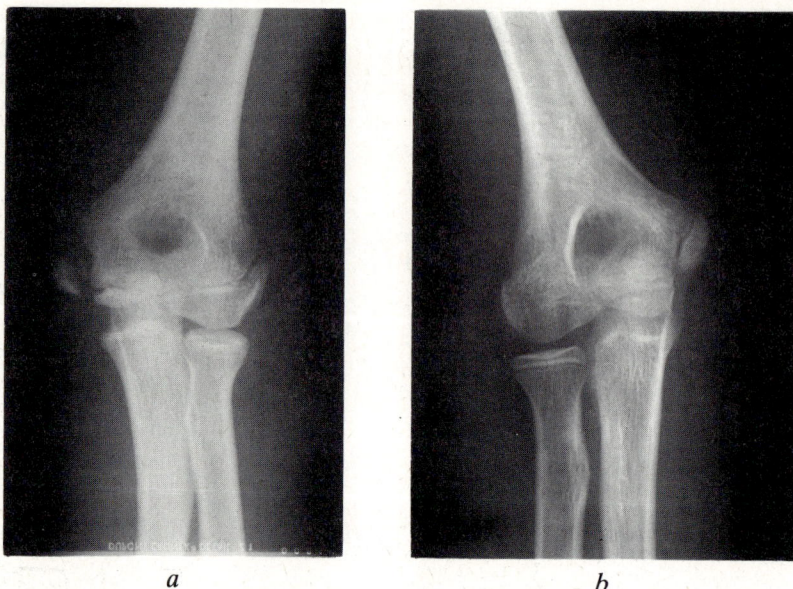

Fig. 1.6. *a*, A fractured L medial epicondyle (15-year-old) with *b*, a comparative film of the other elbow.

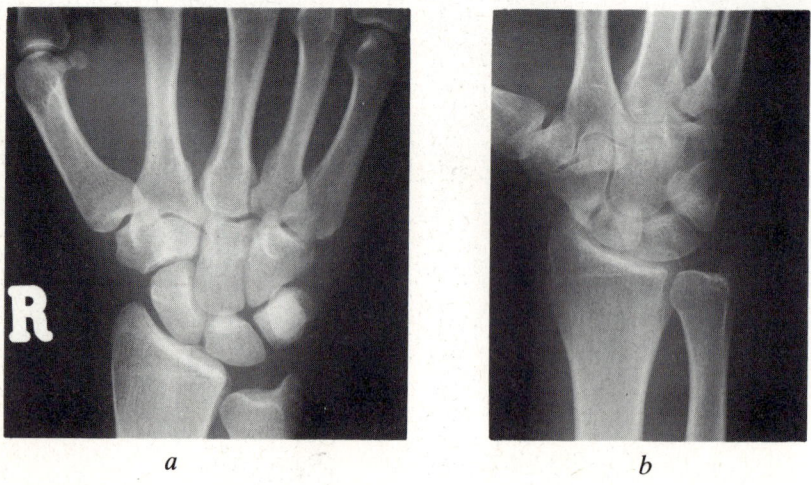

Fig. 1.7. *a*, The first X-ray of a 'sprained wrist' appeared normal. *b*, An X-ray 2 weeks later showed a scaphoid fracture.

9 An introduction to fractures and dislocations

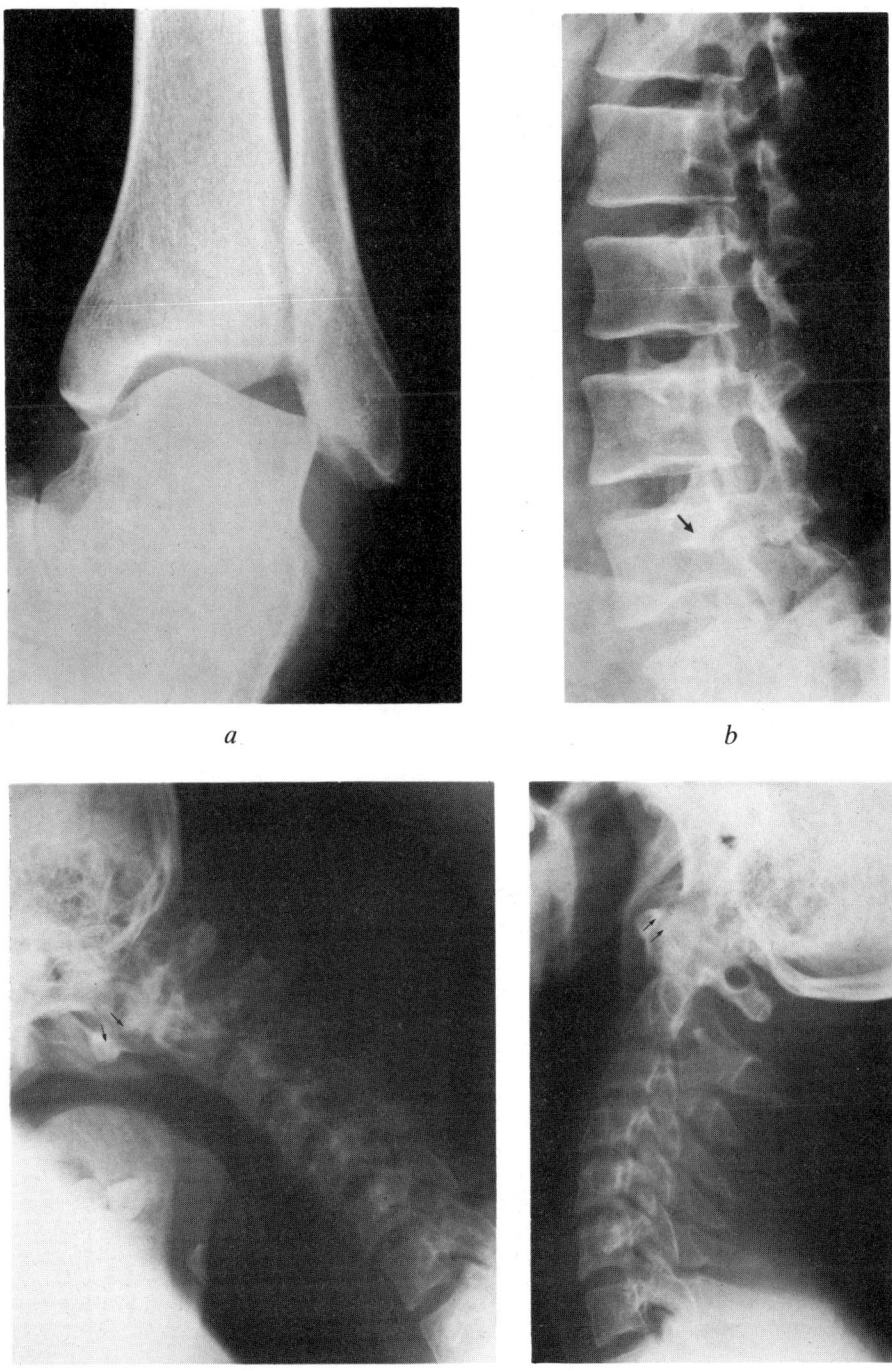

a

b

c1

c2
(*See over for caption*)

10 An outline of fractures and dislocations

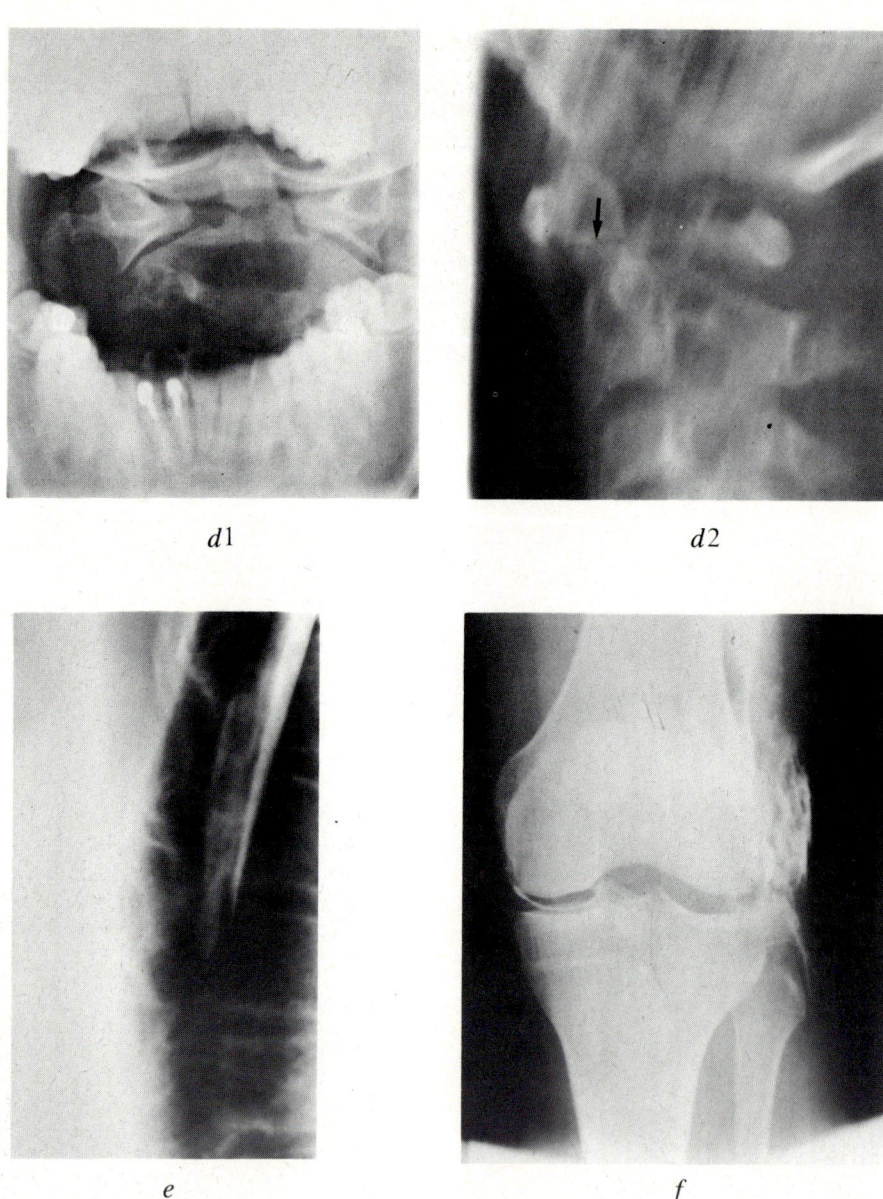

Fig. 1.8. *a*, A stress film (AP) showing disruption of the lateral ligament complex of the ankle in a young rugby player. *b*, An oblique view of the lower lumbar spine showing a stress fracture of the pes interarticularis of L5 in a soccer player. *c*, 1 and 2, Flexion film shows increased anterior movement of the atlas on the axis compared to the extension film (4 mm compared to 2 mm). *d*, 1 and 2, Suspected undisplaced fracture of the odontoid process seen on a tomogram. *e*, A myelogram showing a complete block due to soft-tissue injury and haematoma in the thoracic spine. *f*, An arthrogram indicates the ruptured lateral ligament of the knee following a tibial shaft fracture in a road traffic accident.

11 An introduction to fractures and dislocations

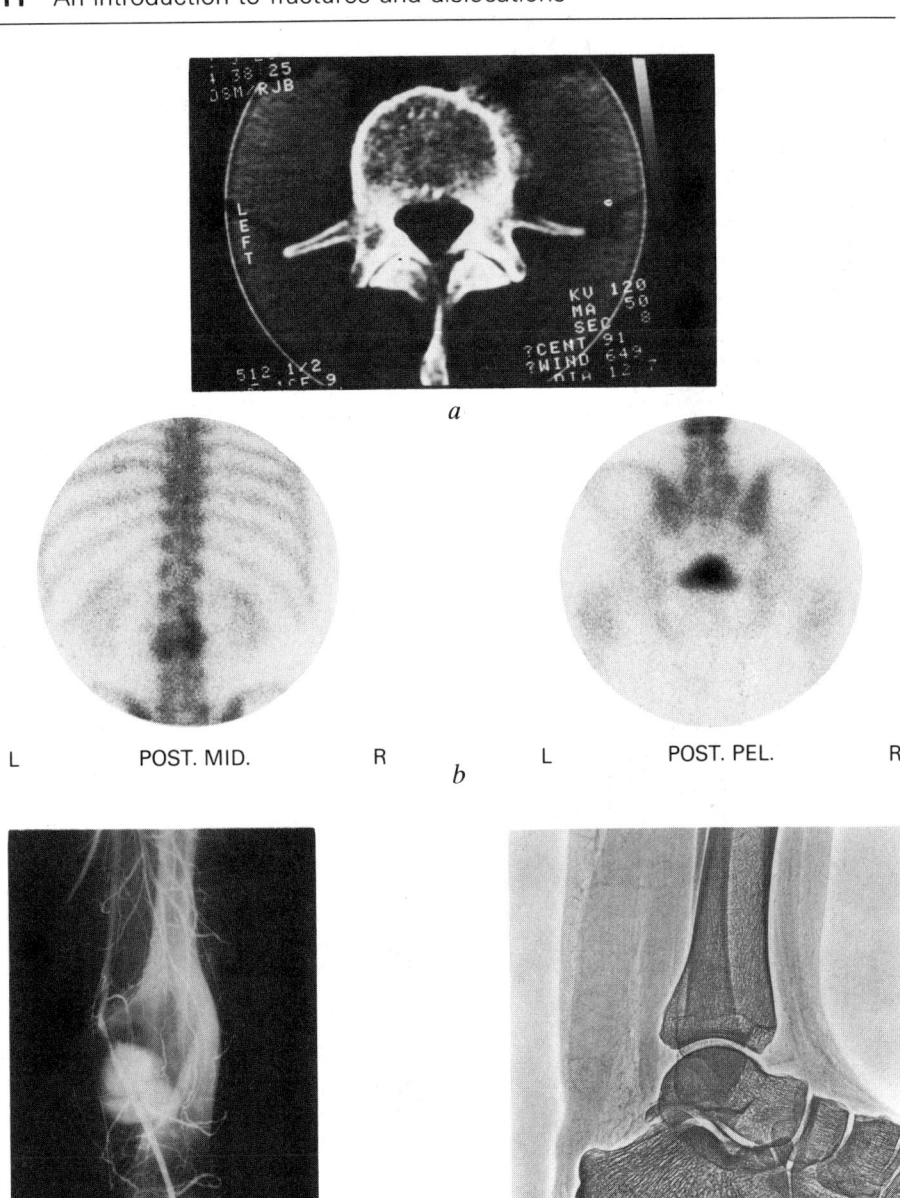

Fig. 1.9. *a*, Computerized tomography (CT) reveals irregular margins of L2 after a crush fracture. No spinal stenosis present. *b*, Technetium 99 isotope uptake in a pathological fracture of L3 body. *c*, An arteriogram reveals an aneurysm of the femoral artery following a femoral shaft fracture in an 8-year-old girl, 1 year previously. *d*, A xerox film showing the soft tissues and bony trabeculae, in this case a chronic thickening of the Achilles tendon in a badminton player.

12 An outline of fractures and dislocations

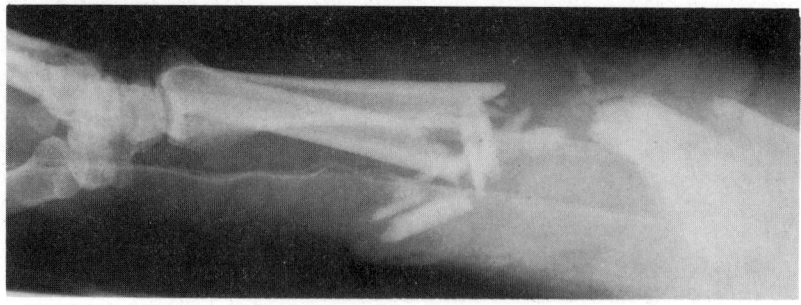

a

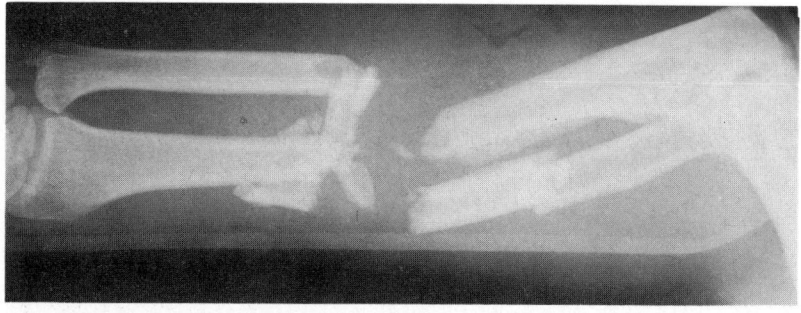

b

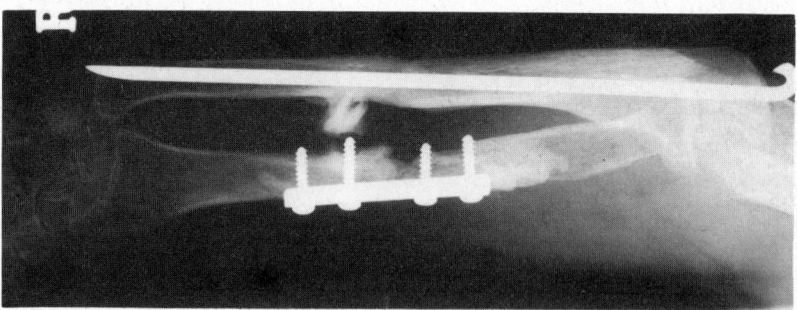

c

Open and Closed Fractures
 • A fracture is *closed or simple* when there is no communication between the site of the fracture and the outside of the body.
 • A fracture is *open or compound* (and thus much more serious) (*Fig.* 1.10) when there is a wound leading down to the fracture site; thus risking contamination by bacteria.

13 An introduction to fractures and dislocations

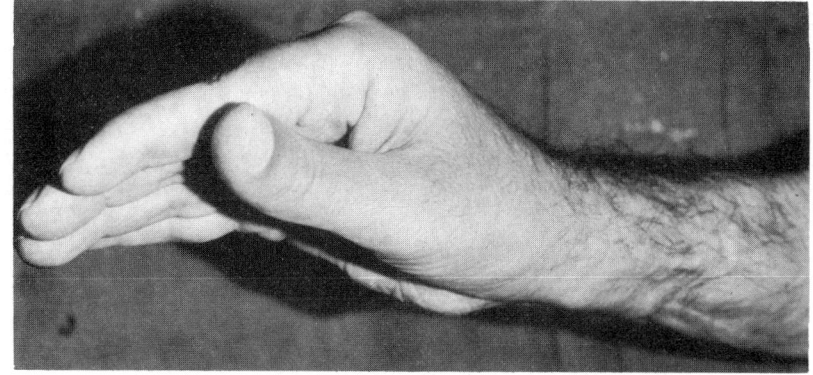

d

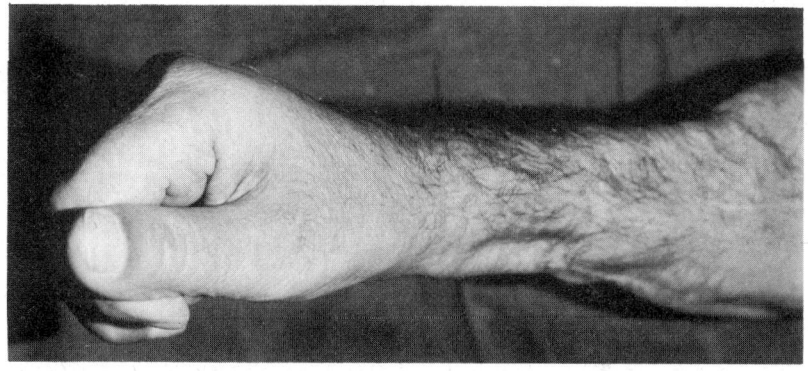

e

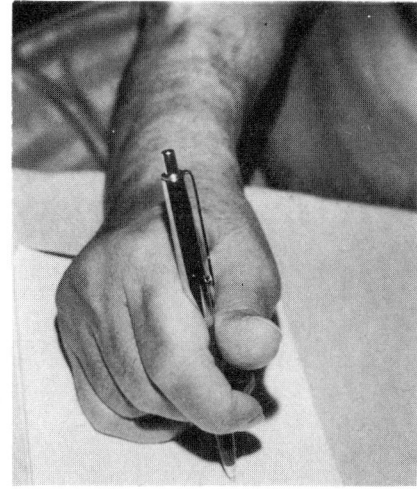

f

Fig. 1.10. The ultimate compound injury. A 34-year-old seaman trapped his R forearm in the stockroom door as a supertanker lurched violently during a North Sea winter's gale. The door locked, the limb lost 6 cm and the attending Captain fainted. Three and a half hours later the man and the severed limb reached hospital by helicopter (*a*) and an immediate vessel and soft-tissue repair was performed by 4½ h (*b*, realigned on a splint). At 6 weeks (*c*) the forearm bones were transfixed; with late nerve and tendon repairs (at 4 months). One year later (*d,e,f*) almost all function had returned, apart from an area of anaesthesia on the dorsum of the index and middle fingers, and a 30° loss of supination. Eventually he returned to sea.

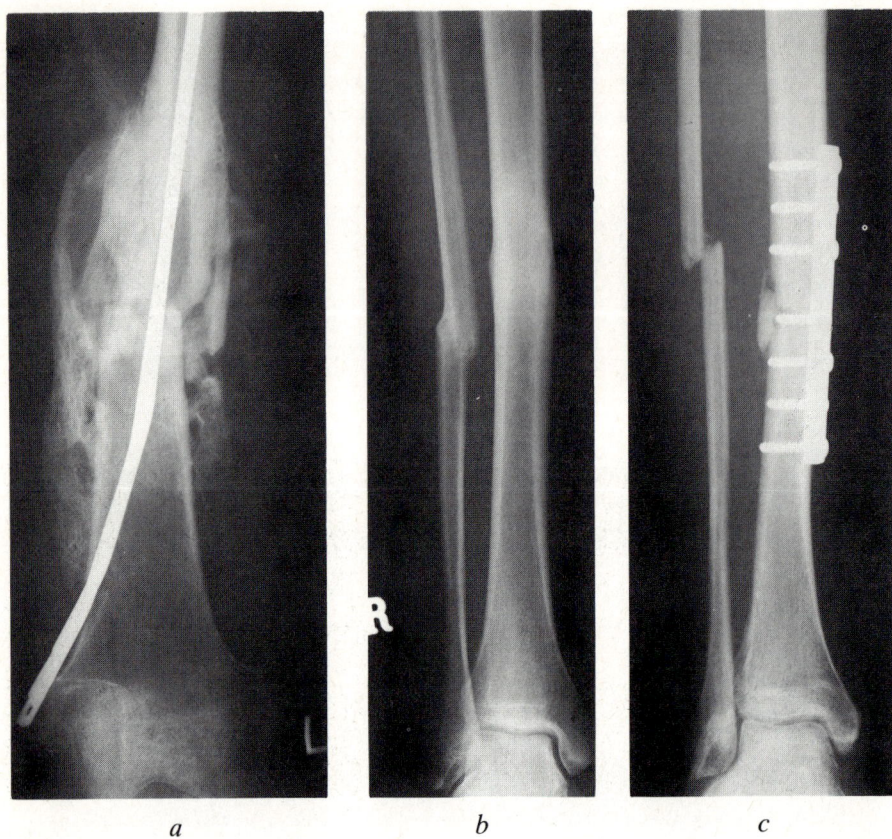

Fig. 1.11. *a*, Abundant callus following Enders' nail fixation (intramedullary fixation) of the femur, indicating movement at the fracture site. *b*, Mature callus with lamellar structure 1 year after a fractured tibia. *c*, By comparison no callus is seen with rigid fixation (AO plating) (although there is callus at the fibular fracture and close to the small segment, at 2 months).

Rate of Union

The time taken for a fracture to unite is very variable and it is difficult to be dogmatic. In the young healing is very rapid and even long bone fractures can be consolidated in 2–4 weeks. In adults such fractures take approximately 12 weeks, although bone remodelling can go on for many months (9–12).

Fractures treated conservatively or by methods which allow some degree of movement (*Fig.* 1.11*a*) at the fracture site are usually associated with abundant callus formation. This temporary bridge of woven bone imparts obvious rigidity to the fracture and can be seen on X-rays and felt. During the stage of consolidation the woven bone is remodelled by the osteoclasts (removers) and osteoblasts (rebuilders) into more mature bone with its typical lamellar structure (*Fig.* 1.11*b*). It is worth noting that when rigid fixation occurs as in AO plating (*Fig.* 1.11*c*) callus formation may be slight or even non-existent. Therefore it is important that the plate is not removed too soon and a delay of 12–18 months is usually recommended so that complete union can occur.

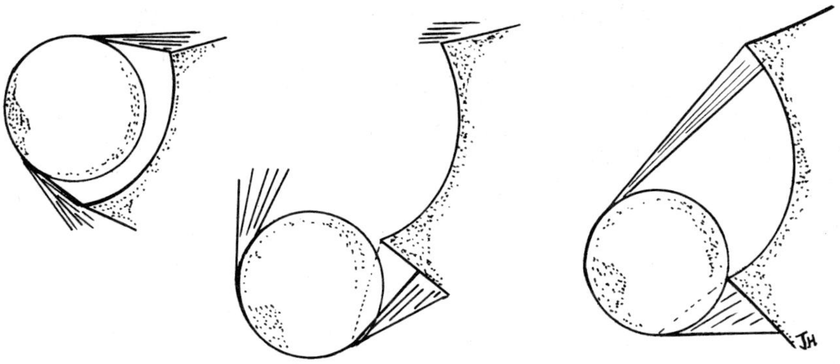

15　An introduction to fractures and dislocations

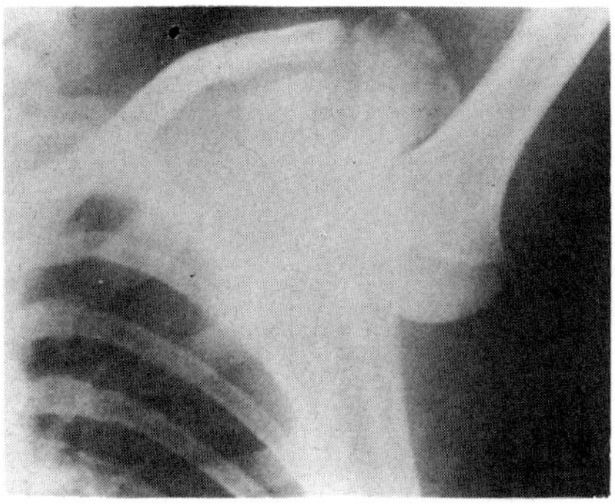

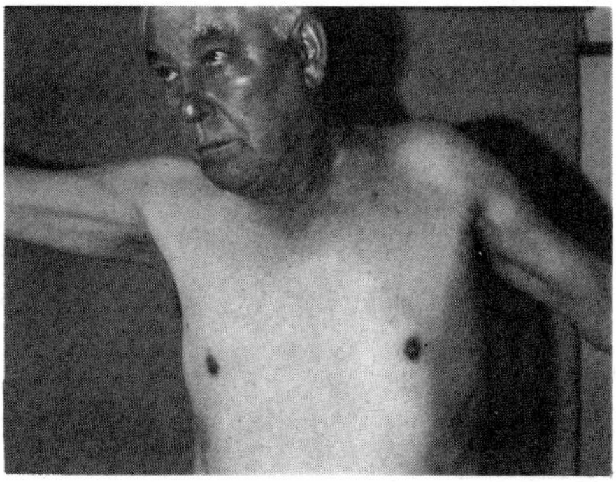

Fig. 1.12. *a*, Normal joint congruity. *b*, The capsule is torn and the joint dislocated. *c*, The capsule is stretched and partial contact is maintained (subluxation). *d*, Anterior shoulder dislocation. *e*, The same patient 2 months after reduction with restricted shoulder movement due to a traumatic pericapsulitis.

- **Dislocations**
  - *A dislocation has occurred when the normally opposed bones of a joint are separated so that the joint congruity is lost. Partial contact is known as subluxation* (*Fig.* 1.12).

Dislocation can only occur with soft-tissue damage—a simple fact which is so often forgotten! Thus either the capsule is stretched, avulsed with a small piece of bone or torn. The surrounding ligaments and muscles may be damaged at the same time, especially if they are blended with the capsule, as for example occurs in the shoulder joint (*Fig.* 1.12*d,e*). Areas of bone may become flattened

16 An outline of fractures and dislocations

on impact (such as the Hill–Sachs lesion in the shoulder (*Fig.* 1.13)) or small bony fragments may become detached and subsequently trapped in the joint as (*Fig.* 1.14), for example, after collateral ligament injuries in the fingers or when there is an avulsion of the anterior cruciate ligament in the knee.

• *Soft-tissue scarring can lead to a marked restriction of joint movement; note the traumatic pericapsulitis shown in Fig. 1.12e.*

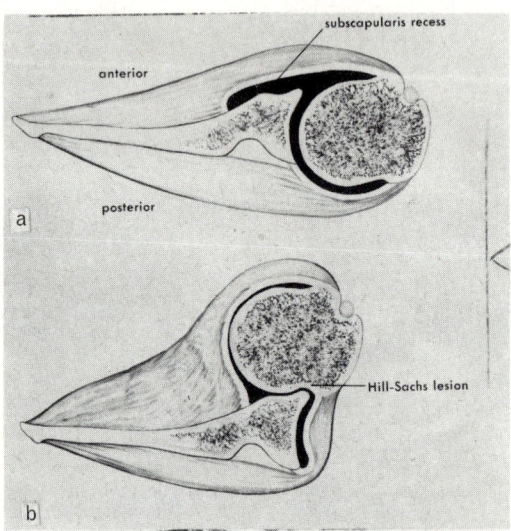

Fig. 1.13. The humeral head is dislocated into the subscapularis recess, repeated trauma to the bone causes a flattening of the head (Hill–Sachs lesion).

Diagnosis

A *dislocation* or *subluxation* is diagnosed by:
1. Pain of a severe or a sickening character near a joint.
2. Fixity of the joint.
3. Deformity of the joint.

Recurrent dislocations may be relatively painless, e.g. in the shoulders or knee (patella) but joint movements are markedly restricted and the associated deformity is obvious both clinically and radiologically.

• *In many cases it is difficult to distinguish between a fracture or a dislocation on clinical grounds alone and X-rays are imperative before reduction is attempted.*

17 An introduction to fractures and dislocations

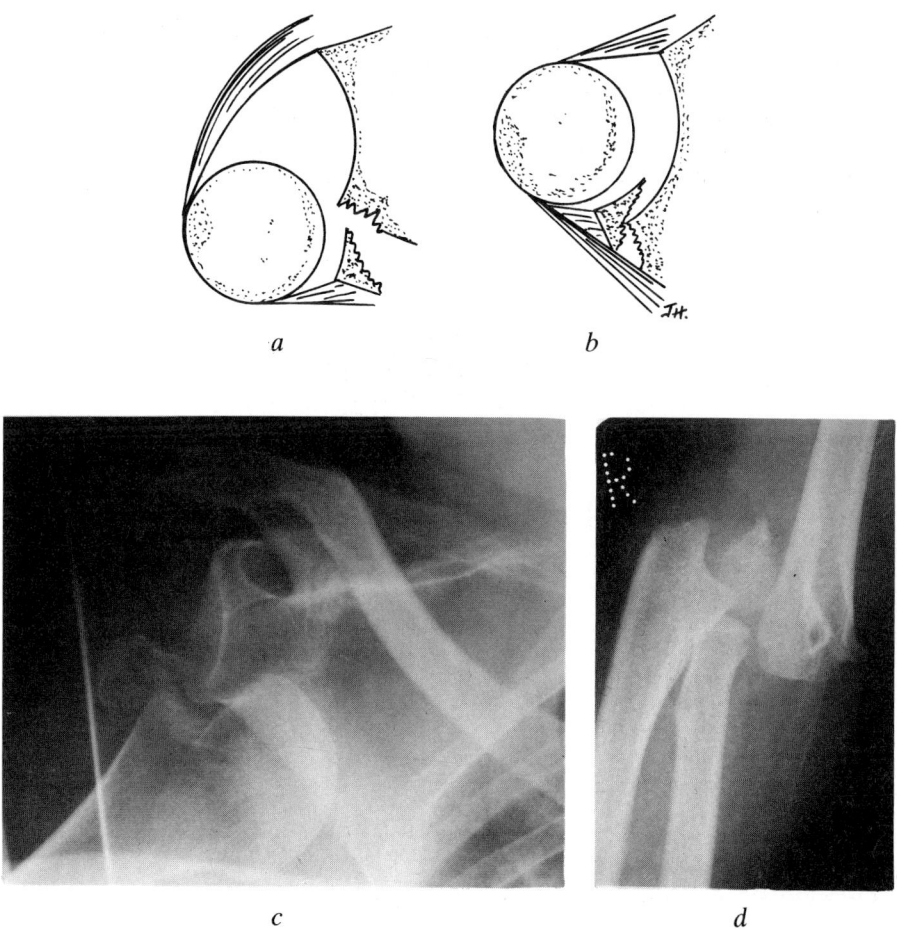

Fig. 1.14. Avulsion (*a*) of bone occurs with the dislocation and the fragment may become trapped in the joint (*b*) after reduction. In (*c*) there is impaction of the humeral head on the inferior margin of the scapula; in (*d*) the lateral condyle is rotated and trapped during a posterior fracture-dislocation of the elbow.

Chronic or Missed Dislocation

Occasionally, especially in the aged and infirm, a patient may present many weeks or months later with a relatively painless but fixed joint due to a missed dislocation. Such a situation happens at the shoulder (especially in patients with hemiplegia), in the knee (patella) and often at the terminal phalanx

18   An outline of fractures and dislocations

of the fingers or toes (*Fig.* 1.15). Congenital dislocation of the hip may be found on routine X-rays in adults, often as the joints become increasingly painful from arthritic changes.

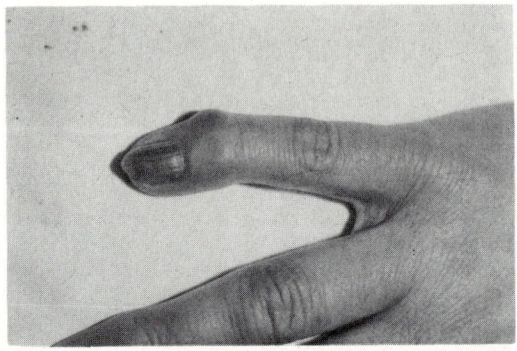

Fig. 1.15. A dislocated TIP joint of 2 weeks' duration.

Treatment
   The acute dislocated joint is reduced either under a general anaesthetic (with complete muscle relaxation) or under local anaesthetic—the latter being used for small joints such as the fingers and toes.
   • *An X-ray is always required to assess reduction and to ensure that a small fragment of bone is not trapped in the joint. As in the case of limb fractures, it is mandatory to check the vessels and nerves below the injured area both BEFORE and AFTER reduction.* Please remember this fact!
   Most joints are stable after reduction but some form of immobilization is desirable for 1–4 weeks to allow soft-tissue healing. Physiotherapy is essential to restore full function and should begin as soon as joint discomfort and swelling have abated.
   In the case of a chronic or missed dislocation the decision has to be made: (*a*) whether to leave the situation alone (especially if the joint is painless in the infirm), (*b*) to arthrodese (if painful), or (*c*) to reduce and hope that some function may return.

X-rays
   The same precautions apply as for fractures (p. 5) but stress films or arthrograms may be required to evaluate joint congruity and ligment continuity.

19 An introduction to fractures and dislocations

- **Sprains and Strains**

A sprain usually refers to a minor disruption in the joint capsule (including ligaments), whereas a strain refers to a tendon injury, as for example in the groin (the ubiquitous groin strain of runners).

A sprain is usually acute and denotes macroscopic tears in the collagen and elastin structure of the joint tissues. It is treated by 1–3 weeks of rest in strapping or plaster-of-Paris with anti-inflammatory tablets to control the pain and swelling. It is often necessary to use ancillary X-ray investigations (as mentioned above) to ensure that a bad sprain is not a partial or complete tear.

Chronic sprains (e.g. ankle ligaments) and strains (e.g. tennis elbow) often respond to local steroid injections, ultrasound and plaster-of-Paris immobilization.

It is worth recalling that one side of a joint may be stretched while the other is crushed, causing bilateral symptoms and signs.

- **Ligament Injuries**

A *sprain* is a minor disruption (as described *above*).

A *partial tear* has more severe pain and the tenderness is accurately localized with joint swelling often present. However, no abnormal joint mobility occurs. If necessary, the joint is aspirated to relieve the haemarthrosis and a plaster used for immobilization for 3–4 weeks.

A *complete tear* has severe pain, excessive joint mobility and a major haemarthrosis. Stress X-rays, an arthrogram or arthroscopy are used to confirm the diagnosis. However, the severity of symptoms may warrant surgical exploration and repair within 48 hours, with plaster immobilization for 4–6 weeks.

- **Acute Tendon Injuries**

These are either *partial or complete*, and can be caused by fragments of bones (e.g. the extensor pollicis longus rupture in a Colles fracture—the so-called 'drummer boy palsy') and by excessive joint movement during a dislocation (e.g. the tibialis posterior tendon may become trapped between the talus and medial malleolus in ankle injuries).

Partial tears are treated by plaster for 2–3 weeks. Complete tendon tears need suture and plaster immobilization for 3–6 weeks.

2
Principles of treatment

- **Fractures**

General
1. Assess the severity of injury, especially look for wounds, nerve and vessel damage.
2. Avoid further injury, i.e. institute first aid and rest the damaged tissues with a sling, splint, plaster, etc.
3. Treat the general condition of the patient, i.e. shock, respiratory problems, head injury, etc.

Specific or Local
1. Reduce the fracture by either closed manipulation or open reduction.
2. Stabilize the fracture by either plaster-of-Paris, continuous traction (e.g. a Thomas splint) or by internal fixation.
3. Treat the soft-tissue injury by elevation, cold compress, anti-inflammatory agents and physiotherapy.

Reduction
- *Closed reduction demands that the fracturing forces be reversed* (*Fig. 2.1*). This requires complete relaxation by either a local anaesthetic (e.g. Biers local forearm block for a wrist fracture) or a general anaesthetic.

The first stage of reduction is to apply *gentle* but *sustained* traction along the longitudinal axis and then, as the fragments are distracted, to reverse the original direction of injury and to interlock the fracture line (*Fig. 2.1c*). The periosteal and muscular soft-tissue bridge ensheaths and usually stabilizes the reduced fracture.

The following points should be noted.
1. Many fractures do *not* require reduction because there is no displacement or only slight displacement (*Fig. 2.2a*). Experience is needed for such judgement. However, rotatory displacement can lead to a marked loss of function, especially in forearm fractures (*Figs. 2.2b, 2.3*) so can angular deformity (*Figs. 2.2c, 2.3*). However, some degree of overlap (*Fig. 2.2d*) with good alignment may prove to be of little handicap although too

21 Principles of treatment

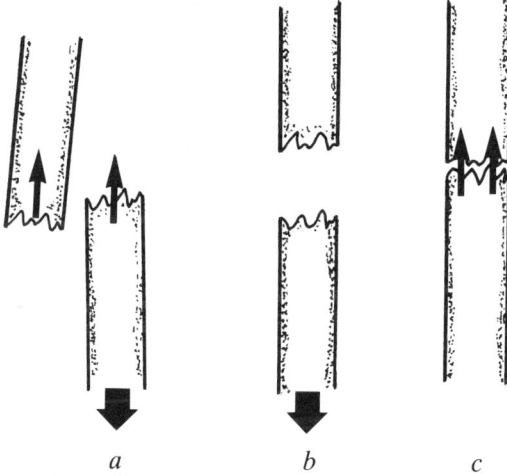

Fig. 2.1. *a*, Traction is applied (large arrow) to overcome the muscle pull (small arrow). *b*, During traction the fracture is correctly aligned (AP, lateral and rotation) and allowed to reduce (*c*) when the periosteal hinge and muscles forces lock the fragments.

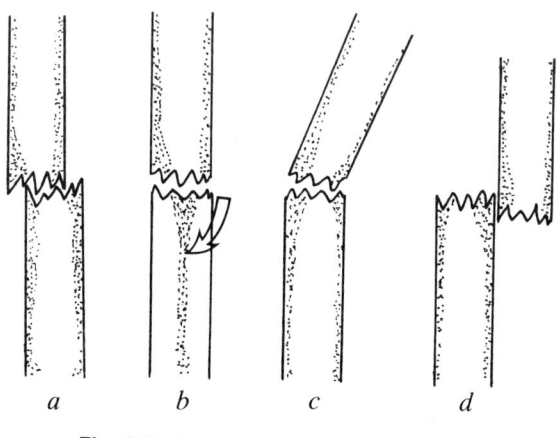

Fig. 2.2. See text.

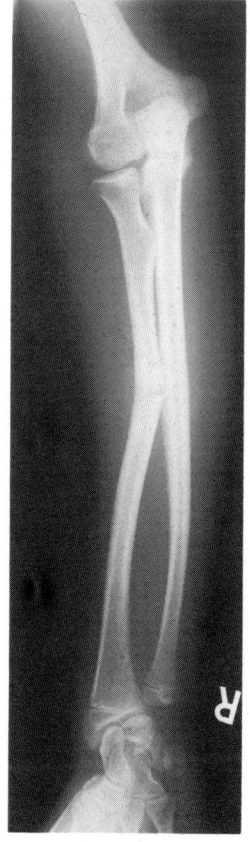

Fig. 2.3. A 15-year-old boy with a fourth refracture of the radius, due to angulation, malrotation and lack of mobility. An osteotomy was later used to correct alignment.

22 An outline of fractures and dislocations

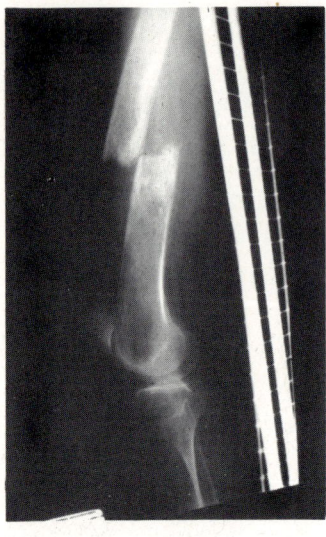

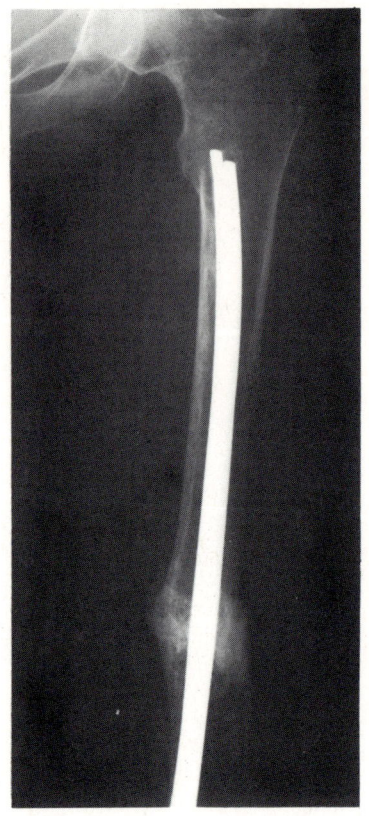

Fig. 2.4. *a*, A 65-year-old lady referred for lower limb amputation with multiple breast secondaries, treated by intramedullary flexible nails (*b*). Well 6 years after surgery. The fracture had healed despite the neoplastic infiltration and a bone texture resembling cheese.

much shortening (over 1·5 cm) could prove troublesome by adding stresses to the joints in the affected limb.
 • *Imperfect alignment is not acceptable, although some loss of bony contact may be.*
2. When the fracture is intra-articular and there is irregularity of the joint outline, the bony pieces must be accurately realigned to lessen the risk of subsequent osteoarthritis.
3. With vessel or nerve injury the fractured area is stabilized to prevent additional movement at the site of repair.
4. Neoplastic fractures will often unite and should be reduced with great gentleness and immobilized by plaster or internal fixation (*Fig.* 2.4).

Methods of Reduction

1. Closed manipulation.
2. Mechanical traction, with or without manipulation.
3. Open reduction.
 Closed manipulation is the method of choice whenever possible (*Fig.* 2.5*a*).

23 Principles of treatment

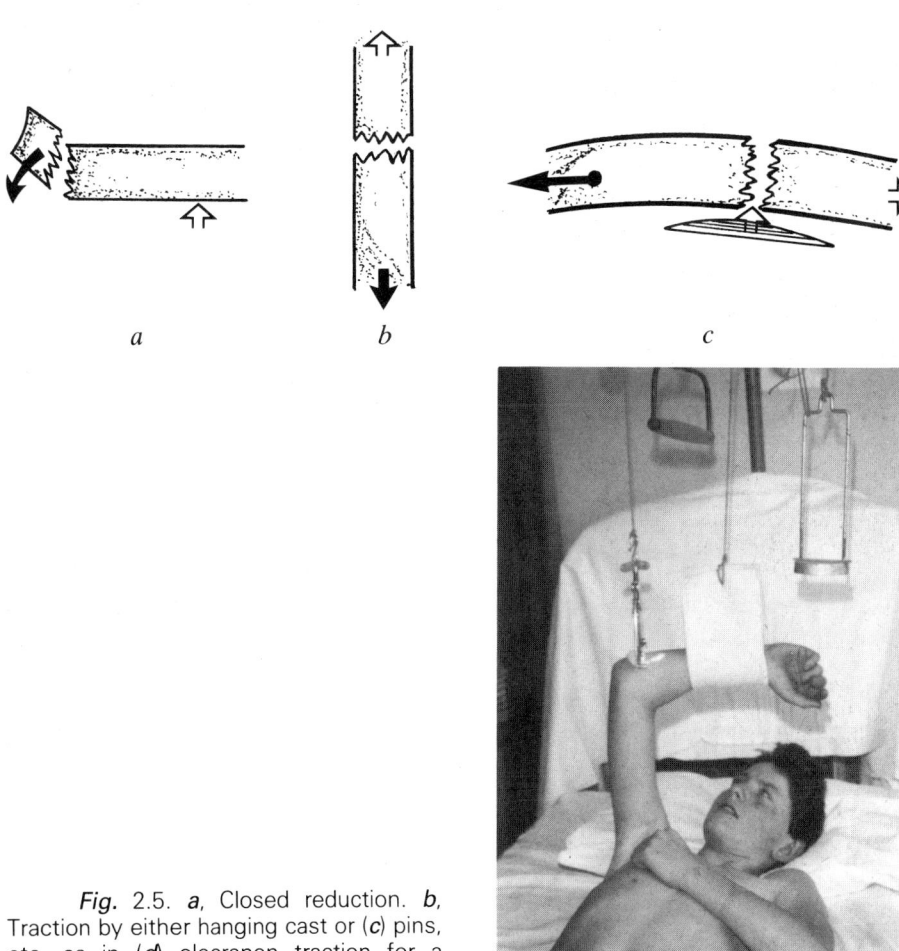

Fig. 2.5. *a*, Closed reduction. *b*, Traction by either hanging cast or (*c*) pins, etc. as in (*d*) olecranon traction for a comminuted lower humerus.

Mechanical traction is required when large muscles exert a powerful displacement force such as occurs in femoral shaft fractures (*Fig.* 2.5*c*). Traction may be applied by weights attached to adhesive strapping, or to pins or screws inserted across the long axis of the bone (*Fig.* 2.5*c,d*). The fracture is reduced under anaesthesia and maintained by weights; as an alternative, when there is only a small amount of displacement reduction is achieved slowly by the suspended weights without anaesthesia, such reduction may take several days.

Open reduction is used when other methods fail or are not directly applicable (such as displaced intra-articular fractures of the elbow). Surgical reduction allows fixation with plates, screws, etc. under direct vision.

Immobilization
● *Once a fracture has been reduced it must be immobilized to allow sound union and to avoid re-displacement.*

This is a general rule! Some fractures heal effectively with minimal splintage such as the clavicle or fibula. However, when the fragile capillary circulation could be impaired by movement the fracture must be rigidly held to avoid avascular necrosis (e.g. scaphoid, talus and femoral neck).

Indications
There are *four* reasons for immobilization:
1. To prevent displacement, rotation or angulation of the fracture fragments.
2. To relieve pain.
3. To rest the soft tissues.
4. To prevent movement that might hamper union.

Plaster-of-Paris
Since it is so commonly used to maintain fractures in a good position and rest the injured area, it is worth discussing this material which can have several important drawbacks. Recently, there have been many proprietary preparations introduced, some designed for lightness (which can be an advantage in the aged) and others for rapidity of setting and robustness.

Plaster must be evenly applied over a soft wool base, and should be free of lumps (like custard) and not be too tight. The length of the plaster should completely immobilize the injured area. This usually involves both joints in relation to the fracture, e.g. an above-knee plaster in tibial shaft fractures extending to the toes.

The *disadvantages* are:
1. It is rigid and *cannot* easily accommodate swelling—one moment too tight and needs splitting, a few days later too slack as the swelling subsides. This fickleness is a major fault.
2. Plaster sores may develop in the skin from indentations, rough edges or plaster crumbs.
3. Muscle atrophy and joint stiffness occur in the immobilized limb.
4. Dependent oedema and Sudeck's atrophy are often found.
5. It stops inspection and needs a window cut if a wound requires dressing.
6. It can cause an alteration in gait due to its weight, bulk, rigidity and the extra limb length (walking heel) which the patient may acquire for several weeks after removal. This feature may be important in sportsmen and women.

Application of Plaster
A thin lining of stockinet or cellulose bandage is needed to prevent the plaster from sticking to the skin or hair. If marked swelling is anticipated then padding with cotton wool is used. The plaster bandages are applied in two forms: rolled bandages or slabs (longitudinal strips) to reinforce an area such as a joint. The plaster roll is soaked in fairly warm water until all the bubbles disappear. The wet bandage is squeezed lightly to expel excess moisture and rolled gently but firmly around the limb, commencing at the fracture area (*Fig. 2.6*). The roll is kept uppermost and applied closely and evenly to the stockinet. Usually 6 to 12 thicknesses are applied according to the limb girth. The edges are trimmed or rolled back and the surface massaged to smoothness.

25 Principles of treatment

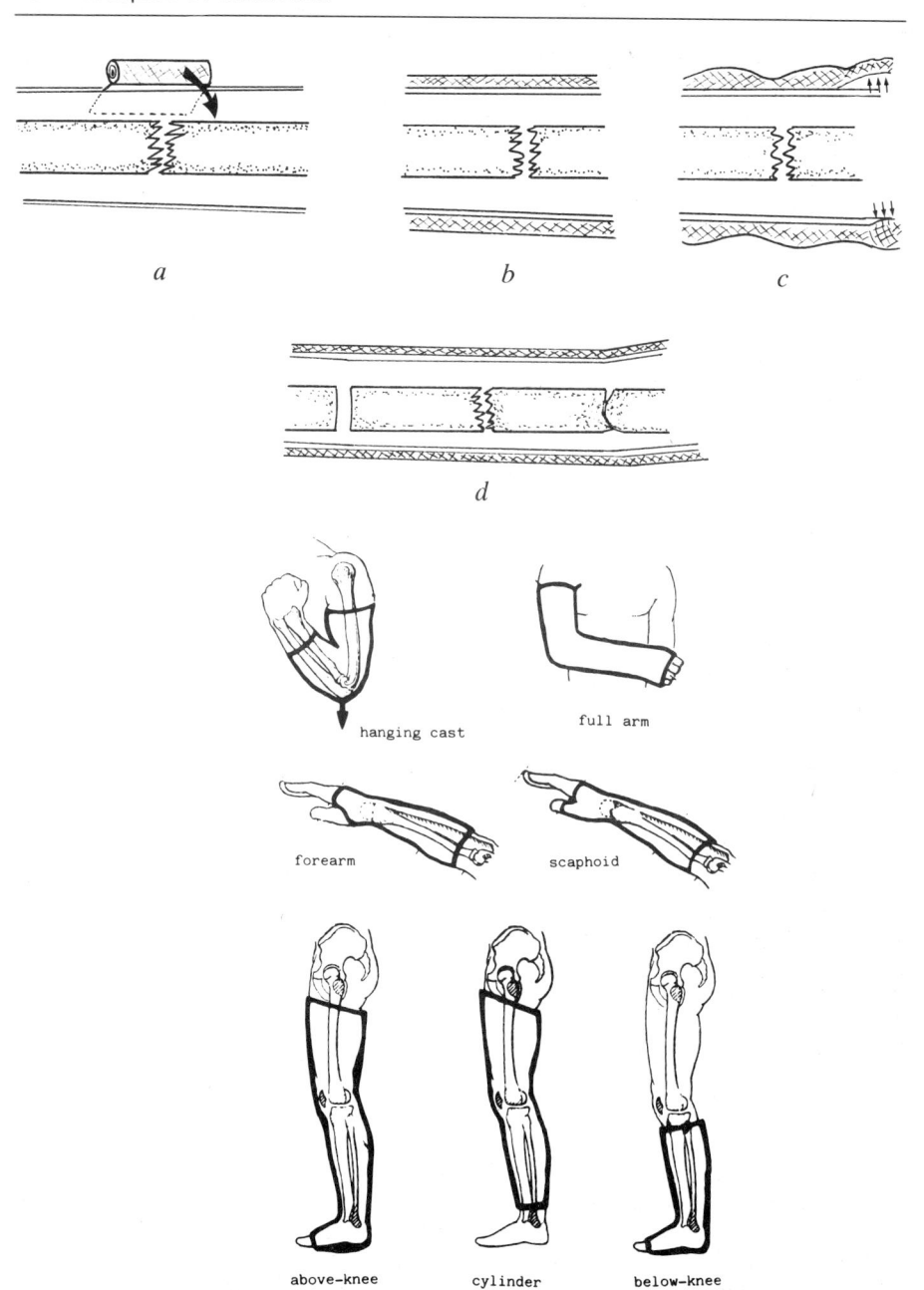

Fig. 2.6. In (*a*) and (*b*) the plaster-of-Paris is evenly applied; in (*c*) lumps and airpockets appear (the 'houseman's plaster'). *d*, The plaster must extend across both related joints (above and below). *e*, A variety of commonly used plasters.

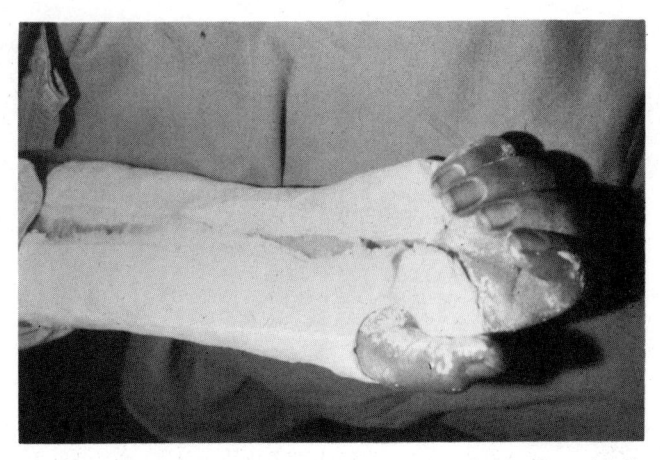

*Fig. 2.7. The plaster and padding must be split **throughout** its length.*

Throughout the procedure the gloved hands must be kept wet and free from plaster 'crumbs'. The plaster is best dried by exposure to air but may not be suitable for bearing weight for 24 h or more.

Removal of Plaster
Plaster shears or an oscillating saw, especially designed, are used to remove the plaster. The line of cut should be over soft tissues and concavities and should avoid bony prominences. It should also be noticed that the point of the shears should slide along between the plaster and the lining, with the base kept horizontal and the cutting edge used to punch away the plaster.

* *If the circulation is impaired as denoted by pain, swelling, cyanosis or pallor then the plaster must be split throughout its length. Dressings and bandages under the plaster should be divided right down to the skin. The plaster is then opened from top to bottom and used as a backslab* (*Fig.* 2.7).

Other Forms of Immobilization
These are shown in *Fig.* 2.8. The figure-of-eight bandage (*Fig.* 2.8*a*) is used for clavicular fractures, a collar-and-cuff (*Fig.* 2.8*b*) for undisplaced fractures of the humeral neck, a sling (*Fig.* 2.8*c*) for shoulder or elbow injuries, a wrist support for wrist injuries and a mallet splint for finger fractures (*Fig.* 2.8*d*), a Thomas' splint (*Fig.* 2.8*e*) for femoral shaft fractures, crêpe-and-wool (*Fig.* 2.8*f*) for knee or calcaneal injuries, a cervical collar for neck injuries and a plaster jacket or lumbosacral support for lower spinal problems (*Fig.* 2.8*g*).

Immobilization by Continuous Traction
This type of traction is used for long-bone fractures. The humerus can be re-aligned by a heavy plaster U-slab and a collar-and-cuff around the wrist. Gravity reduces the fracture vertically (*Fig.* 2.9). Femoral shaft fractures in young children can be treated by 'gallows' traction (*Fig.* 2.10) (when the child, lying on the back, is suspended from an overhead beam by strapping along the lower limbs), whereas the Thomas' splint (*Fig.* 2.8*e*) or its modifications are used

27 Principles of treatment

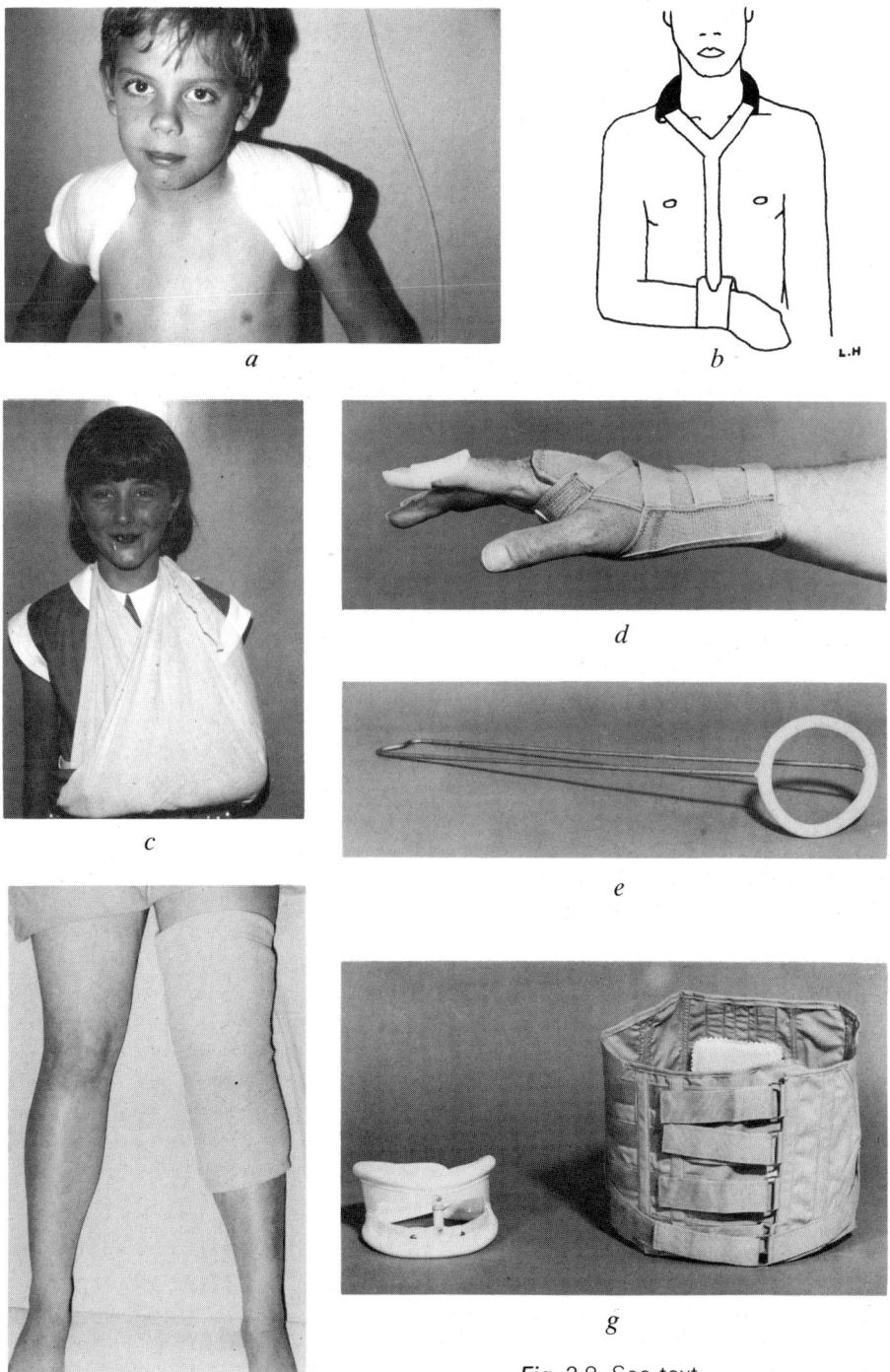

Fig. 2.8. See text.

28 An outline of fractures and dislocations

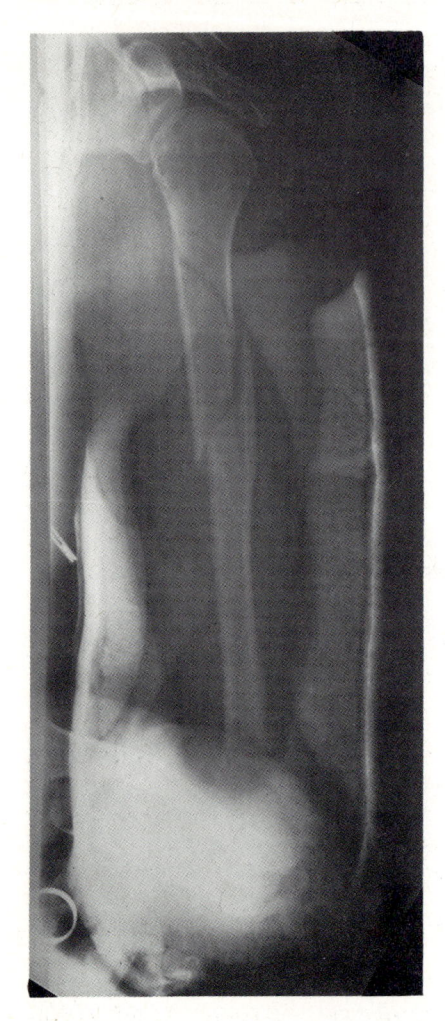

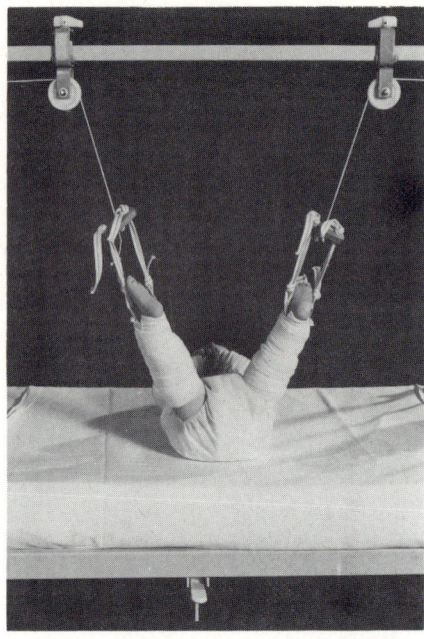

Fig. 2.10. Gallows traction. The knees should be slightly flexed (with a light splint) and the circulation watched in the foot. The buttocks should be just off the bed.

Fig. 2.9. A hanging plaster cast giving excellent reduction of a humeral shaft fracture (note the plaster can be assessed on X-rays).

for femoral shaft fractures in older children and adults. Counter traction is often through the tibial shaft just below the tibial tubercle. Weights counterbalance the pull of the muscles which would cause over-riding of the bony fragments. Cervical spine injuries can be immobilized by traction through tongs inserted into the skull.

Duration of Immobilization
There is no set time for each fracture but arabic numerals dictate 3, 6, 12 weeks etc. (with decimalization 5, 10, 15 weeks may become the norm). However, usually within 4 weeks fibrous union has occurred, by 4–8 weeks early callus, by 2–6 months mature callus, and by 9 months sound union is established.

Thus small fractures (e.g. wrist, ankle malleoli) can be mobilized at 4–6

29 Principles of treatment

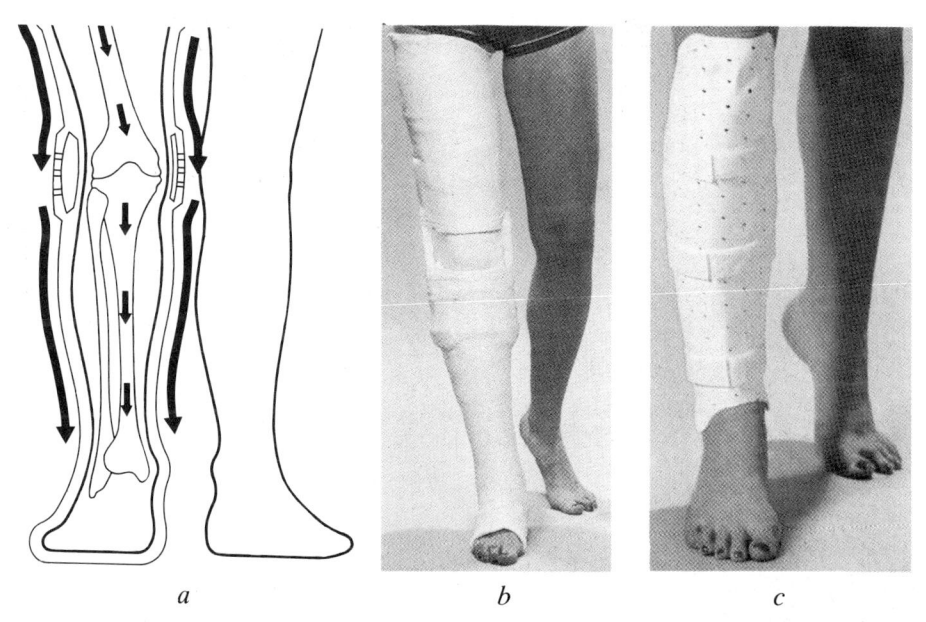

Fig. 2.11. Cast bracing. *a*, The principle of forces. *b*, Femoral brace with knee hinge. *c*, Patellar tendon-bearing cast for tibial fractures.

weeks; tibial and humeral fractures at 6–9 weeks; and femoral shaft fractures at 9–12 weeks.
* *It is important to assess the fracture regularly according to the age of the patient, the bone involved and the type of fracture.*

Functional Bracing
A concept of fracture treatment which has rightly gained in popularity during the last decade is functional bracing. This technique utilizes close-conforming, lightweight materials (usually either a plaster-of-Paris or one of the new resins or plastics) and hydraulic compression (*Fig. 2.11a*) of the soft tissues to hold the fracture and transfer weight from the injured bone to the brace. Early ambulation and joint movement are possible.
1. The femoral cast-brace (*Fig. 2.11b*) is a total contact cast with the plaster-of-Paris closely moulded to the thigh, extending from the groin to 4 cm or so above the knee. Polycentric hinges made of polyethylene allow flexion of the knee and are attached to a well-fitting below-knee plaster. This cast can be hinged at the ankle to a shoe or a further small plaster. A femoral shaft fracture is treated in this way and the cast-brace can be applied at 3–4 weeks and used for a further 6–10 weeks depending on the rate of union.
2. The patellar tendon-bearing cast or Sarmiento plaster depends upon total contact which compresses the soft tissues so that the vertical load of ambulation is transferred to the brace, thus bypassing the fracture. This treatment is used for a tibial fracture and can be applied from 2 weeks onwards and used for 4–6 weeks (*Fig. 2.11c*).

Fractures of the humerus, radius and ulna can also be treated by functional bracing.

The slight movement which occurs at the fracture site is not detrimental to fracture healing.

Test of Union

Whether a conventional plaster or a cast brace is used it is necessary at certain appropriate intervals to assess the state of union. This is especially important in long bone fractures such as the femur and tibia which are going to be subjected to the stress of weight-bearing. There are *three* clinical tests of union:
1. Absence of mobility between fragments.
2. Absence of tenderness on deep palpation of the fracture site.
3. Absence of pain when an angular or rotatory stress is applied to the fracture area.

Radiological Assessment of Union

Generally X-rays are used to assess bony union but should not replace the clinical appraisal. There are *two* principal features that suggest union:
1. Visible callus bridging the fracture site blending with both fragments (*Fig. 2.12a*).
2. Continuity of bone trabeculae across the fracture (*Fig. 2.12b*).

Callus implies early woven-bone whereas bony trabecular continuity suggests a more mature union and stability. Old callus is both mature and strong and remains permanently at the fracture site.

Open Reduction

Closed reduction may fail if:
1. The fragments are too small to be manipulated.
2. They are trapped in a joint.
3. There is interposition of soft tissues.
4. The area is unstable due to comminution.
5. Or is unstable due to associated ligamentous injuries.
6. There is marked swelling.

Under these circumstances *open reduction* (with internal fixation in most cases) is required, especially in the following injuries:
1. In fractures involving joint surfaces.
2. Where rigidity is needed to prevent avascular necrosis, such as femoral neck fractures.
3. When damaged arteries, veins or nerves have to be repaired and bone stability is essential.
4. If accurate reduction is impossible due to soft-tissue trauma, etc.
5. When the fracture is unstable.
6. With multiple fractures, especially when occurring in the same limb.
7. When nursing care can be greatly aided, e.g. unstable spinal fractures with bed sores and bladder problems.

31 Principles of treatment

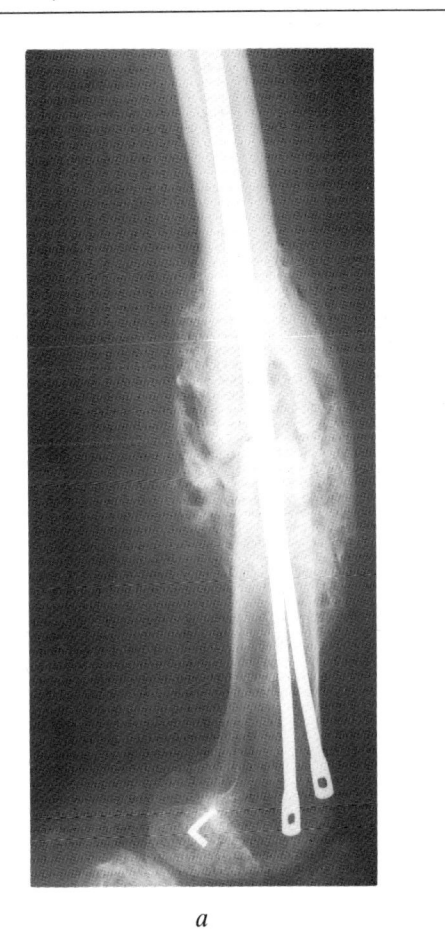

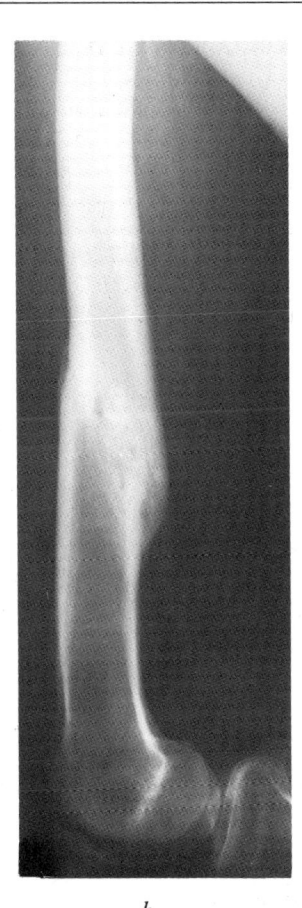

Fig. 2.12. Indicators of bony union. *a*, External callus. *b*, Continuity of bone trabeculae.

Methods
The choice of fixation device depends upon the extent and location of the fracture.

Metal screws and plates (usually made of a special stainless steel, titanium or alloys, e.g. containing chromium, cobalt and molybdenum) are most often used in a variety of forms. Fixation by ordinary plates has the disadvantage that the bone fragments are not forcibly pressed together. Indeed, if the fractured area reabsorbs slightly due to avascular changes then the plate tends to hold the fragments apart and induce non-union.

In the AO technique (Association for Osteosynthesis, developed in Switzerland) special cortical, cancellous and lag screws—with the corresponding plates and compression apparatus—have been developed (*Fig.* 2.13*a,b*) to produce firm compression at the fractured area, thus circumventing the necessity for rigid plaster immobilization. Early movement of the injured area is encouraged with less joint stiffness.

32 An outline of fractures and dislocations

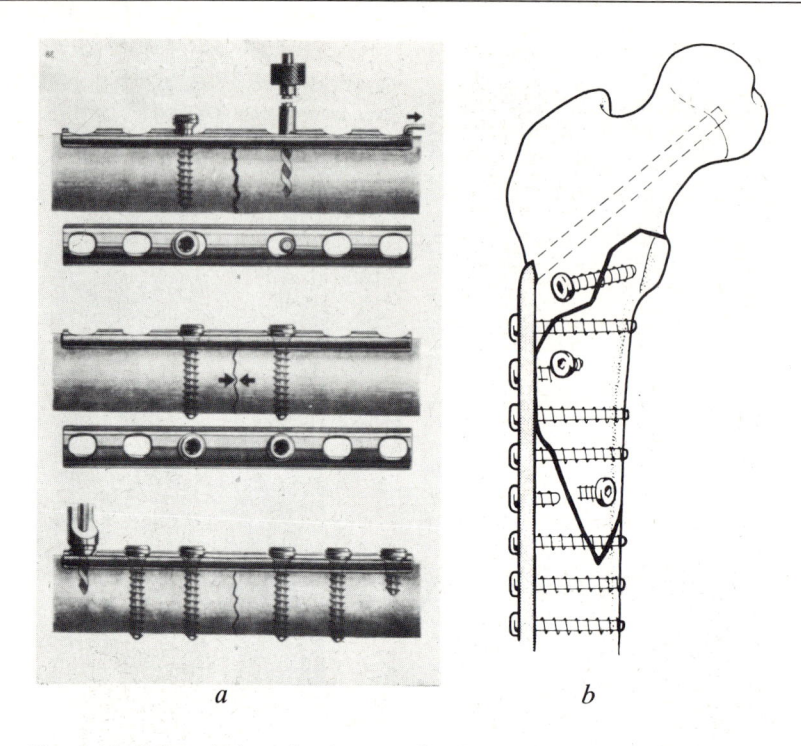

Fig. 2.13. AO technique for fracture fixation. *a*, Long bone. *b*, Subtrochanteric fracture.

When there is a defect in the fractured bone a bone graft should supplement the fixation plate—the graft may be taken from a local site or the pelvic crest. Under certain circumstances a muscle-pedicle-bone graft can be used or a fibular graft inserted.

Plates and screws crossing bone may produce resorption locally and subsequent weakness, and they may cause a stress gradient at the bone/metal interface leading to a refracture after a blow or a fall (*see* Chapter 3). Thus intramedullary techniques (*Fig.* 2.14) using a single strong nail (such as the Küntscher or AO) or multiple nails (such as the Enders) have been developed for a long bone fracture, especially when it occurs near the middle of the shaft. This form of treatment is popular in young adults with fractures of the femur, tibia, humerus and ulna. The soft-tissue dissection is much smaller than required for open plating and the weight distribution down the long axis of the bone is good.

Wires can be used around oblique fractures of long bones or as a figure-of-eight (*Fig.* 2.15) at the olecranon or medial malleolus. Nylon bands can also be used for cerclage techniques. Special plates and pins of carbon have recently been developed.

33 Principles of treatment

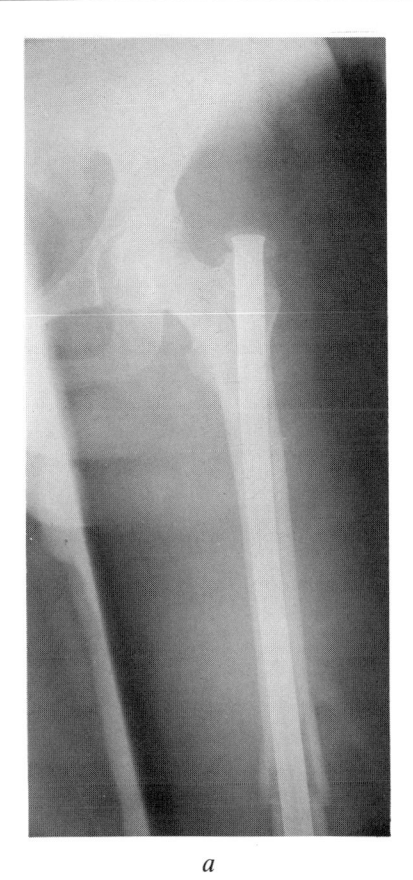

Fig. 2.14. A 33-year-old woman with bilateral fractures—shaft of femur. *a*, The L side treated by close nailing. *b*, The R side required open reduction due to soft tissue interposition (note the drain). AO nail.

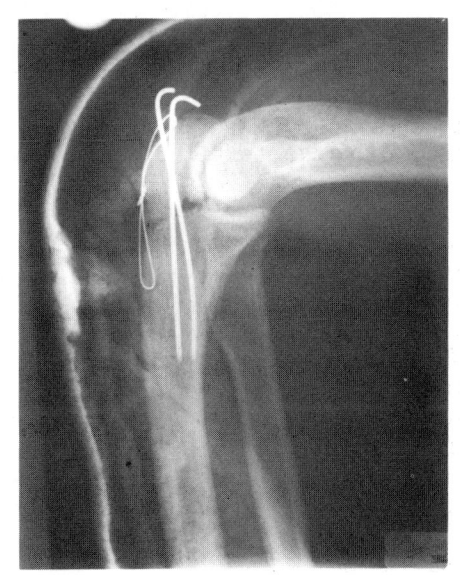

Fig. 2.15. Tension band wiring of an olecranon fracture.

34 An outline of fractures and dislocations

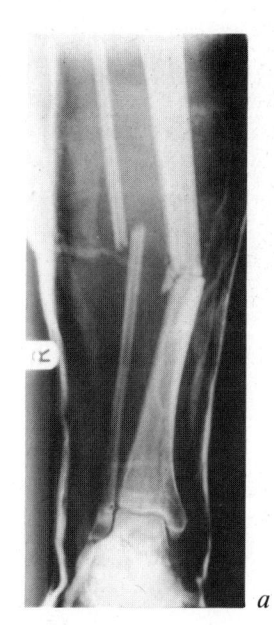

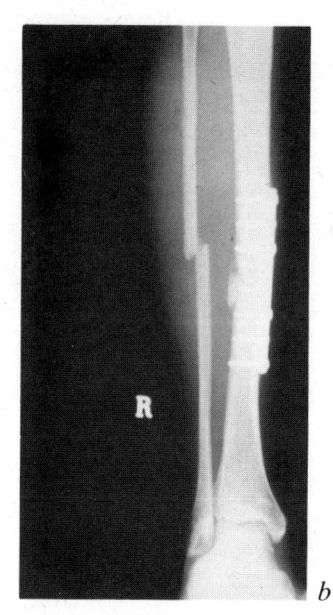

Fig. 2.16. *a*, Unstable tibial shaft fracture in plaster. *b*, Treated by compression plating.

Advantages of Internal Fixation
Since the radiological and clinical picture after internal fixation is often excellent it is worth recalling that *not* all fractures demand surgery, although many centres now adopt a more vigorous approach to fracture management, especially in young adults (*Fig.* 2.16). The advantages are:
1. Excellent reduction and strong fixation.
2. Less time in hospital.
3. More rapid and often better function of the limb.
4. More rapid mobilization out of bed—good for the elderly.
5. Less non-union and mal-union.

However, there are disadvantages. These are related to surgical intervention, i.e. blood loss, wound infection, deep vein thrombosis, chest infection, stripping of soft tissues (leading to adhesions or avascular changes hindering bony union), misplacement of screws and fixation devices, erosion through the skin by metal plates (when used subcutaneously) and acute or chronic osteomyelitis. (The complications are fully outlined in Chapter 3.)

External Fixation
During the recent decade many of the advantages of internal fixation have been met by the use of external fixation devices (*Fig.* 2.17) which give excellent fixation and can be adjusted in three planes to achieve reduction once the rigid pins have been inserted. Little surgery is required—the fractures being reduced by closed methods and then transfixed by pins that are attached to metal frames. The device is worn until union has occurred (usually 2–4 months) and the limb can be mobilized early.

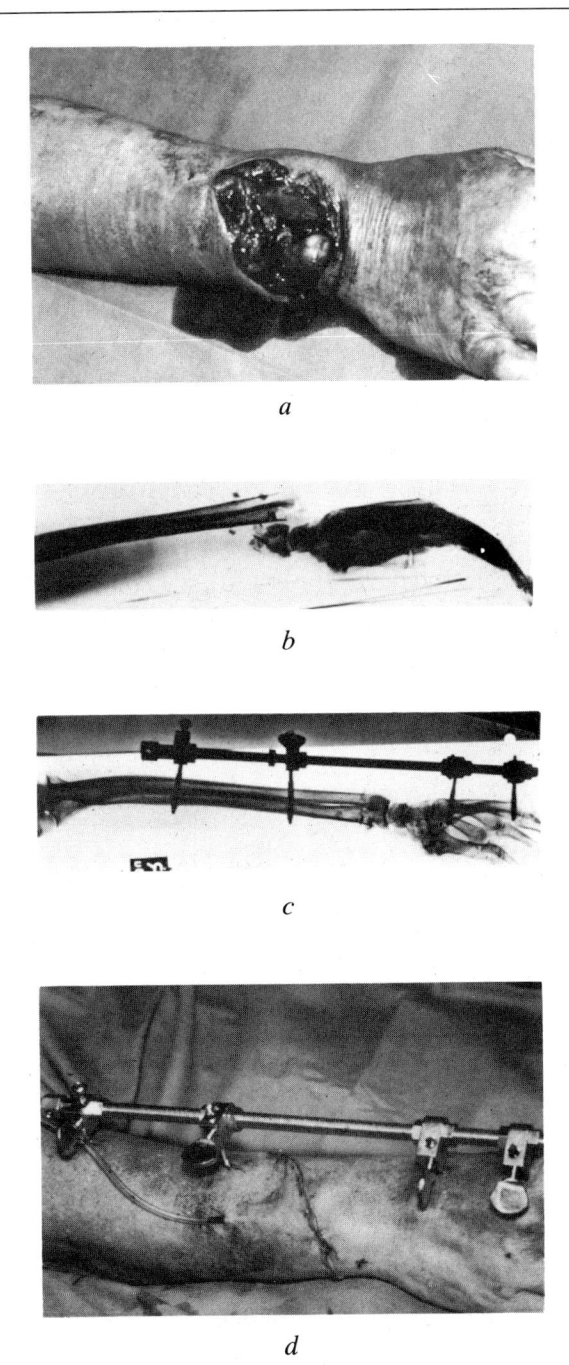

Fig. 2.17. The use of an external fixation device in (*a*), compound, comminuted lower radial fracture (*b*); *c*, X-ray and (*d*) clinical appearance.

• Dislocations

Treatment

The first principle of treatment is to reduce the displacement. When this has been achieved it is then important to deal with the soft-tissue injuries, especially to the capsule and its ligaments. Most heal spontaneously but a few, e.g. ankle or knee, will demand operative repair.

An anaesthetic is needed for reduction in order to overcome muscle spasm. In the case of a finger a local anaesthetic will suffice, but with the shoulder, hip or elbow, relaxation under general anaesthesia is required.

Once the soft tissues are relaxed and the muscle spasm gone the joint surfaces are gently pulled apart and by directing the applied force in the opposite direction to the dislocating force the joint usually spontaneously reduces. For example in the hip the dislocating force is often a blow on to the flexed knee (dashboard injury) and the femoral head is whacked posteriorly (through or over the acetabular rim). Thus, with the patient lying on his back the flexed hip is pulled firmly forward with a rotatory movement inwards and the hip will reduce with a satisfying 'clunk'.

Certain points mentioned in Chapter 1 require re-emphasis: never attempt to reduce a dislocation without an X-ray (*Fig.* 2.18) because an associated fracture may be present or indeed may be the only injury. Check all reductions with X-rays before the patient wakes up.

Immobilization

A sling is used for shoulder injuries, while with stable elbow injuries a collar-and-cuff can be employed, or if there is any instability a plaster backslab is applied. Finger dislocations can be immobilized in malleable splints or by strapping adjacent fingers. A hip dislocation is usually very stable but the lower limb can be rested on a Thomas' splint or in a foam-trough for two or more weeks depending on the associated bony damage. Knee, ankle and foot dislocations usually require a plaster. Toes are treated by strapping.

The period of immobilization will vary from 1 to 2 weeks in shoulder and finger injuries, to 4 to 6 weeks after hip and knee dislocations. Generally early movement is encouraged but not when the tissues are swollen and painful. Special precautions such as slow mobilization and very rigid splintage are needed when an important ligament is torn (e.g. the collateral ligaments of the knee and ankle), or when early movement might encourage further swelling or bleeding and thus encourage excessive fibrosis or even myositis ossificans (e.g. the elbow and hip).

Recurrent Dislocations

When the capsule is permanently stretched or torn the joint may redislocate after minor trauma or even after normal forces, such as yawning and stretching the arm. The joints most often affected by recurrent dislocations are the shoulder, sternoclavicular, elbow, and patellofemoral (*Fig.* 2.19).

Surgery is required for recurrent dislocation not only to avoid the pain and discomfort but also to prevent damage to the lining hyaline cartilage and thus osteoarthritis.

37 Principles of treatment

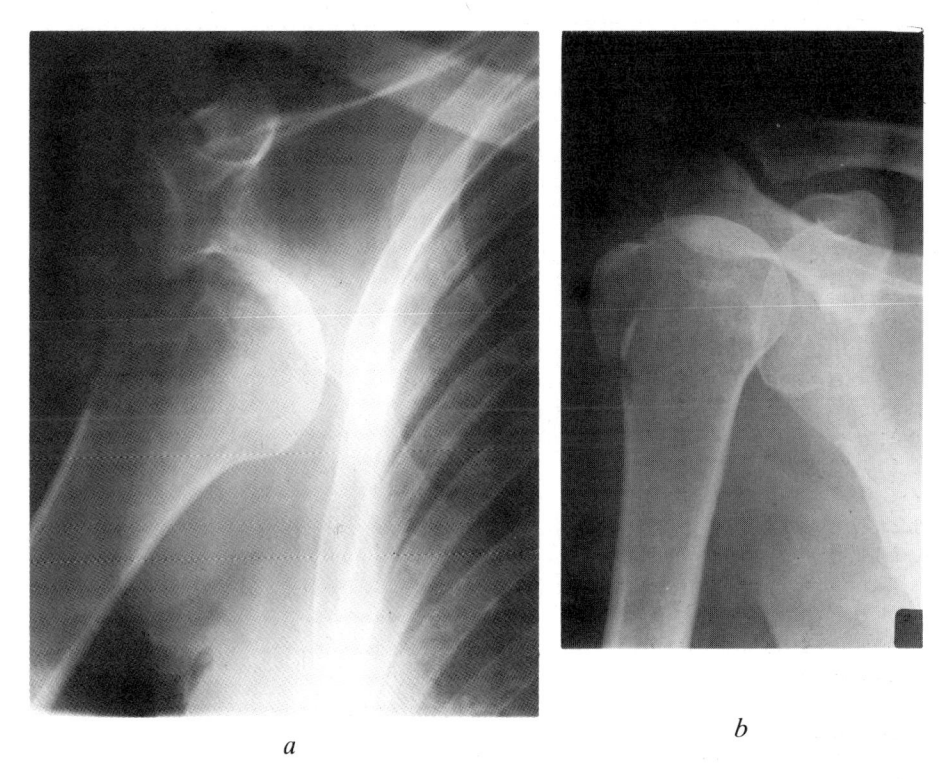

Fig. 2.18. A fracture–dislocation of the R shoulder (*a*); after reduction showing good apposition of fragments (*b*).

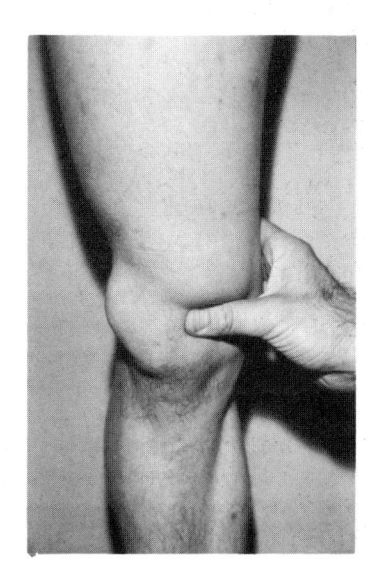

Fig. 2.19. A 14-year-old with recurrent dislocation of the patella (easily subluxed) due to familial joint hypermobility.

Unstable Joints

Many patients feel their joints to be 'unstable' or 'dislocating' when in fact joint movement is hampered only by miscellaneous soft tissue or bony causes. Such examples are snapping shoulders or hips (due to fascial bands which emit a disturbing 'clunk'), chondromalacia patellae (when reflex stumbling or 'giving way' may occur during certain painful movements at the patellofemoral junction), tendons impinging on a bony exostosis or subluxing at the ankle (peroneal tendons). Pain from fibrotic areas in a healed lateral ligament of ankle often causes reflex ankle instability. To treat such miscellaneous problems attention is directed towards the underlying cause and the appropriate surgical measures taken, e.g. removal of the exostosis or repair of the retaining retinaculum over the peroneal tendons.

An unusual joint problem occurs in young adults, especially teenage girls, who complain of 'dislocating joints', usually the shoulder or hip. Some have the ability to sublux the shoulder as a party piece. Usually the hip concern is due to the staccato clunk from the fascia moving abruptly over the greater trochanter. There is often an underlying psychological problem which should be treated. It is also worth noting that epileptics may regularly dislocate a certain joint (previously injured) during an attack.

Physiotherapy and Rehabilitation

Rehabilitation, it used to be said at the Radcliffe Infirmary, Oxford, begins at the scene of the accident. The recently injured area is disturbed as little as possible. Once the fracture or dislocation has been treated the first 48–72 h of rest allows the soft-tissue biochemical tide to settle. However, that is not to say that the patient should not fully and vigorously exercise the other limbs—professional soccer players have shown the marked advantages of such continuous therapy by a more rapid return to sport. For example, a patient with a forearm fracture can successfully carry out weight exercises with the unaffected limbs, e.g. cycle in the gymnasium.

Rehabilitation has the following purposes:
1. The preservation of function while the fracture is uniting.
2. The rapid restoration of function once union has occurred.
3. The maintenance of a good level of patient fitness.

Although not intending to cover fully the whole of physiotherapy or usurp the later details given in the ensuing chapters, the following principles apply:
1. Apart from minor injuries the patient should be under the care of a *qualified* physiotherapist or doctor.
2. Exercises initiated in hospital must be continued at home. Self-help is encouraged.
3. Exercises should be graduated and not induce undue pain or discomfort.
4. Electronic apparatus (e.g. short-wave diathermy and ultrasound), although of great benefit, is no substitute for skilled remedial therapy.
5. The physiotherapist should encourage the patient by a mixture of coercion and muted optimism: a nihilistic attitude breeds discontent.
6. Full activity (especially in sport) should not be allowed until the muscles are powerful, flexible and coordinated and joint movements should be full, stable and pain-free.

Principles of treatment

Exercises are usually *passive* or *active*. Passive exercises occur when the therapist gently moves the limb; active therapy occurs when the muscles are clenched without joint movement (isometric), or used against gravity or resistance (such as weights) (isotonic). During the final stages of activity pool therapy (hydrotherapy), swimming, running (first in a straight line and then turning) and gymnasium work are encouraged.

3

Complications: local and general

- *Most fractures unite with only minor residual problems and little, if any, permanent disability.* However, in a few cases complications do occur. They are broadly divided into:

1. Local (at the fracture site).
2. Regional (in the affected limb).
3. Systemic (throughout the whole body).

- **Local**

Delayed Union
When a fracture remains mobile after 3 months union is said to be delayed, although there is no absolute time for union to occur and certain estimations (as for example 6 weeks for a Colles fracture) are purely arbitrary (*see* Chapter 1). Generally speaking, femoral shaft fractures (the biggest long bone injury) feel firm by 12 weeks and thus 3 months becomes the limit of normality. Definitely by 16 weeks fracture union should have occurred. If delayed union persists for 2–3 months then non-union usually follows.

The causes of delayed union and non-union are essentially the same (*Fig. 3.1*). Thus the treatment of delayed union (*see* 'non-union') is a combination of continued immobilization, general physiotherapy and the eradication of an underlying cause such as infection or osteomalacia. Internal fixation and bone grafting may be needed.

Non-union
Many factors influence the speed of union. They include the age of the patient and the type of injury. Union may be hindered or even prevented by an impairment of blood supply or by movement of the fragments. However, not all fractures require strict immobility, e.g. fractures of the ribs, humerus and clavicle can heal without plaster or internal fixation. But movement in the forearm bones, scaphoid, talus or femoral neck may lead to non-union because of damage to the delicate capillaries in the bone, bridging callus and soft tissues.

41 Complications: local and general

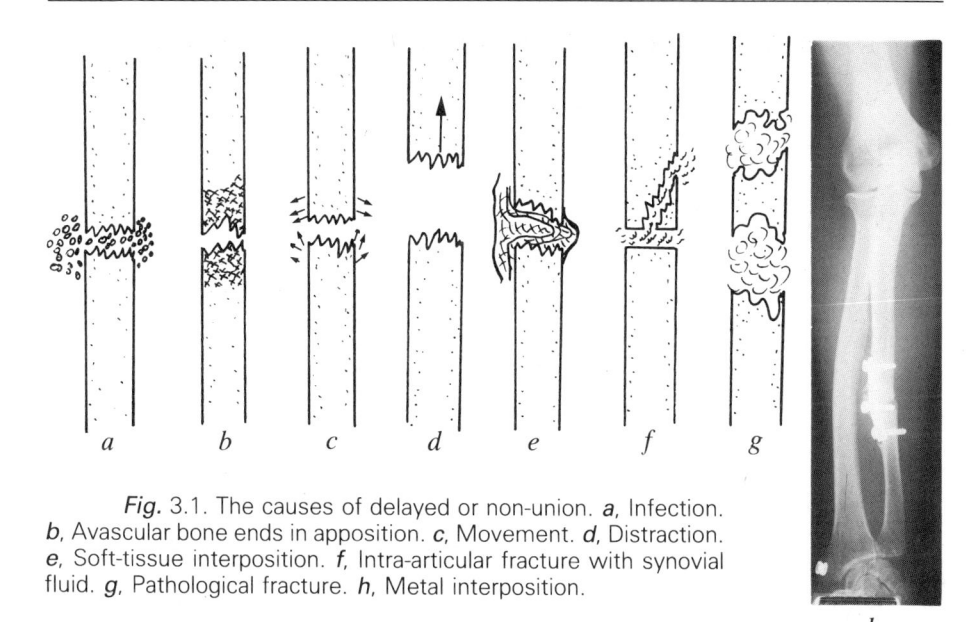

Fig. 3.1. The causes of delayed or non-union. *a*, Infection. *b*, Avascular bone ends in apposition. *c*, Movement. *d*, Distraction. *e*, Soft-tissue interposition. *f*, Intra-articular fracture with synovial fluid. *g*, Pathological fracture. *h*, Metal interposition.

Other prime factors which may retard union are infection, interposition of soft tissue such as muscle, and pathological changes in the bone, including osteomalacia and neoplasia. When a fracture occurs in an intra-articular situation non-union is a possibility, probably due to the presence of synovial fluid hampering the formation of osteogenic tissue at the fracture site.

Thus, in summary, the causes of non-union are (*Fig.* 3.1):
1. Loss of apposition.
2. Movement.
3. Soft-tissue interposition.
4. Infection.
5. Impaired blood supply.
6. Synovial fluid bathing the fracture.
7. Destruction of bone by disease.
8. Loss of contact due to metal plates or screws.

Diagnosis
The fracture is freely mobile and may be relatively painless. On X-rays the bone ends become dense and rounded, so that the fracture line is readily apparent (*Fig.* 3.2). Callus formation stops and often reabsorption occurs leaving a fibrous bond. In some cases a false joint (a pseudarthrosis) develops.

Treatment
This depends upon the bone involved, the nature of the fracture, the cause of the non-union and the residual disability.
1. *Internal Fixation with Bone Grafting or External Fixation*
This treatment is most suitable for long bones. The graft is usually obtained from the pelvic crest or locally. Sometimes such autogenous grafting is supplemented

42 An outline of fractures and dislocations

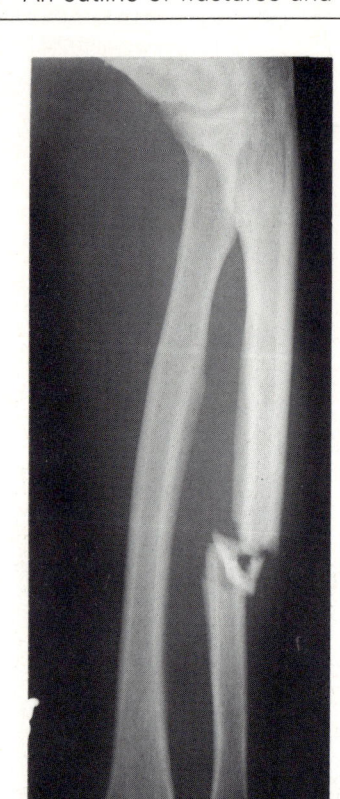

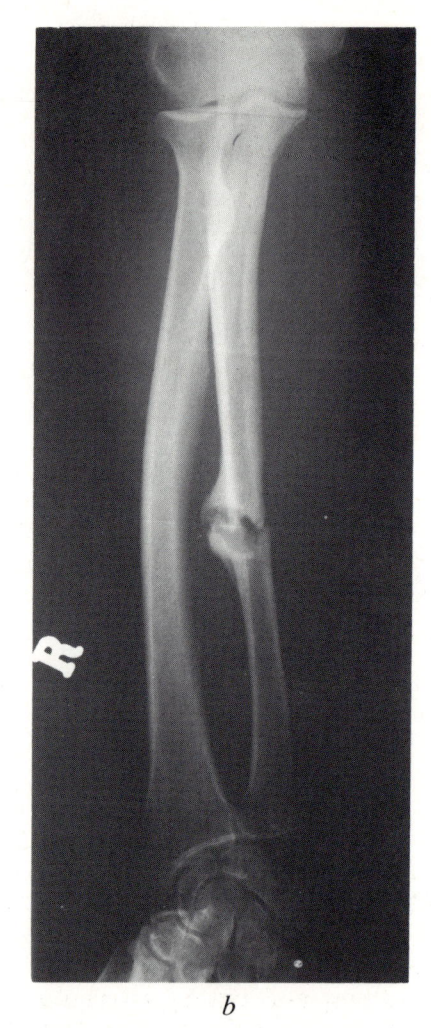

Fig. 3.2. Non-union of the ulna—a frequent site (*b*, taken 1 year later).

by bone from a 'bone bank' (a homograft). Bone, specially prepared from animals, is also used (a heterograft). The purpose of all types of graft is to serve as a scaffolding upon which new bone is deposited and to provide local calcium and phosphate, etc.

2. *Non-treatment*

In certain cases the fracture may cause little or no disability (e.g. sometimes in the carpal bones, 5th metatarsal, etc.) and no treatment is given.

3. *Excision of the Painful Fragment*

In certain instances, especially when the fracture is within a joint, the damaging fragment may be excised, e.g. with collapse of the proximal pole of the scaphoid or with an avulsed fragment in the terminal joint of the great toe.

43 Complications: local and general

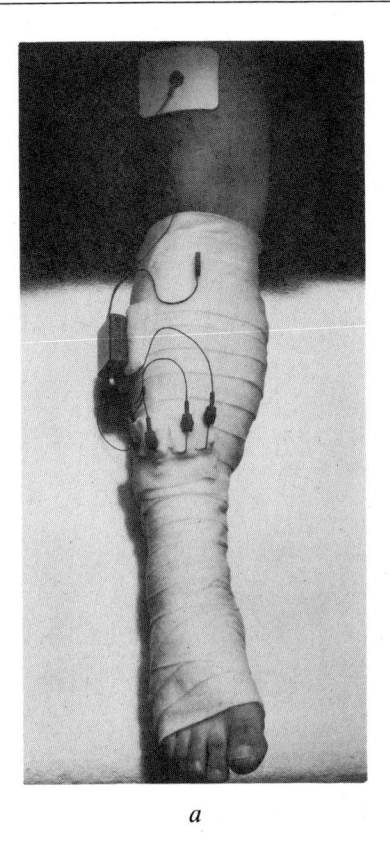

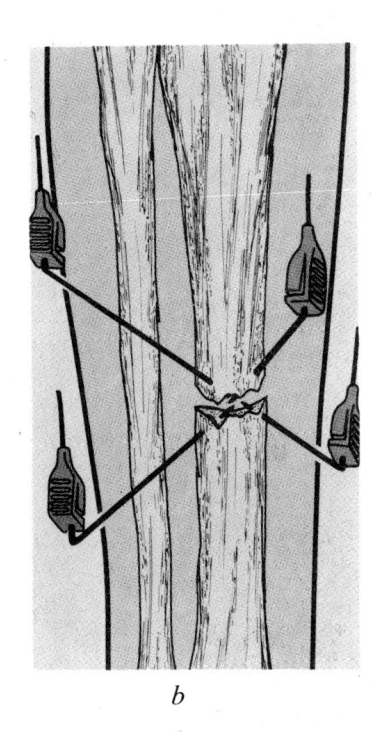

a   *b*

Fig. 3.3. Induction of new bone by minute electric currents passing from the four cathodes placed in the fracture area; the anode is attached to the skin.

4.   *Treatment of Cause*
Infection is eradicated with antibiotics; movement at the fracture line inhibited by a firm plaster incorporating the joints above and below the fracture; restoration of contact by releasing traction when the distracting force is too strong; or by removing interposed soft tissues and metal plates. Avascular segments need excision and a fresh cancellous graft applied. Intra-articular fractures need accurate fixation and drainage of excess synovial fluid for a time with a suction drain. With pathological fractures radiotherapy and chemotherapy will be required; while metabolic problems such as osteomalacia demand medical therapy, in this case vitamin D.
- *Several factors can coexist and all need complete rectification* (*Fig.* 3.1).

Established Non-union
When bone grafting and internal fixation have failed or (more recently) as a primary procedure, *electromagnetic therapy* can be used (*Fig.* 3.3).
    A case of non-union of the tibia was first treated with electricity in 1812. Minute currents around the cathode (negative pole) of 5–20 microamperes can induce bone formation when applied for 12 weeks or so. In some techniques the

limb is placed in a plaster while in others free unrestricted weight-bearing can be carried out, although usually the former method is preferred. The applied current is usually direct, although alternating currents have been used to induce a constant electromagnetic field.

The two methods employed are *invasive* and *non-invasive*.

With *invasive* methods the metal electrodes (cathodes) (usually four) are inserted directly into the fracture site while the anode and power pack are placed subcutaneously; or the cathodes are passed subcutaneously and positioned by X-rays and the anode and power pack remain externally.

A simpler *non-invasive* method uses inductive coupling through electromagnetic coils placed on the skin around the fracture area and applied for 10–12 h at night. This is also a popular method. All three methods give a 70–80% success rate in a 3–6 month period. However, before treatment a synovial pseudarthrosis must be excised and a large gap apposed; mild infection or metal implants are not always a contraindication.

Avascular Necrosis

Bone stripped of its blood supply dies. The cut-off in vascularity is often immediate (*Fig.* 7.10, p. 149) but X-ray changes can take several months or even a year or more to appear.

Avascular necrosis occurs most frequently in the head of the femur (*Fig.* 3.4*a*), the proximal half of the scaphoid (*Fig.* 3.4*b*), the body of the talus and in the lunate.

The salient and common feature in these injuries is a fracture close to the articular surface (often devoid of soft tissues and thus vascular attachments) with the bone depending for its nutrition almost entirely upon intra-osseous vessels. These are torn or compressed at the moment of injury (or shortly afterwards). Tearing is an obvious cause, but compression from swelling (such as may occur in a distended joint, e.g. hip following a children's hip fracture) is often forgotten; under these circumstances aspiration is worthwhile.

The bone cells die, the trabeculae soften and compress, while the bone crumbles and distorts under the stress of weight-bearing. To add to the sorry picture the overlying hyaline cartilage eventually shows necrosis (*Fig.* 3.4*a*) and osteoarthritis supervenes.

Radiological Diagnosis

• *The affected segment appears more dense on X-rays.* Why? Because the inflammatory processes of injury cause local osteoporosis which cannot involve the avascular area due to the impaired blood supply. In addition, within the collapsed area forces compress the weakened trabeculae while new bone may be added to cause trabecular thickening (a late feature if the blood supply returns).

Treatment

It is wise to recognize the fractures which may suffer from avascular necrosis and treat them by rigid plaster immobilization. When in doubt internal fixation with a screw may be needed, e.g. the scaphoid waist fracture or the subcapital fracture of the femoral neck. Once established the avascular bone should be excised if causing symptoms and, if necessary, replaced by a metal or plastic/metal prosthesis, e.g. total hip replacement.

45 Complications: local and general

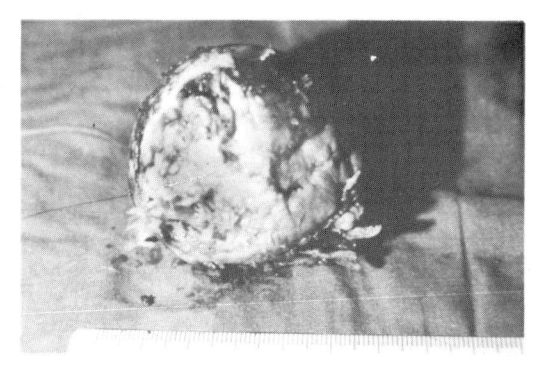

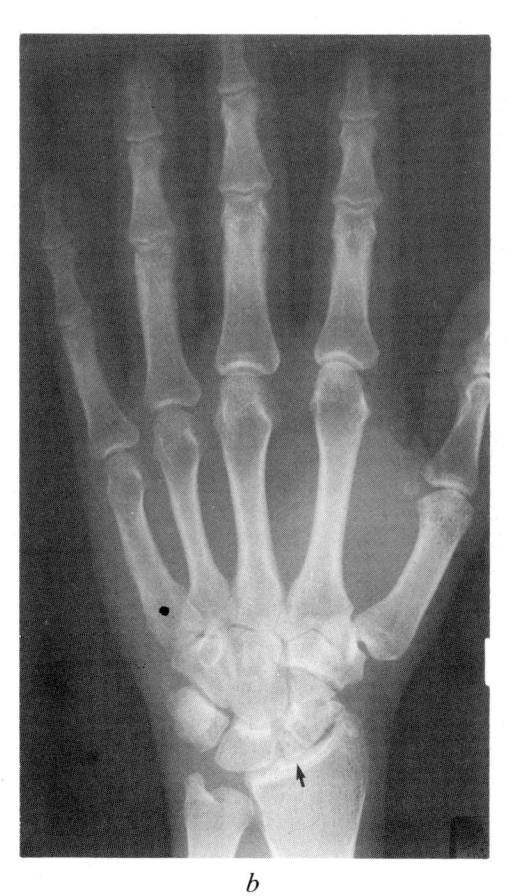

Fig. 3.4. *a*, An avascular femoral head following a femoral neck fracture 9 months previously: note hyaline cartilage necrosis. *b*, Avascular necrosis of the proximal pole of the scaphoid.

46 An outline of fractures and dislocations

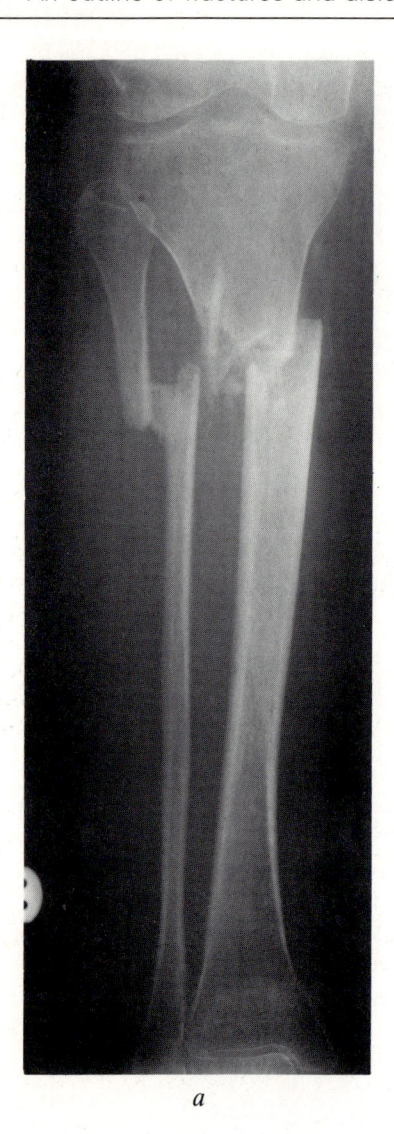

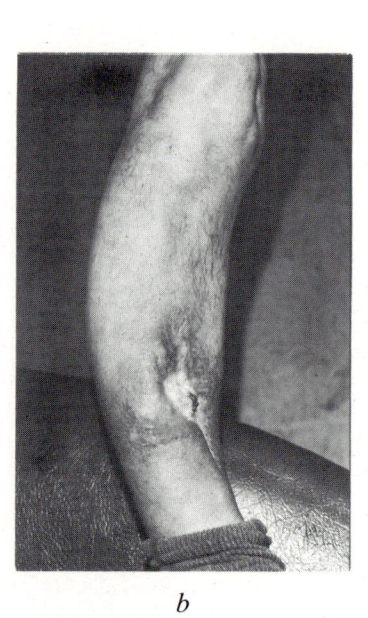

Fig. 3.5. Mal-union: *a*, Tibia and fibula following a 'bumper fracture'. *b*, After gross infection.

Mal-union

Mal-union signifies imperfect alignment (*Fig.* 3.5), at its worst a 'dog's leg' deformity. This complication is usually preventable and commonly caused by imperfect reduction, inadequate immobilization, or a failure to recognize non-union before weight-bearing begins.

Treatment
The fracture may be mobile enough for re-manipulation or the bone may have to be divided surgically (osteotomy) and internally fixed with a plate.

Infection

● *This usually follows open (compound) fractures or when surgery has been performed* (*Fig.* 3.6). The infection may be:
1. In the skin or soft tissues (cellulitis).
2. In the bone (osteomyelitis).

Bone infection can last for life, with a chronic discharge, skin sinuses and dead bone fragments (sequestra). Metal plates add to the problem and potentiate the infection; usually they have to be removed. The drawback is that a stable infected fracture may be converted to an unstable infected fracture.

Treatment

Prevention is, as always, better than cure. Every effort must be made to avoid infection in orthopaedics by fastidious theatre techniques, prompt and meticulous excision of all dead and contaminated tissue and the appropriate selective antibiotic cover.

With the acute soft-tissue infection (cellulitis) antibiotics will suffice with complete rest in a plaster backslab, for joint and muscle movements disturb the inflamed tissues; an abscess needs incision and drainage. Dead bone is removed along with any plates, screws or wires. Antibiotics are given for 6 weeks and a regular wound swab taken.

Chronic infections rarely respond to long-term antibiotics and more radical surgery may be needed with deroofing of the cavity, wide excision of necrotic bone and prolonged plaster immobilization (8–12 weeks). Swab cultures are often negative or show a mixed bacterial growth. Special laboratory culture media may be required.

Refracture

Refracture is very demoralizing for the patient and the underlying cause may give problems for the orthopaedic surgeon.

Refracture can occur:
1. With a *normal* force when the callus is immature (i.e. walking on a comminuted tibial fracture at 6 weeks).
2. With a *normal* force when the bone is weak from other causes such as infection or tumour.
3. With a *normal* force when delayed or non-union union is apparent.
4. With a *slightly abnormal* (stronger) force when mal-union has occurred (*see Fig.* 2.3).
5. With a *slightly abnormal* force when the fracture has been fixed internally but reabsorption of the bone ends has occurred (*see Fig.* 3.1*b*).
6. With an *abnormal* force during the re-modelling phase (e.g. a heavy fall onto the outstretched hand 4 months after a forearm fracture).
7. With an *abnormal* force after internal fixation when the stress forces are channelled to bone/metal interface (*Fig.* 3.7).

Treatment

Usually the refracture is treated conservatively with plaster but an underlying cause such as infection requires appropriate therapy. If the metal implant has broken it may need taking out but often the bone ends accurately appose and union begins in the newly formed haematoma. Sometimes the metal device

48 An outline of fractures and dislocations

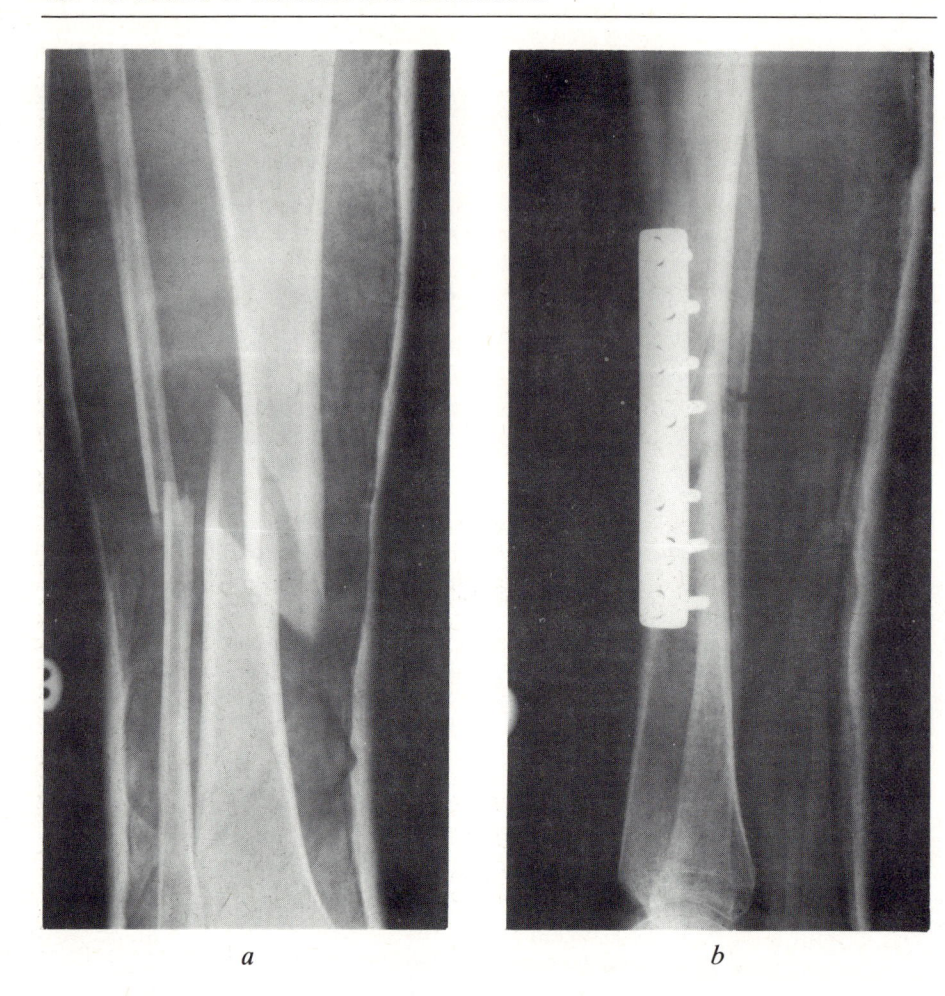

           a   *b*

Fig. 3.6. A 60-year-old alcoholic with a spiral fracture of the tibia (and fibula) (*a*); treated by internal fixation (*b,c*); marred by living rough, early weight bearing and gross infection (X-ray 2 years later) (*d*).

requires removal and if avascularity and non-union are apparent then a bone graft is used (as described under non-union).

In summary, the *local* complications are:

Delayed union
Non-union
Avascular necrosis
Mal-union
Infection
Refracture

49 Complications: local and general

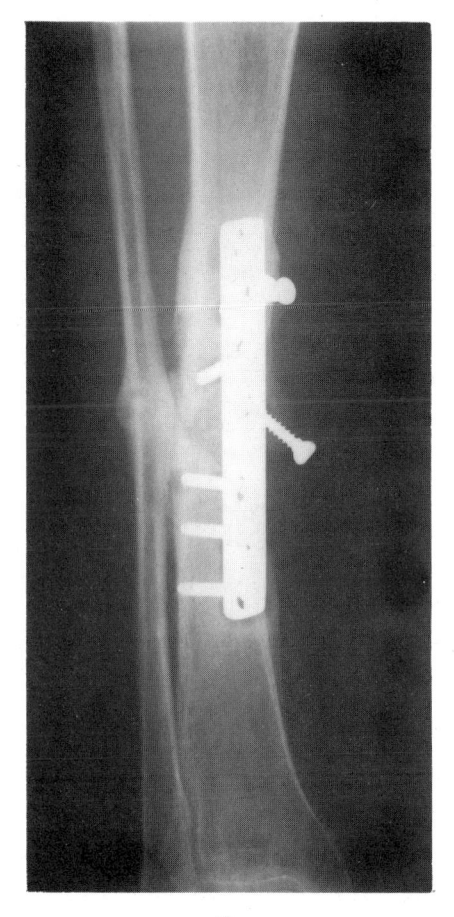

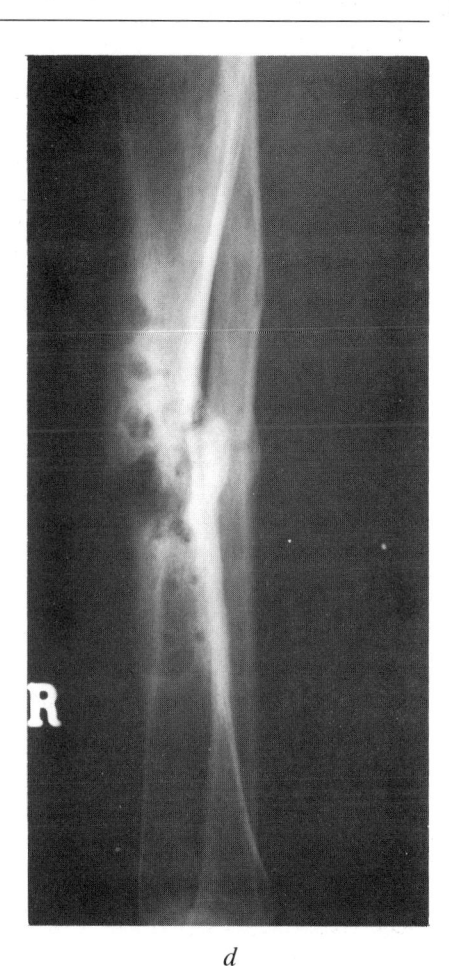

c *d*

Fig. 3.6. (*cont.*)

- **Regional Vascular Injury**
  Occasionally an important artery or vein is damaged due to:
1. Crushing or nipping by the fracture (supracondylar at the elbow affecting the brachial artery) or by a dislocation (e.g. popliteal vessels at the knee) (*Fig.* 3.8*a*).
2. Laceration by the bone ends (*Fig.* 3.8*b*).
3. Intimal thrombosis.
4. The wound extending through the vessels in compound fractures or dislocations (*Fig.* 3.8*c*).

The late effects of vascular injuries are:
1. Gangrene.
2. Ischaemic muscle or nerve damage.

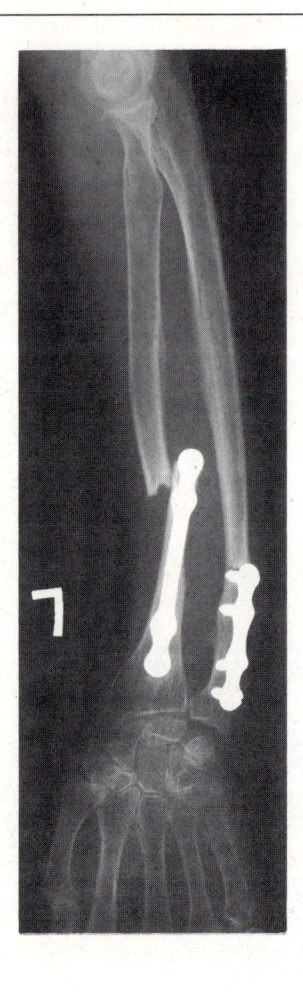

Fig. 3.7. A fracture at the weak point, i.e. metal/bone interface.

3. Refractory oedema.
4. Intermittent claudication.
    ● *Do not forget that a tight plaster or bandage can occlude the limb circulation* (Chapter 2).

Diagnosis
The *signs of avascularity* are:
1. Pain.
2. Pallor.
3. Cyanosis.
4. Swelling.
5. No pulse below the injury.
6. No bleeding below the injury.
7. Nerve tingling and muscle spasm.
    ● *All occur in the affected limb below the damaged area.*

51 Complications: local and general

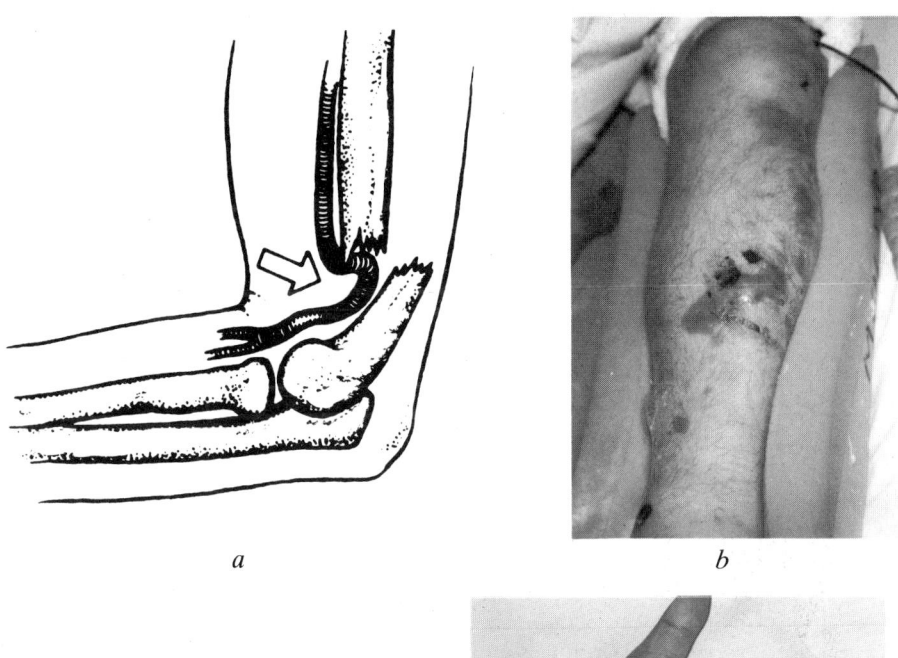

Fig. 3.8. Vessel injury. *a*, The brachial vessels with a supracondylar fracture. *b*, Femoral artery damage due to a femoral shaft fracture (direct injury) in a 20-year-old motorcyclist. Gas gangrene and renal failure followed but the patient (and the leg) survived. *c*, Ischaemic changes in the fingers in a child with axillary artery severance (and repair).

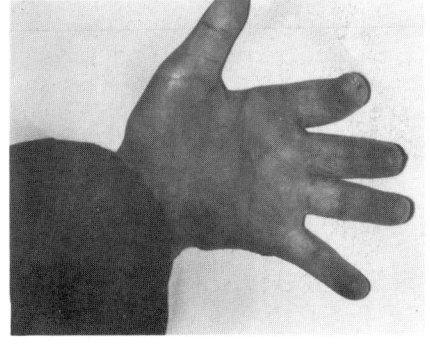

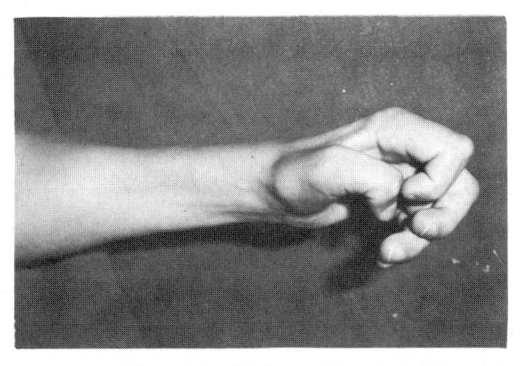

Fig. 3.9. Volkmann's ischaemic contracture following a supracondylar fracture.

Treatment

• *This is urgent because the effects of ischaemia can rapidly become irreversible.*

If there is impaired circulation at the beginning the fracture (or dislocation) *is reduced as quickly as possible*. If there is no response to an adequate reduction an emergency arteriogram is arranged. Prompt surgery is performed to release external pressure from bone and soft tissues (by dividing the overlying fascia as in the compartmental syndromes of the tibia) or to remove internal pressure from clots and subintimal thrombi. Any damaged vessel is usually excised and replaced with a vein graft, sometimes a synthetic material is used for large vessels. The fracture is usually fixed internally to prevent further vascular damage by bone movement or displacement.

Two major complications which occur with arterial injury are gangrene and Volkmann's ischaemic contracture of the forearm, although other muscles (especially the tibial muscles after tibial shaft fracture) can develop these ischaemic changes.

Gangrene

Once the arterial circulation has been cut off for several hours the limb becomes gangrenous and local amputation will have to be carried out. Sometimes only the toes or fingers are affected (*Fig. 3.8c*) but on other occasions a larger area may be involved (e.g. a mid-thigh amputation with femoral artery damage). Such a serious complication is rare nowadays and usually the affected vessels are repaired either directly or by a grafting operation.

Muscle Ischaemia

Damage to the brachial artery (or the radial or ulnar arteries) (supracondylar humerus or forearm fractures) can result in ischaemia of the forearm muscles and the later sequel of Volkmann's contracture (*Fig. 3.9*). The forearm becomes atrophic and the hand and fingers clawed with the wrist flexed. Surgery is needed to release the origins of the flexor muscles and to elongate or transfer tendons.

Ischaemia of the *hand* may follow forearm injuries and the intrinsic hand muscles fibrose and shorten, flexing the fingers at the metacarpophalangeal joints but straightening the interphalangeal joints; while the thumb is adducted across the palm. Similar intrinsic injuries can occur in the *foot*, leading to clawing of the toes. Ischaemia of the *tibial* and foot muscles will require operations described under forearm ischaemia; femoral shaft and tibial fractures can cause lower limb ischaemia; intracompartmental pressure can be monitored.

Nerve Damage

The common sites of nerve damage are shown in *Fig. 3.10*. With mild nerve bruising, usually from compression (*Fig. 3.11a*), the damage is slight and recovery occurs within a few days or weeks. With nerve severance (*Fig. 3.11b, d*) recovery is only possible after resuture (*Fig. 3.11c*) or by repairing the defect with a nerve graft.

53 Complications: local and general

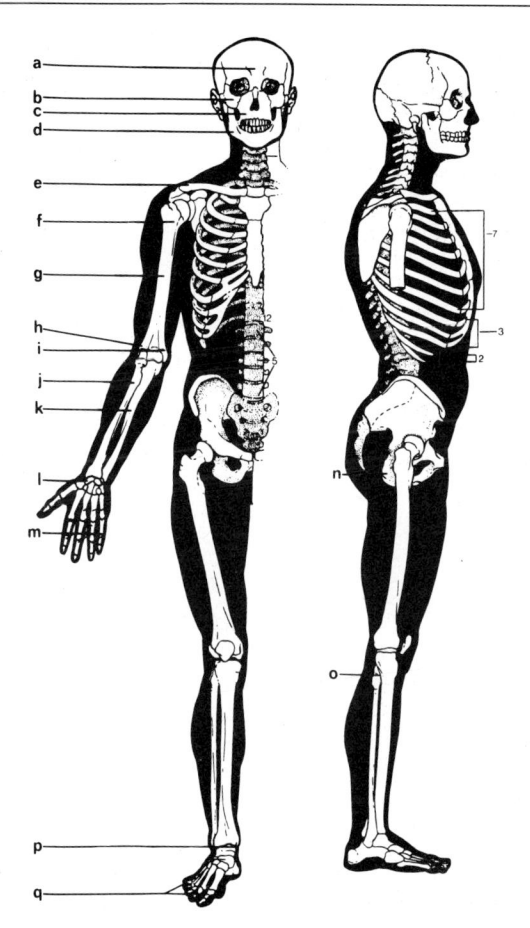

Fig. 3.10. Principal areas of nerve injury. **a**, Supraorbital; **b**, Infraorbital (zygoma); **c**, **d**, Dental nerves (facial fractures); **e**, Brachial plexus; **f**, Axillary (shoulder dislocation); **g**, Radial (humerus fractures); **h**, Median (elbow injuries); **i**, Ulnar (elbow); **j**, Posterior interosseous, and **k**, Anterior interosseous (forearm injuries); **l**, Median (wrist); **m**, Digital nerves (finger injuries); **n**, Sciatic (pelvic or hip injuries); **o**, Lateral popliteal, and **p**, tibial nerves with tibial fractures; **q**, Digital nerves (foot).

Diagnosis
The *signs of nerve injury* are:
1. Pain.
2. Loss of sensation.
3. Loss of movement.
4. Tingling or altered sensation.
5. Weakness of muscle power.
6. Absent reflexes.

- *All occur in the affected limb below the damaged area.*

54 An outline of fractures and dislocations

a

b

c

d

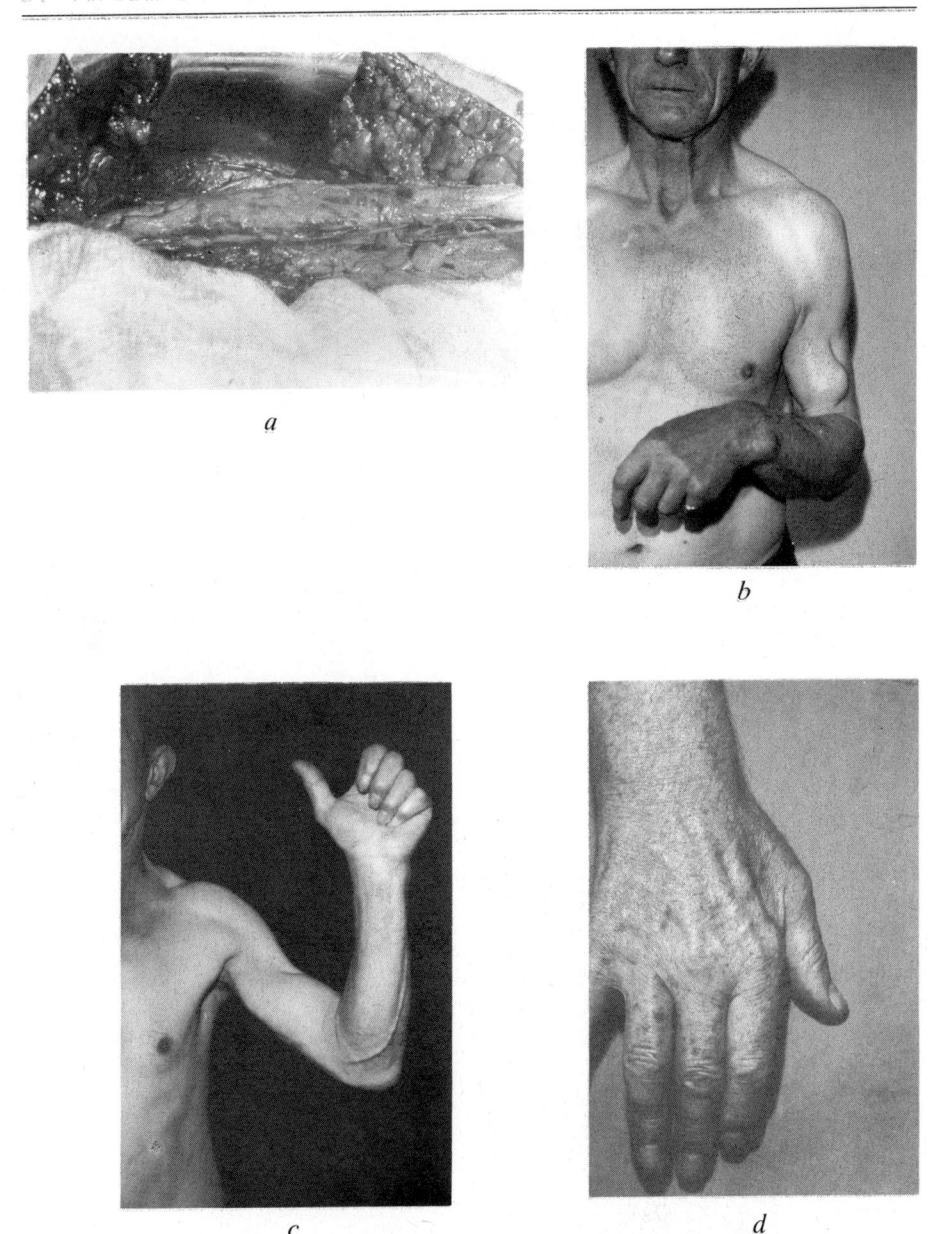

Fig. 3.11. Nerve damage. *a*, Contusion of the sciatic nerve following a posterior dislocation of the hip. *b*, A 75-year-old village cricketer from the North Yorks Moors referred as a ruptured long head of biceps due to a blow at cricket. Note the wrist drop. Radial nerve repair was performed and 18 months later (*c*) he is giving the thumbs up sign (radial nerve function) after returning to cricket. *d*, Ulnar nerve injury at the elbow (fractured lower humerus) reflected in interosseous wasting.

Treatment

With closed injuries the nerve is usually assumed to be in continuity, but if there is no recovery by 2–3 weeks then the nerve conduction studies are performed. However, in the presence of a marked defect (such as a foot drop after a blow over the lateral popliteal nerve on the outer aspect of the knee) then early studies or even an exploratory operation might be carried out. When there is gross comminution, a major dislocation or a compound injury it should be assumed that complete severance has occurred and an immediate repair instituted by surgery. Usually nerves regenerate at the rate of 2·5 cm (1 in) per month. Sometimes marked scarring around a fracture can cause compression or traction on a nerve and lead to problems. Under these circumstances the scar tissue is excised and the nerve freed.

Tendon Injury

Tendons can be torn by direct laceration in compound injuries or by sharp bony fragments (e.g. in the wrist). Direct suture is usually carried out.

Joint Injury

Damage to the hyaline articular cartilage, menisci, ligaments and capsule are all involved in intra-articular and peri-articular injuries and surgical intervention is required.

Post-traumatic Ossification

Sometimes when a joint has been injured or when a fracture has occurred with stripping of the periosteum, the induced haematoma slowly converts to bone (myositis ossificans) (*Fig.* 3.12). With a large mass of bone, joint or muscle

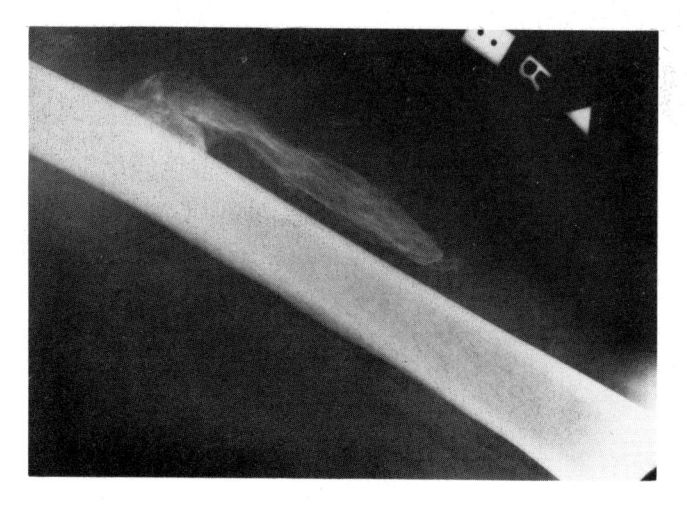

Fig. 3.12. Myositis ossificans in the thigh muscles.

movement may be restricted and the lump may be painful. The mass of callus on X-ray may be mistaken for a bone tumour, but isotope studies will indicate when the lump is quiescent and it can be excised. The commonest sites are the elbow

56 An outline of fractures and dislocations

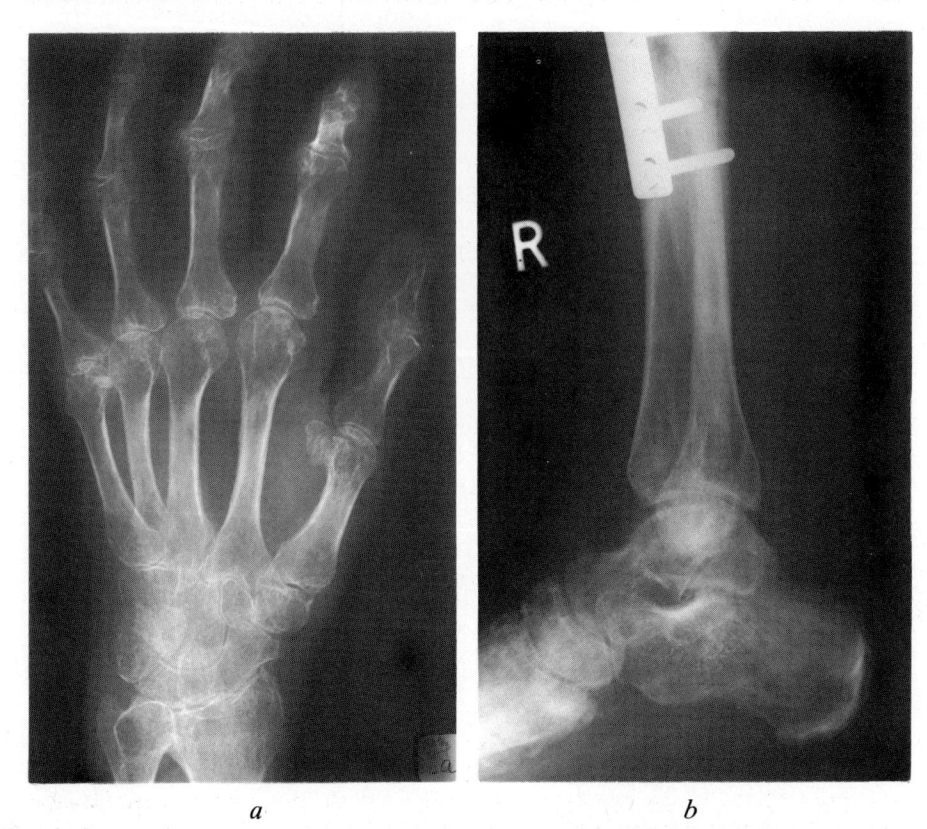

Fig. 3.13. *a*, Sudeck's atrophy; the hand is painfully swollen and the bones show patchy osteoporosis. *b*, Disuse osteoporosis of the ankle and foot following a tibial shaft fracture.

after a fracture-dislocation, the anterior thigh muscles, gluteal muscles and hip. Patients with a prolonged period of unconsciousness or paraplegia often develop widespread myositis ossificans in several muscles of the hips, knees or shoulders.

Treatment
Rest in the early stages when the lump is forming and the avoidance of manipulation, massage and heat (which add to the formation); with late excision, as mentioned.

Sudeck's Post-traumatic Atrophy

Diagnosis
The painful osteoporosis which occurs in the bones of the affected limb, usually after a fracture, is called Sudeck's atrophy or osteodystrophy. It is characterized by pain, swelling and marked joint stiffness in the hand or the foot of the injured limb, usually accompanied by a mottled bluish-pink discoloration and shiny skin, which is very painful to touch. X-ray shows a patchy osteoporosis (*Fig.* 3.13*a*).

57 Complications: local and general

Although all limbs immobilized for a long period show atrophic changes (*Fig.* 3.13*b*) in this condition the clinical picture is so clearcut as to make it a distinct entity.

Treatment
Most cases respond slowly to progressive, gentle mobilization, wax baths, with anti-inflammatory agents given in fairly high dosage.

Osteoarthritis

Post-traumatic osteoarthritis (*Fig.* 3.14) (or osteoarthrosis) occurs:
1. When there is an irregular joint surface.
2. Lack of joint apposition.
3. Loose bodies.
4. Restricted joint movement.
5. Ligamentous laxity.
6. Avascular segment.
7. Mal-alignment or mal-union.

Treatment
If the cause can be corrected by realignment of the affected bones by osteotomy (e.g. marked bowing of the tibia causing undue stress on the medial compartment of the knee) the prognosis is good and the arthritic change may be halted—the same can be said if ligamentous instability is removed. However, when the joint surfaces are markedly disorganized a fusion (arthrodesis) or a joint replacement (arthroplasty) is performed. With only minor osteoarthritic change, physiotherapy designed to strengthen the associated muscle groups, anti-inflammatory tablets, restricted activity (e.g. the use of a stick or support) are prescribed.

Shortening

Limb shortening is due to:
1. Overlapping of the fragments.
2. Mal-union.
3. Loss of bone or crushing.
4. Loss of bone growth in children due to epiphyseal injury.
5. Collapse of the avascular head in femoral neck or hip injuries.
6. Loss of limb growth after cord or major nerve injury in a child.

Treatment
Shortening is most important in the lower limb but up to 2 cm (¾ in) is not significant in adults. Above this level a shoe raise is supplied (it might be prudent to correct all discrepancy in athletic persons). Since marked shortening causes stress in the related joints, especially the hip and low back (with some scoliosis), it may be advisable to correct the leg length in children by an elongation operation and in adults by shortening the opposite limb (although most people do not like to lose height unless very tall).

58   An outline of fractures and dislocations

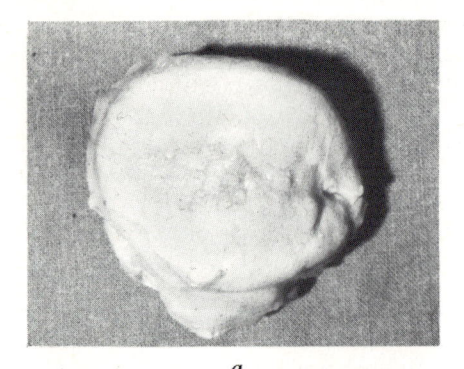

Fig. 3.14. *a*, Patellar osteoarthrosis due to direct impact following a road traffic accident 3 years previously. *b*, Slight malalignment in the ankle following fracture with osteoarthritic change. *c*, Loose body in the elbow.

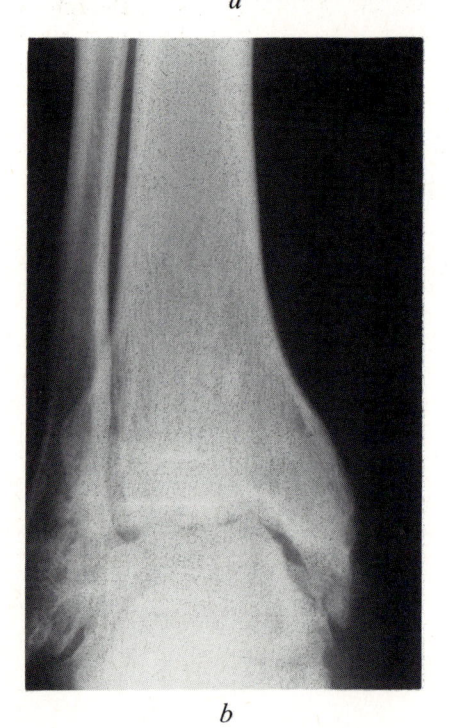

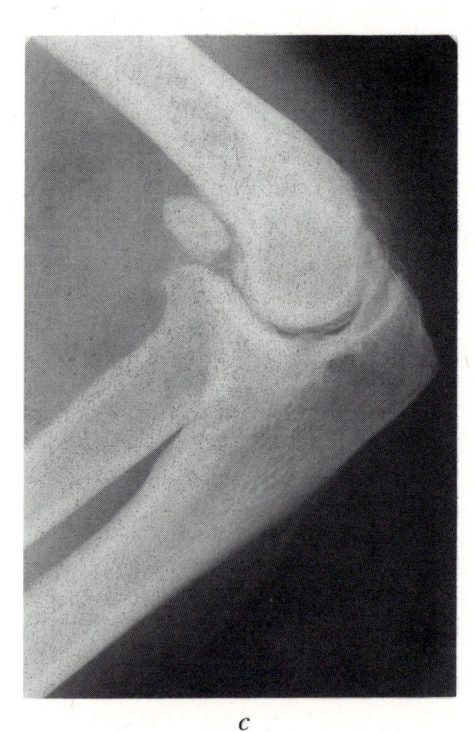

Injury to Viscera
Viscera may be damaged either by the forces causing the fracture (or dislocation) or by impalement upon a sharp fragment of bone, e.g. rib fractures may penetrate lung tissue or liver; pelvic fractures may cause rupture of the bladder, urethra, colon or rectum.

Treatment
Immediate attention is given to the serious complications listed above and the patient is referred to a general surgeon. Fracture treatment follows after surgical intervention but there is always a risk from blood-borne or local bacteria if internal fixation is used.

Intra-articular and Peri-articular Adhesions

Joint stiffness from adhesions is common after fractures and dislocations, with some joints, such as the knee, elbow, fingers and toes, being more vulnerable.

Bleeding within the joint causes *intra-articular* adhesions; whereas *peri-articular* adhesions due to fibrosis in the surrounding capsule, ligaments and muscles are a greater and more common problem. They are due to a combination of injury, oedema and immobilization (especially if plaster has been used for long periods). Muscle tissue may also become directly adherent to the fracture site.

Treatment

Joint stiffness usually responds to graduated physiotherapy, although a manipulation can be carried out under a general anaesthetic if there is marked initial stiffness or there has been no response to 4–6 weeks of therapy. Reverse slings and traction can be used slowly in hospital to restore the range of movement.

Rarely is surgery required to free adhesions except when the muscles are bound down to the fractured area, as for example sometimes occurs in the lower thigh.

In summary *regional* complications are:
Vascular injury
Nerve damage
Tendon injury
Joint injury
Post-traumatic ossification
Sudeck's atrophy
Osteoarthritis
Shortening
Injury to viscera
Intra-articular and peri-articular adhesions

- **General**

Bronchopneumonia

Pyrexia with chest discomfort and purulent sputum may indicate a bronchopneumonia, although in the elderly pyrexia may be absent with confusion or apathy a presenting factor; the clinical examination with a chest X-ray showing consolidation, will clinch the diagnosis (*Fig. 3.15a*).

Treatment
Antibiotics and chest physiotherapy.

60 An outline of fractures and dislocations

a

b

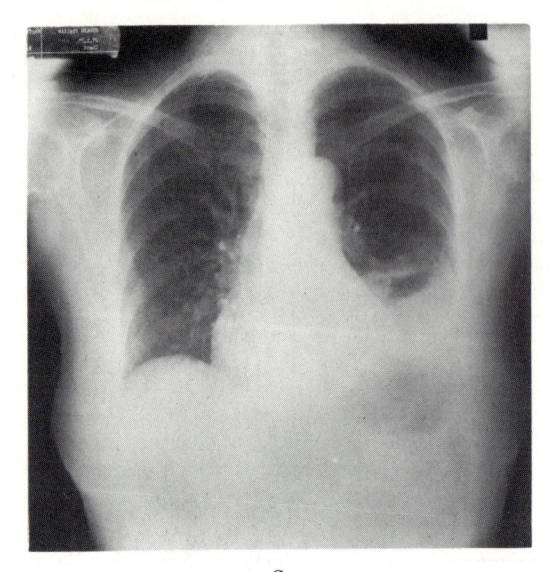

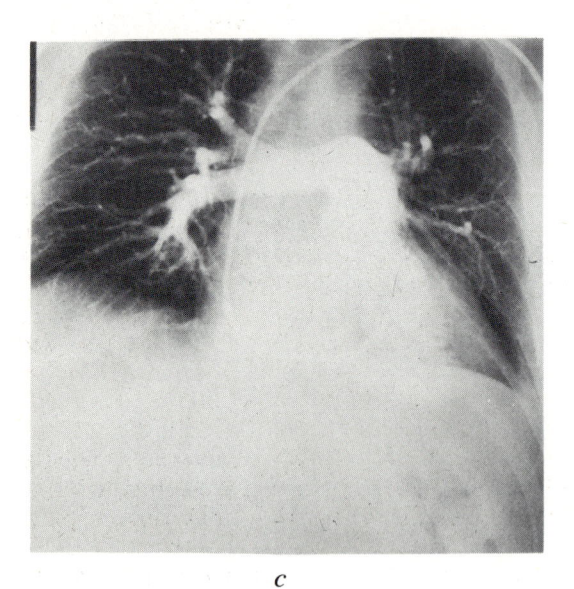

c

Fig. 3.15. *a*, Consolidation of the L lower base due to infection. *b*, A venogram showing an occluding thrombosis in the femoral vein. *c*, The arteriogram shows the pulmonary embolus (absent vascular markings). *d*, Isotope uptake after multiple pulmonary emboli (patchy perfusion denoted by lighter areas).

Deep Vein Thrombosis and Pulmonary Embolism

For many years local signs in the legs, a spike of temperature or a pulmonary embolus were the only ways of diagnosing a deep vein thrombosis. More sophisticated methods now include phlebography (*Fig.* 3.15*b*) (when a radio-opaque dye is injected up the vein), isotope uptake (usually ^{125}I-labelled fibrinogen) or ultrasound.

61 Complications: local and general

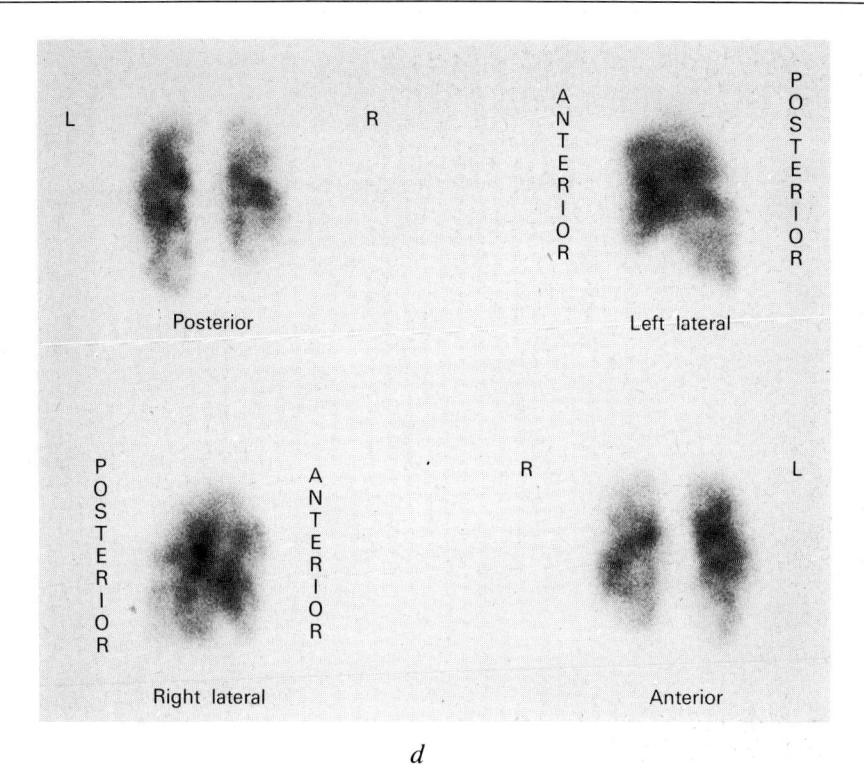

Fig. 3.15. (cont.)

When a fragment of the vein thrombosis breaks free and occludes the pulmonary circulation a pulmonary embolus is said to have occurred. Minor emboli present with haemoptysis and pleurisy: major embolism is heralded with collapse, chest pain, hypotension, dyspnoea and a rapid pulse. The ECG patterns are complex and reflect right ventricular strain, while the chest X-ray, retrograde arteriogram (*Fig. 3.15c*) or a lung scan (*Fig. 3.15d*) will give the diagnosis.

Treatment
Deep vein thrombosis can be prevented by early mobilization, passive compression of the limb from elastic supports and intermittent compression of the calves from pneumatic bags or electrical stimulation during surgery. Subcutaneous heparin is the method of choice, although some centres advocate plasma expanders, such as Dextran 70 or oral anti-inflammatory agents which affect platelet function (e.g. soluble aspirin, flurbiprofen etc.).

Once a deep vein thrombosis is established oral anticoagulants for 3 months are required. Since such agents take 2–3 days to affect the coagulation factors in the blood, heparin is given immediately by intravenous injection and oral anticoagulants (warfarin, etc.) commenced. Later the dose of the oral anticoagulant is varied according to blood coagulation estimations and the heparin ceased.

62 An outline of fractures and dislocations

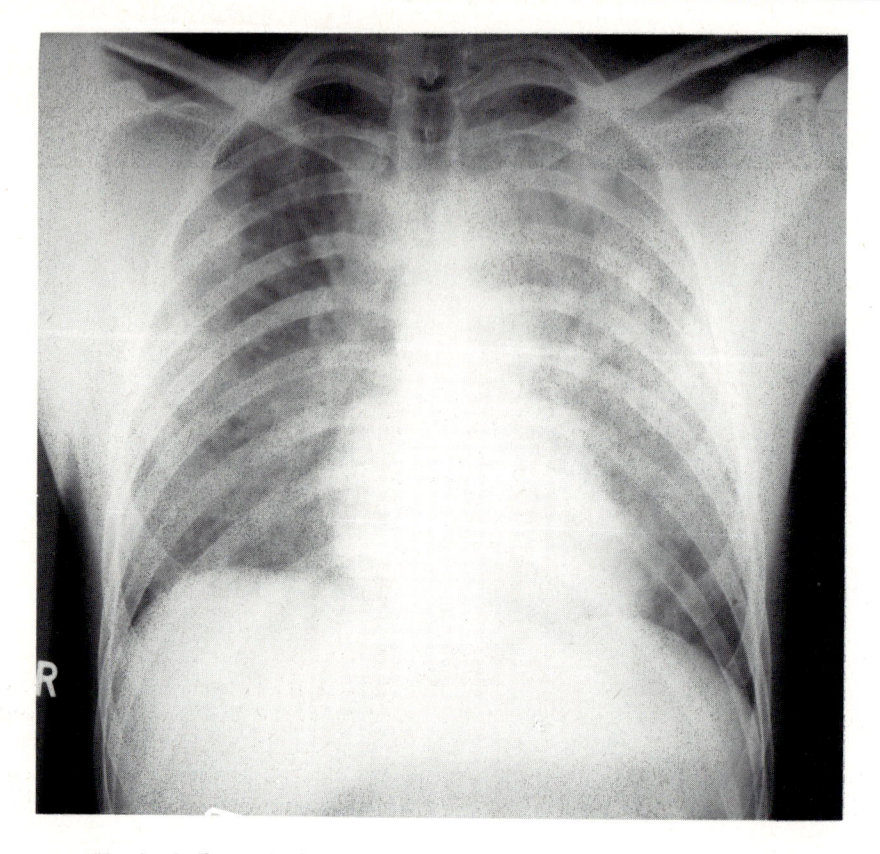

Fig. 3.16. Fat embolism on X-ray: typical 'snow storm' appearance.

With a minor embolus anticoagulants are given as for deep vein thrombosis; a massive embolus may need thrombolytic therapy with fibrinolytic agents or bypass embolectomy.

Fat Embolus
Five per cent of long bone fractures suffer this major complication, although fulminating fat embolism is rare. It is defined as the blockage of blood vessels by fat globules of 10–40 μm. Cases present with a rapid onset of pyrexia, coma, fast pulse and breathing (*Fig.* 3.16) and a petechial rash characteristically located on the chest and neck. Hypoxaemia can be severe. The exact relationship between fat embolism and hypoxaemia is difficult to determine since many patients with major fractures (e.g. femur) have low plasma oxygen levels on admission.

Treatment
Oxygen is given by mask or nasal tube and Po_2 and Pco_2 are regularly estimated. Heparin and steroids have also been used in this condition, without much effect.

63 Complications: local and general

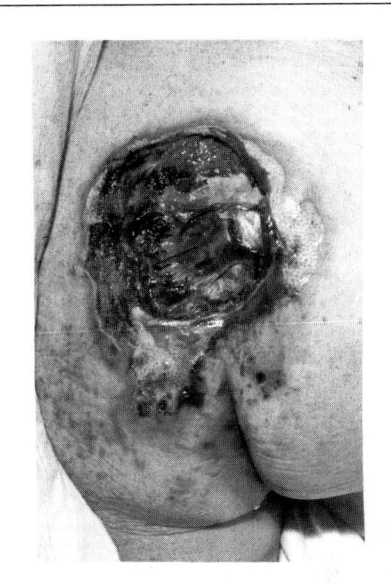

Fig. 3.17. A huge sacral sore in an 80-year-old lady who fell down stairs, fracturing her femoral neck; her husband was afraid to summon help for 10 days, respecting her wish not to be sent to hospital.

Pressure Sores

The projection of bony points can cause a disproportionate amount of body weight to be carried on the heels, trochanters, ischial and sacral regions. After several days of immobility, especially in the elderly or when there is impaired sensation due to a nerve injury, erythema and blistering occur, followed by a coagulum and skin necrosis down to bone or tendon (*Fig.* 3.17).

Treatment
Pressure sores are prevented by good nursing care with strict attention to detail such as a 2-hourly cycle of turning, clean and crinkle-free sheets and the application of bland ointments to the pressure areas. A small blanket of sheep's wool also helps. Any ulceration is treated by lavage with sterile saline, mild antiseptics and de-sloughing agents. A wound swab is taken and the correct antibiotics given. Sometimes the ulcer can be excised (where the skin is lax, e.g. the elbow) or may need a skin graft. Every effort is made to mobilize the patient as soon as possible. Other general measures include ripple beds, heel and sacral rings and foam or air mattresses.

Other Medical Conditions

The blood should be checked after a serious injury for anaemia, uraemia (from renal shutdown), liver failure, protein loss, diabetes and thyroid dysfunction.

In summary general complications are:
Bronchopneumonia
Deep vein thrombosis and pulmonary embolism
Fat embolism
Pressure sores

- **Multiple Injuries**

The treatment of multiple injuries and the principles of intensive care will only be briefly mentioned, since this subject would involve a whole textbook on its own.

The management of the severely injured patient is both urgent and complex. First, check for respiratory problems from airway obstruction, from weakness of the respiratory muscles (as in head injuries) or from insufficient lung ventilation (with a chest injury). Second, look for circulatory failure and shock. Assess the patient for head injury, and other injuries, including abdominal.

Treatment
1.   *Respiratory Obstruction*
The airway may be occluded by the tongue, false teeth, blood, vomit, mucus or water. The obstruction must be removed immediately. The jaw is elevated or the tongue grasped and pulled forward. Fluid is cleared with a sucker using laryngoscopy or bronchoscopy. Any chest wound is covered with a moist sterile dressing and strapping to prevent a valvular effect. A pneumothorax requires release with a drain inserted through the second intercostal space on the affected side and connected to an underwater seal. In more severe cases with crushed ribs and marked ventilation problems oxygen is given and endotracheal intubation, or a tracheostomy, is performed. Acute changes in intrathoracic pressure during deceleration in a road traffic accident can cause marked haemorrhage and oedema (wet lung or haemorrhagic lung).
2.   *Shock*
Blood loss may be external or internal and if 2 or more litres are lost then an infusion pump is needed for rapid replacement—up to 26 units (13 litres) have been given by the author within 3 h of admission but fresh frozen plasma and calcium ions are also essential to prevent massive oozing from coagulation problems. Accurate blood grouping takes time but an emergency grouping is often available within 30 min; if desperate, 'O' Rh-negative blood may be used. Plasma and plasma substitutes are of much less value. If the patient is not responding to transfusion it is probable that there is concealed haemorrhage within the chest or abdomen.

Painful injuries may cause neurogenic shock. Often the patient is very emotional. Usually this form of shock responds to pain relief and rest. *N.B.* Cups of tea should never be prescribed until it is quite certain that the patient will not need a general anaesthesia.
3.   *Head Injury*
Is the patient conscious and orientated; semiconscious; unconscious and responding to pain; or deeply unconscious and thus not responding? The head is inspected for wounds, depressed fracture and a cerebrospinal fluid leak, usually from the nose. If the pupils are unequal in size and there is inequality of limb movement in one half of the body, localized brain damage may have occurred. With a generalized increase in intracranial pressure breathing becomes laboured and the pupils dilate and become fixed. With all head injuries a clear airway is essential and oxygen is given to lessen anoxia which increases cerebral congestion. A simple airway (such as a Brook's airway) is used unless the

65 Complications: local and general

severity of unconsciousness demands endotracheal intubation, especially if there are airway problems due to an associated chest injury. A brain scan and urgent craniotomy are undertaken with a marked deterioration of conscious levels.

4. *Abdominal Injuries*

The abdomen is inspected for wounds, rigidity, tenderness, masses and absent bowel sounds. Rectal and pelvic examination, gastric intubation, bladder catheterization, and peritoneal aspiration may clinch the diagnosis.

When in doubt the abdominal viscera are explored and the necessary surgical measures taken.

5. *Burns*

Shock is an essential feature due to fluid loss through the burnt area into the swollen tissues, and from red cell damage, electrolyte and renal problems. Infection adds to these problems later. The accurate estimation of the burnt area (Rule of Nines) and the volume of fluid needed every hour is made and the appropriate antibiotic therapy given, either systemically or in a cream or paste to the damaged skin. Blood volume, red cell mass and renal output are charted continuously by estimations of pulse, blood pressure, haematocrit, serum profile, etc. The treatment is adjusted accordingly. The care of burns requires a unit specializing in this treatment and the injured patient may have to be looked after on such a unit and transferred to an orthopaedic ward later.

6. *Crush Syndrome*

Renal failure can follow a crush injury with massive muscle necrosis, or after too prolonged use of a tourniquet. It also accompanies fat embolism, gas gangrene and tetanus. Thus in all cases of multiple injury renal function is carefully monitored (urinary output is best estimated in the early stages by continuous catheterization) with serum urea and electrolyte estimations regularly taken. Advice must be obtained from renal physicians since haemodialysis may be required.

7. *Severe Infections*

These include tetanus, gas gangrene, abscess formation (often staphylococcal), and a spreading cellulitis (often streptococcal). A subphrenic abscess is often missed. The appropriate antibiotics are given with surgical drainage of the abscess.

8. *Skin Problems*

The loss of skin may require a split skin graft or a pedicle full-skin transfer (especially when skin loss occurs over subcutaneous bone, such as the tibia). Microsurgery has revolutionized the transfer of flaps with the microcirculation intact and re-anastamosed to the new donor area. Fracture blisters may occur due to elevation of the superficial layers of the skin by oedema but are rarely a problem and simply need covering with a sterile dressing; however, skin necrosis due to plaster pressure (plaster sores) requires the plaster to be trimmed or a window cut and the area regularly dressed (as described under pressure sores).

- **Special Problems**

Under this heading will be discussed *fractures around metal implants* and *fractures in children*.

66 An outline of fractures and dislocations

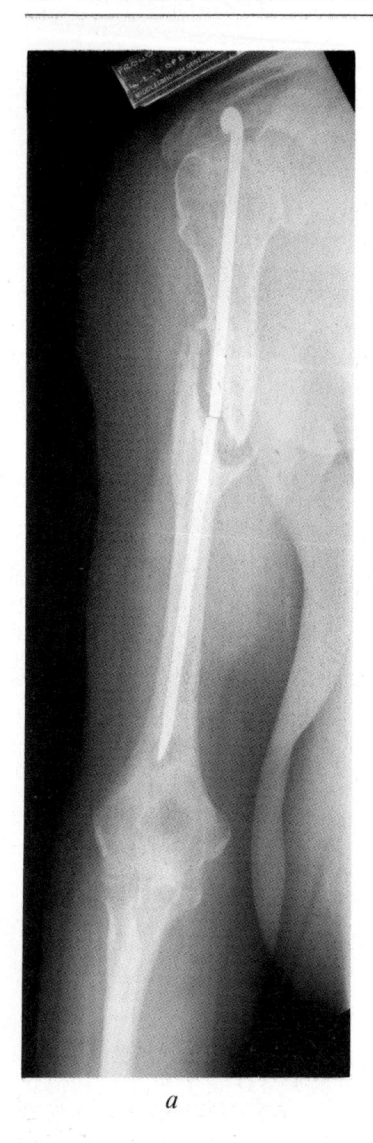

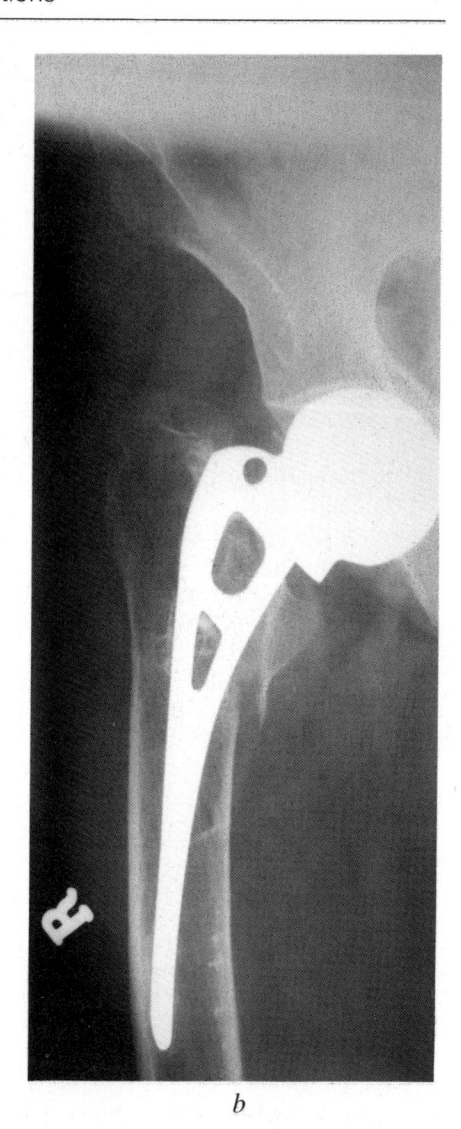

a *b*

Fractures around Metal Implants
These occur either during insertion or later when the patient falls or knocks the affected area and thus produces a stress gradient at the metal/bone interface (*Fig.* 3.18).

Treatment
When the fracture occurs at the time of surgery (i.e. during insertion) the bone can be held with metal cerclage wires, extra screws, longer plates (covering the

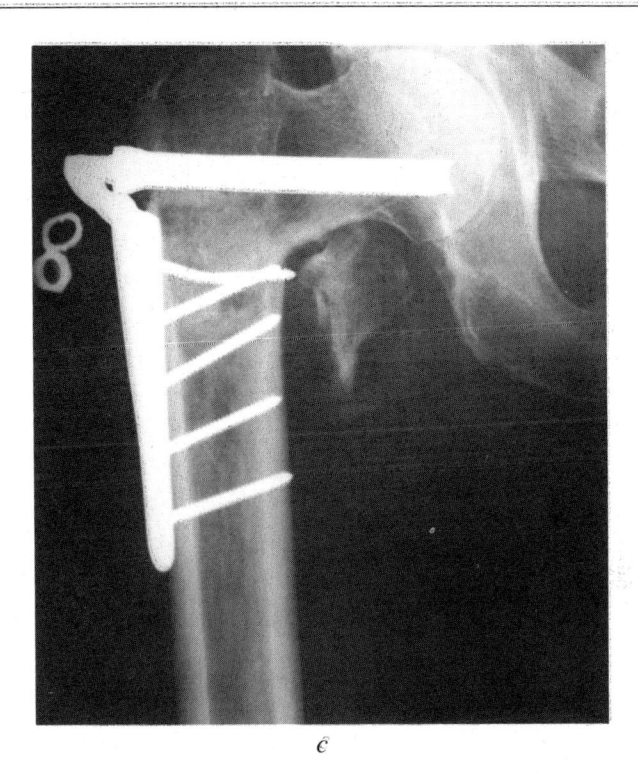

Fig. 3.18. Metal/bone failure. *a*, Rush nail in the humerus. *b*, The osteoporotic bone around a Moore prosthesis. *c*, Collapse of a pin and plate following too early weight bearing and poor stability (note the varus neck).

new fractured area) or with bone cement (as in a total hip arthroplasty). Late fractures can be treated conservatively (i.e. by plaster-of-Paris) or a new fixation device can be inserted at the time of removal of the fractured metal.
* *No metal fixation device will withstand the inherent biological forces of the body if the fracture is not correctly reduced and the fragments are not stable to weight-bearing* (Fig. 3.18c).

Fractures in Children
Although the bones of children are more malleable they have a weak spot in the growth plates which occur at the ends of the long bones. Epiphyseal injury is classified in *Fig.* 3.19. Thus children's fractures differ from adults because:
1. They can stand greater deflection without fracturing, thus producing a greenstick fracture.
2. The epiphysis is a weak point and may 'slip'; arrested growth may occur later.

68 An outline of fractures and dislocations

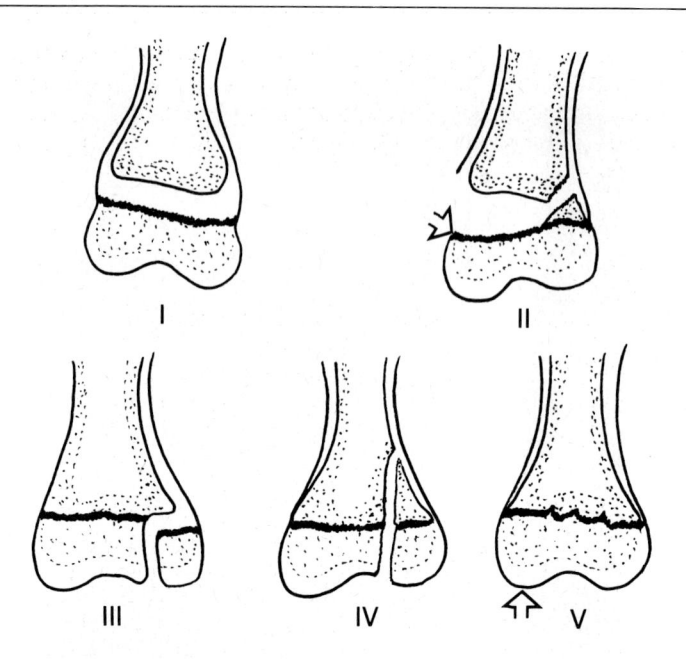

Fig. 3.19. Epiphyseal injury. Types I to V. Note that minor injury (I) and the severe crush injury (V) are not seen on X-rays.

3. The periosteum, although relatively thick, is only loosely attached to the shaft (diaphysis) and is thus stripped off a large area, explaining widespread callus formation.
4. They unite very rapidly.
5. Remodelling is a feature.
6. Diagnosis may be difficult due to no history of injury, absence of deformity and no abnormal mobility.
 - *If the injuries vary in time (separate intervals) and space (i.e. areas of the body), exclude the battered baby syndrome.*

The Battered Baby Syndrome

One of the amazing features of our society is that parents can wilfully damage their children and then conceal the fact with preposterous tales of the infant falling downstairs, or from high chairs and prams (perhaps onto thick carpets in order to explain the lack of bruising) at regular intervals.

Often it is the first child of young parents (sometimes unmarried or divorced), with a poor income in an equally poor environment. The child may be irritable, commonly crying a great deal and awakening the parents at night, thus explaining the frequent assertions of 'falls from a cot' or 'trapping the legs between the cot bars'.

The child commonly presents with a long bone facture (usually tibia, humerus or femur) and a total body X-ray survey reveals previous fractures (usually skull, ribs and long bones) with mature callus. Hospital procedure dictates detailed paediatric and orthopaedic consultation with involvement of the social services and the law.

4

Injuries to the shoulder, arm and elbow

- **Fractures of the Shoulder Girdle**
The shoulder girdle consists of the clavicle, scapula and their related ligaments. Forces from the upper limb are transmitted anteriorly through the clavicle and its muscles and ligaments to the anterior chest wall, and posteriorly via the scapula and its associated muscles and ligaments to the posterior chest wall and spine. Thus fractures of the shoulder girdle can occur *indirectly* from falls on to the upper limb or *directly* (for example, in the body of the scapula when a horse rolls over on its rider).

Fractures of the Clavicle
The clavicle fractures in three areas: *middle, outer* and *inner thirds*.

Fractures of the *middle* third are the *most common* and frequently occur in children (*Fig.* 4.1). They are usually undisplaced, although in adults a more severe force may produce a segmental injury. Blows transmitted through the shoulder from a fall often cause a spiral fracture in the middle third.

Fractures of the *outer* third of the clavicle are usually due to a direct blow and occasionally they extend into the acromioclavicular joint and the coracoclavicular ligaments (conoid and trapezoid) are torn, thus producing a fracture-dislocation. The humeral head may be fractured also (*Fig.* 4.2).

Fractures of the *inner* third of the clavicle are commonly undisplaced.

Diagnosis
The deformity is obvious due to the subcutaneous position of the clavicle—the sternomastoid muscle pulls the inner end upwards, while the weight of the arm depresses the outer end.

Treatment
In children the traditional figure-of-eight bandage can be used but it needs regular tightening and many centres now use a broad-arm sling for the relief of pain. After 2–3 weeks mobilization begins.

The management of adult clavicular fractures is a good deal more difficult because there is often wide separation of the fragments and abundant callus

71 Injuries to the shoulder, arm and elbow

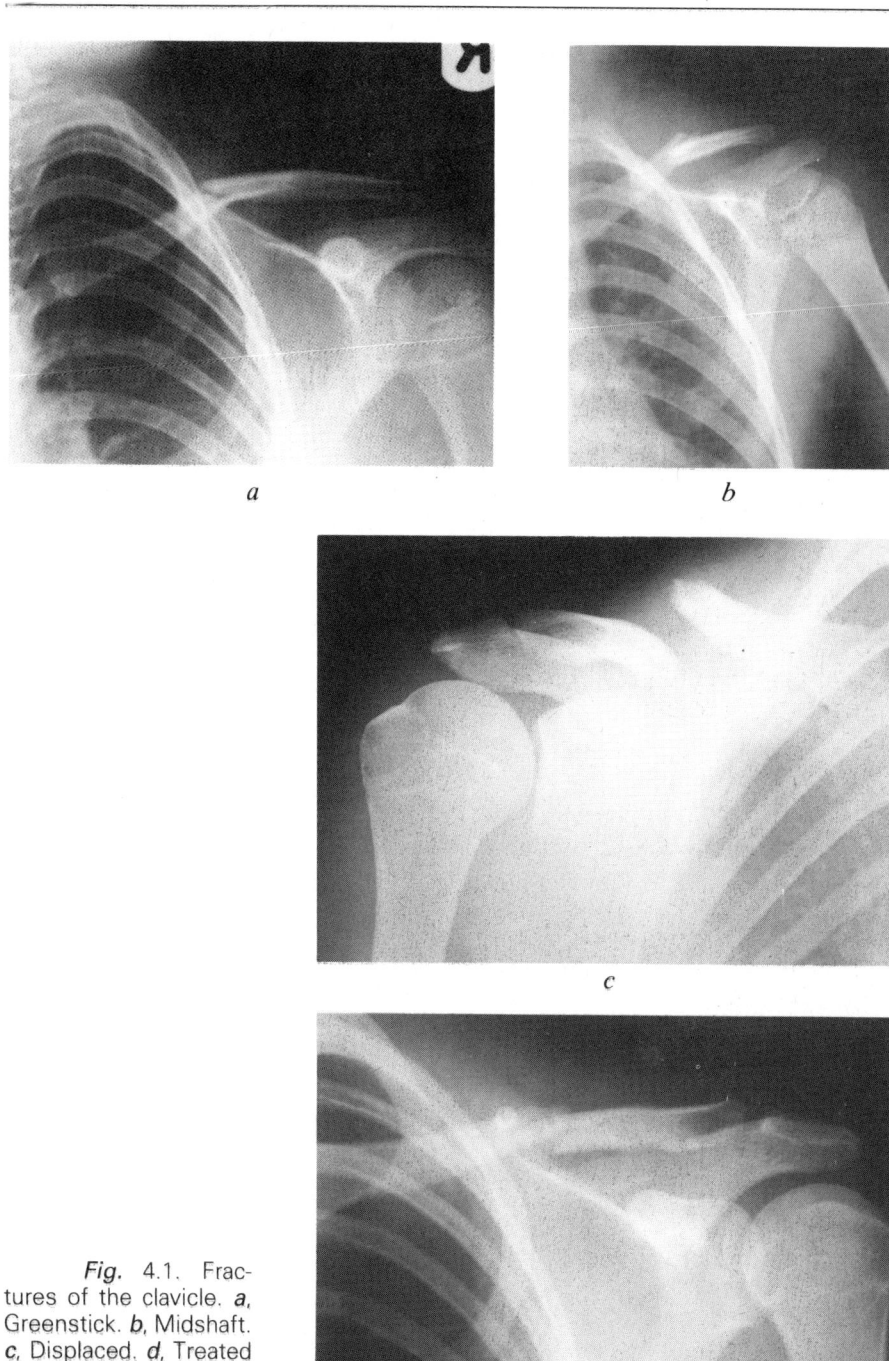

Fig. 4.1. Fractures of the clavicle. *a*, Greenstick. *b*, Midshaft. *c*, Displaced. *d*, Treated by open reduction and pull-out nylon suture on two beads.

72 An outline of fractures and dislocations

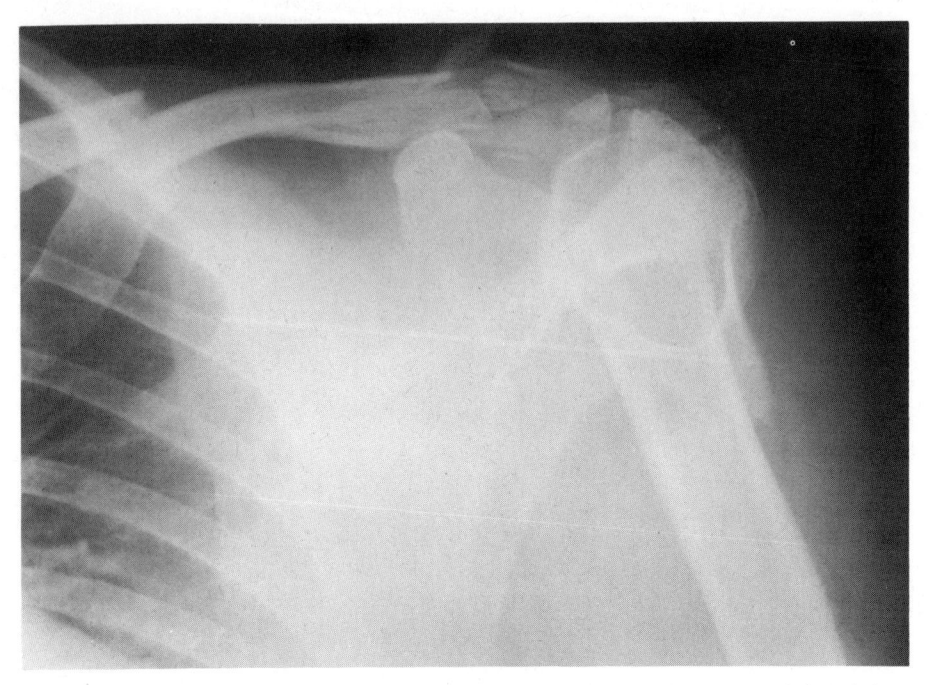

Fig. 4.2. Combined midshaft, outer third clavicle and humeral head in a 40-year-old man hit by falling masonry.

formation. Usually a sling is used and the overlap of the fracture is accepted. Active mobilization of the shoulder, elbow and hand is encouraged as soon as comfort allows.

Open Reduction

This is *rarely* indicated, except (*a*) in comminuted fractures with wide displacement, (*b*) when there is compression of vessels or nerves, (*c*) with disruption of the related ligaments, and (*d*) when there is established non-union.

After open reduction internal fixation with a compression plate (usually 4-holed), a Knowle's pin, a pullout wire or nylon suture is required—a thin Kirschner wire is completely ineffective and usually fractures or migrates. Following surgery a sling and body-bandage are used for 3–4 weeks.

Any ligamentous repair is carried out at the time of internal fixation.

Complications
- Check for injuries to the brachial plexus, the subclavian or axillary vessels, the lungs and pleura.
- Check for associated fractures in the upper limb.

Abundant callus can compress the subclavian vessels and emerging nerves against the first rib causing a thoracic outlet syndrome. The callus is removed or the clavicle displaced by osteotomy. Rarely the supraclavicular nerves are involved in the callus causing chest wall pain. Late thrombosis of the axillary artery has also been reported.

73 Injuries to the shoulder, arm and elbow

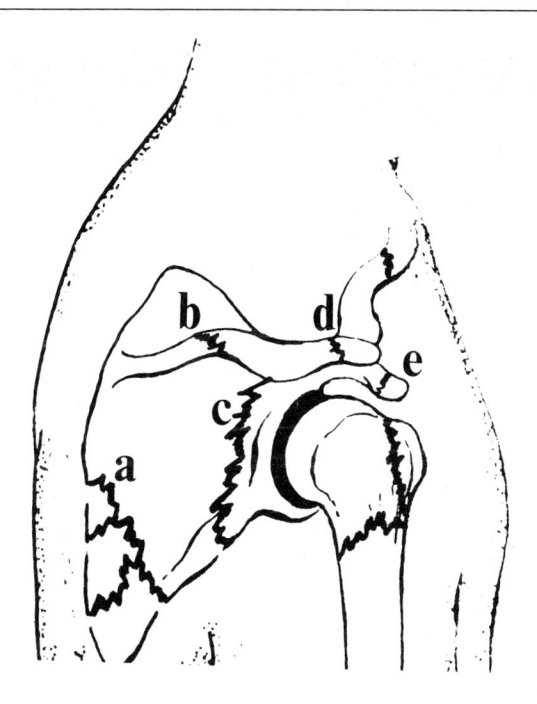

Fig. 4.3. Fractures of the scapula. **a**, Body. **b**, Spine. **c**, Neck. **d**, Acromion. **e**, Coracoid.

Fractures of the Scapula

- *Direct violence fractures the scapula, and the ribs and lungs may be involved.*

Scapular fractures are divided into: body; neck; spine; acromion; and base of coracoid (*Fig.* 4.3).

Usually there is minimal displacement. Muscle pull may cause an avulsion injury to the spine of the scapula.

Diagnosis
There is usually severe pain and an extravasation of blood into the soft tissues.

Treatment
All fractures can be treated with a sling for 3–4 weeks. The only exception is the acromial injury affecting its related joint which may need fixation with a stout pin.

Complications
Rib fractures, pneumothorax, associated spinal injuries, shoulder fractures and dislocations may be found. Occasionally damage to the suprascapular or serratus anterior nerve occurs.

- **Dislocation of the Sternoclavicular joint**

Usually the inner end of the clavicle is displaced forwards but in an extremely uncommon (albeit serious) injury the displacement is backwards (retrosternal) and may press on the trachea and great vessels.

Diagnosis
The displacement, especially anterior, is clearly visible.

Treatment
Anterior displacement is reduced by direct pressure over the inner clavicle and an adhesive strapping placed across the medial end for 3 weeks. *Posterior dislocation* can be reduced by firmly grasping the clavicle and pulling it upwards and forwards. Sometimes open reduction is needed.

Complications
Recurrent dislocation usually requires no treatment unless there are symptoms; then excision of the affected inner 2 cm is performed. Usually stabilizing the medial end with fascial or ligamentous slings gives poor results.
Pan-clavicular is a rare dislocation of both sternoclavicular and acromioclavicular joints—treated by internal fixation of the latter.

- **Dislocation of the Acromioclavicular Joint**

Injuries of this joint are fairly frequent in sport due to a fall on to the shoulder. In *subluxation* the joint capsule is torn but the *conoid and trapezoid ligaments remain intact*. Thus the tip of the clavicle is more prominent than usual. However, *when the above ligaments tear* the outer end of *the clavicle is dislocated* upwards (*Fig.* 4.4 a,b).

Diagnosis
The prominent part of the clavicle can be easily seen (*Fig.* 4.4c) and felt. The raised bone may be freely mobile. Displacement is often confirmed on X-rays and, when there is a doubt, the patient can hold a heavy weight in the affected limb and this will accentuate the gap (*Fig.* 4.4d).

Treatment
Sprains and *subluxations* are treated by a sling for 7 days and then shoulder exercises begun in order to strengthen the local muscles. Strapping encircling the outer shoulder and elbow is not usually effective. However, with a *dislocation* the decision has to be made whether to accept the situation (if causing little symptoms) or whether internal fixation is required. It is preferable to stabilize the joint in active persons with repair of the damaged conoid and trapezoid ligaments. The joint can be transfixed with a Knowle's pin through the acromion and into the clavicle; or a vertically placed screw can be inserted through the clavicle and into the coracoid process. A sling is worn for 3 weeks. Then active mobilization begins. The wire or screw can be removed at 6–12 weeks.

75 Injuries to the shoulder, arm and elbow

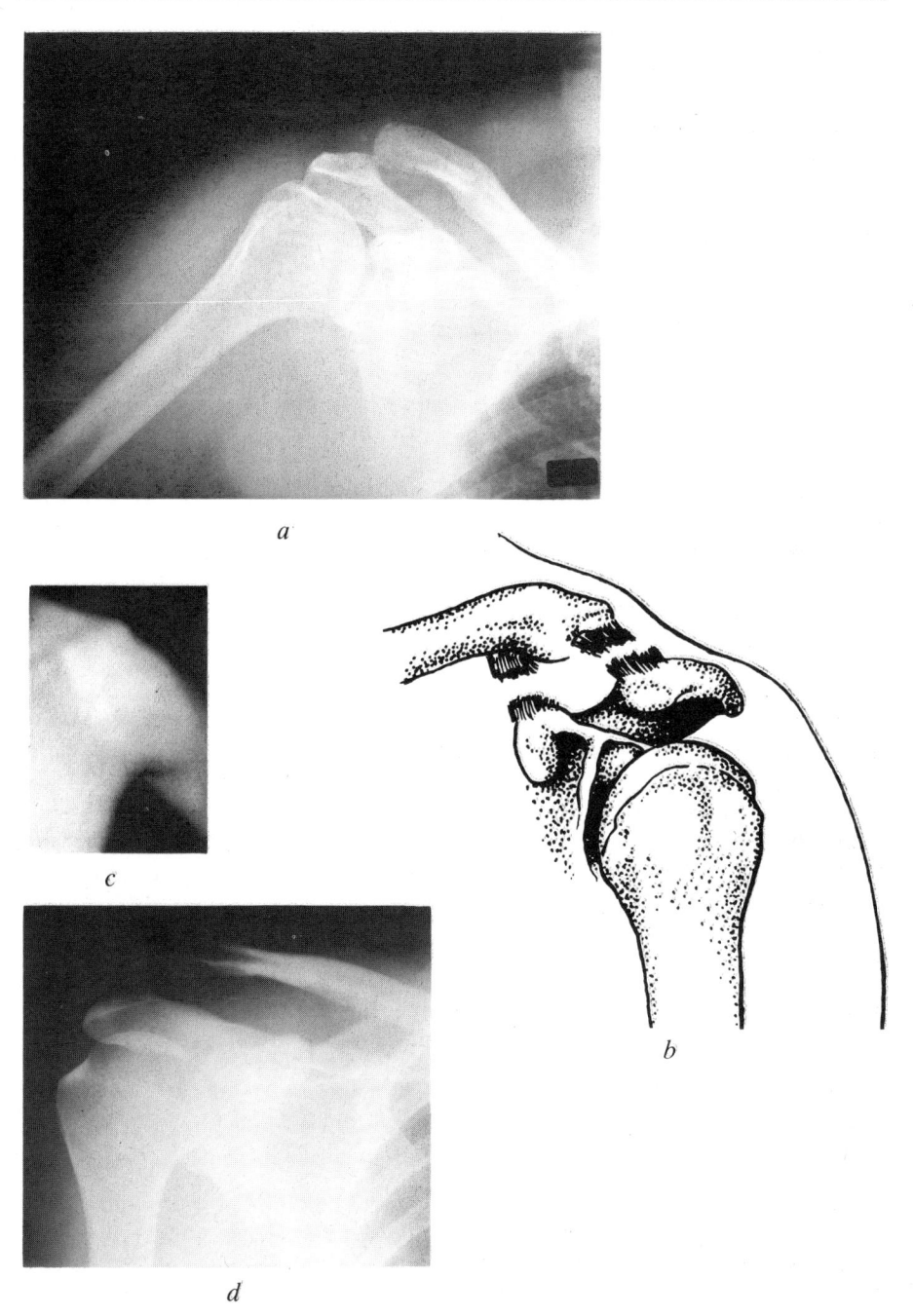

Fig. 4.4. *a,* Dislocation of the acromioclavicular joint. *b,* Rupture of the acromioclavicular and coracoclavicular ligaments. *c,* Prominent outer aspect of clavicle. *d,* There is upward subluxation of the outer clavicle when a weight is held in the affected limb.

Another procedure that can be carried out in young athletes is to detach the coracoid process (with the short head of biceps and coracobrachialis intact) and fix it to the outer end of the clavicle. Muscle forces hold the joint in position, but this procedure is not suitable if there is marked osteoarthrosis present. It can also be used for recurrent dislocation.

Complications
Osteoarthritis may develop with a *chronic dislocation* and the joint can be arthrodesed or, more commonly, the outer end of the clavicle excised leaving a pseudarthrosis.

With a *chronic dislocation* (painless) no surgery is required.

With *recurrent dislocation* the joint is stabilized by pin fixation or muscle-pedicle transfer (*above*).

- **Subluxation and Dislocation of the Shoulder**
  - *The shoulder is a joint within a joint (three layers) acting in conjunction with other joints (three joints).*

The *outer* layer consists of the deltoid and related muscles. The *innermost* layer consists of the glenohumeral articulation (shoulder joint) which has a loose capsule inferiorly and anteriorly (where there is an anatomically large subscapularis bursa). The capsule is intimately blended with the rotator cuff muscles. Between these two layers lie the *subdeltoid* (or subacromial) *bursa*, the overhanging *coraco-acromial ligament* and the *supraspinatus tendon* (whose anatomical insignificance belies its importance).

However, the global range of shoulder movement is only achieved by a summation of movements with the sternoclavicular, acromioclavicular and the thoracoscapular articulations—the three other joints. A special constant delicate relationship exists between the humerus and the scapula during elevation and abduction of the arm. Through the first 30° of abduction the scapula remains fixed but then for every 10° of humeral motion an additional 5° occurs by scapular movement. The sternoclavicular joint contributes 40° and the acromioclavicular joint 20° to full abduction of the arm. Thus, after a shoulder injury all joints must be fully mobilized by thorough physiotherapy.

Subluxation of the Shoulder

Subluxation can be *inferior, anterior* and *superior* (rarely *posterior*). With forceful *abduction* (as in rugby football) the *inferior* capsule may be stretched; when an *external rotation* component is added the disruption occurs *anteriorly*; while *superior subluxation* can occur when the *body weight is suspended* from the upper limb (e.g. hanging from a tree with one arm).

A special type of inferior subluxation occurs in patients with a hemiplegia (*Fig. 4.5a*). In an epileptic seizure the arm may be adducted and internally rotated causing the rare *posterior* subluxation.

77 Injuries to the shoulder, arm and elbow

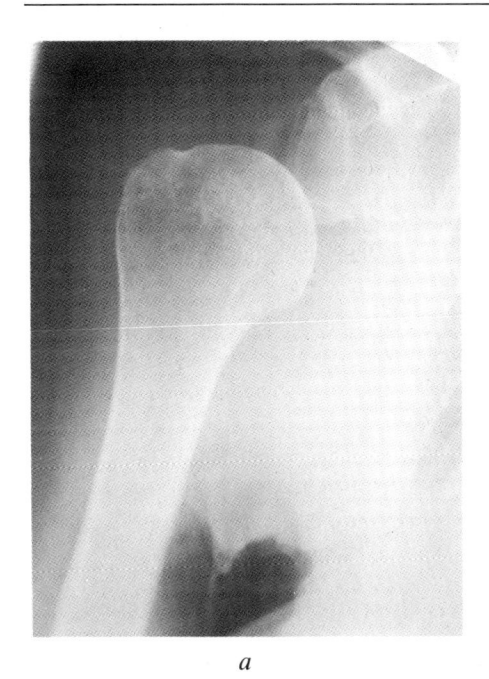

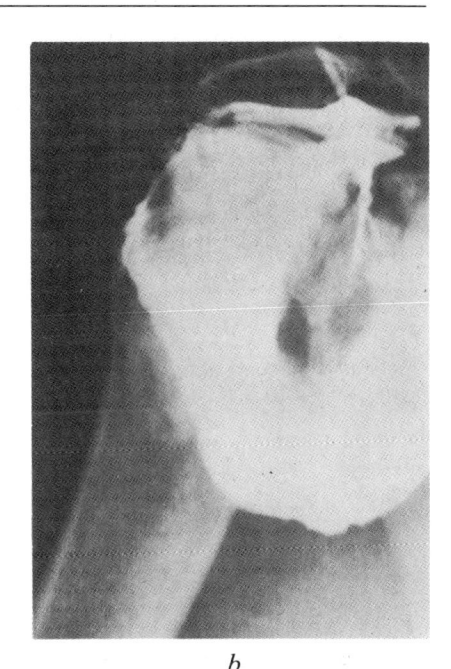

Fig. 4.5. *a,* Subluxation of the R shoulder in a hemiplegic patient. *b,* An arthrogram shows pouching of the shoulder capsule.

Diagnosis
The patient has a short, severe pain in the shoulder, leaving a more chronic discomfort but a tendency for the shoulder to 'give way' in certain positions of the joint, often during sports such as squash. Tenderness may be found on palpating the affected area of the capsule. An arthrogram may reveal pouching of the capsule (*Fig.* 4.5*b*).

Treatment
A sling is worn for 7 days and active shoulder exercises begun designed to strengthen the controlling muscles.

Complications
Acute pericapsulitis may follow these injuries in patients over 40 years. This condition demands intensive physiotherapy with ice-facilitation exercises and intermittent short-wave diathermy as well as anti-inflammatory agents.

   Recurrent subluxation can become a problem and may need surgery (*see* Shoulder Dislocation).

   Tears in the rotator cuff muscles, especially the supraspinatus, may require operative intervention and repair. Such injuries are also more frequent in the elderly.

- **Shoulder Dislocation**

Anterior (95%) Subcoracoid; Subglenoid (or inferior); Subclavian (*Fig.* 4.6).

Posterior (5%).
- *These bald facts give the anatomical breakdown of the body's most troublesome dislocation, which so often becomes recurrent despite the apparent ease of the initial treatment.*

Anterior Shoulder Dislocation

Diagnosis
With an anterior dislocation the arm is fixed in slight abduction and the shoulder contour is flattened; while the acromion process is unduly prominent.

Treatment
- *The dislocation should be reduced as quickly as possible.* If there is a delay in giving a general anaesthetic the Stimpson technique can be used. The patient is placed prone on the edge of the table and a 10 kg weight attached to the affected limb for 10–15 min. Gentle rotation of the shoulder may then produce a reduction in this position.
  Under an anaesthetic *two* manoeuvres can be carried out. In the *Hippocratic* method traction is maintained on the upper limb while counter axillary pressure is produced by the physician's stockinged foot. The shoulder is gently rotated and adducted. In the *Köcher manoeuvre* the arm is gently externally rotated until 80° is achieved, the elbow being held flexed. The elbow is brought across the midline of the trunk and then internal rotation is carried out.
- *As mentioned previously (Chapter 1) all suspected dislocations of the shoulder must have an X-ray before and after reduction.* This ensures that there is no associated fracture. A sling is worn for 2 weeks, followed by shoulder exercises. In the elderly a collar-and-cuff can be used to promote earlier mobilization to prevent pericapsulitis (frozen shoulder).

Complications
Anterior dislocation of the shoulder is associated with many problems:
1. *Damage to the axillary nerve*, shown by deltoid weakness and a small area of numbness on the lateral aspect of the upper arm.
2. The *posterior cord* or other parts of the *brachial plexus* may be injured.
3. *Vascular injury*—damage to the axillary vessels.
4. An *associated fracture* of the *upper humerus* or *glenoid*, in 25% of cases.
5. *Tearing of the rotator cuff*, usually the supraspinatus, especially after marked displacement of the humeral head with occasional impaction below the glenoid fossa.
6. The *dislocation is irreducible* due to interposition of the rotator cuff or the tendon of the long head of biceps.

79 Injuries to the shoulder, arm and elbow

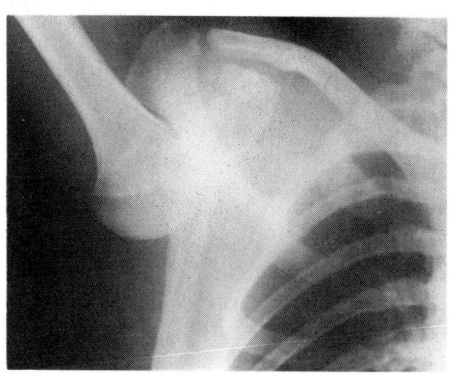

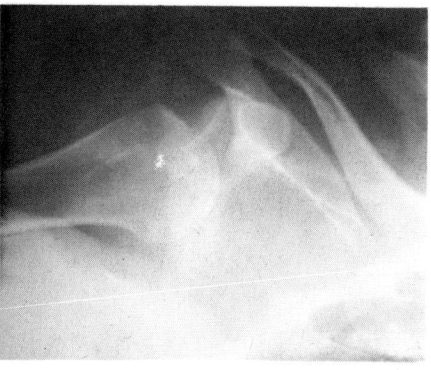

Fig. 4.6. *a,* An anterior (subglenoid or inferior) shoulder dislocation. *b,* Subcoracoid anterior dislocation.

7. *Recurrent dislocation*—in sportspeople may approach 60%. Paradoxically, recurrence is much less common (5%) when there is an associated fracture.
8. *Missed dislocation.* In *elderly patients* often with a hemiplegia there may be a longstanding anterior dislocation; closed reduction is usually impossible and risks a fracture or nerve injury. Thus surgical intervention is needed if the patient has symptoms. However, with a *young patient* it is wise to attempt open reduction although the joint may have suffered areas of hyaline cartilage necrosis. The joint is opened from behind which allows excision of the scarred posterior capsule and transfer of infraspinatus to hold the head in position. The results are often much better than expected, although a shoulder replacement (metal/plastic) may sometimes be required.
9. Joint stiffness.

Posterior Shoulder Dislocation

- *This lesion is commonly missed.* Why? Because the anteroposterior X-ray looks almost normal (*Fig.* 4.7*a*); axillary views are essential (*Fig.* 4.7*b*).

The dislocating force is a blow to the front of the shoulder, as in boxing or karate, a fall from a height or during an epileptic seizure. Some children with joint laxity can habitually dislocate posteriorly.

Diagnosis
The arm is held in internal rotation and the greater tuberosity is prominent.

Treatment
Reduction is performed under general anaesthesia with traction applied to the arm with the elbow adducted. Pressure is exerted over the humeral head posteriorly and gentle external rotation reduces the fracture. A sling is *never* used because the arm would be held internally, i.e. the forearm across the chest,

80   An outline of fractures and dislocations

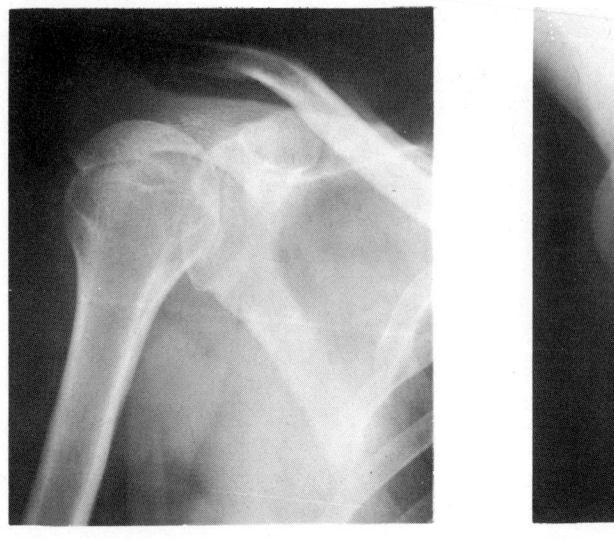

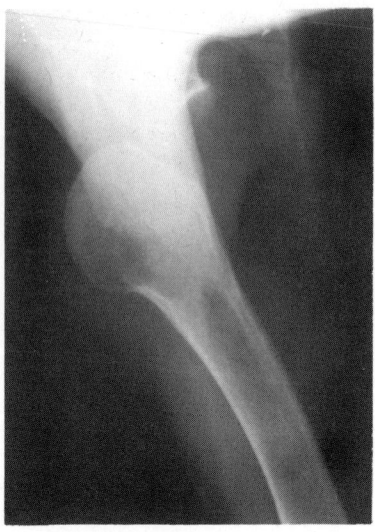

Fig. 4.7. *a,* This AP film of the shoulder could be considered normal at first inspection but there is marked internal rotation, i.e. the head points backwards. *b,* The posterior dislocation is confirmed in an axillary view.

thus risking redislocation. The arm is placed in the neutral position (palm forward) and bandaged to the side for 2–3 weeks.

Complications
This dislocation is commonly missed and late cases will require an open reduction with excision of the scarred anterior capsule and repair of the torn posterior labrum.

Fracture-dislocation of the Shoulder
● *One in four of all shoulder dislocations are associated with a fracture.* They commonly occur in the greater tuberosity (from impingement against the acromion) or across the humeral neck. They may be *undisplaced* or *displaced*. Sometimes marked comminution is found in the humeral head or the acromioclavicular joint (e.g. when masonry falls on to the tip of the shoulder).

Diagnosis
In the young there is severe pain and swelling, but in the elderly the symptoms may mimic a simple dislocation.

Treatment
Attempts should be made at closed reduction, often the fragments spring into position as the joint reduces. However, if closed reduction fails then surgery with internal fixation is preferred. A body bandage and sling are worn for 6 weeks. Physiotherapy should be intensive, especially with regard to regaining abduction and external rotation.

Recurrent Anterior Dislocation of the Shoulder
The factors involved are:
1. Detachment of the glenoid labrum (Bankart lesion).
2. Pouching of the anterior capsule.
3. Defects in the humeral head (Hill–Sachs lesion).
4. Injury to the related muscles, especially subscapularis.
5. Anatomical factors such as a large synovial recess or unusual arrangements of the glenohumeral ligaments.

Diagnosis
As for dislocation but pain may be slight when there have been several episodes and often the shoulder can be easily reduced by the patient. However, the same precautions regarding an associated fracture apply.

Treatment
If attacks occur at intervals of 1 year or so the patient may elect to continue with certain restrictions in activity, but after two or three dislocations per annum many wisely accept surgery which offers a 90% cure.

Techniques
1. The *Bristow procedure* (*Fig. 4.8a*) when the coracoid process is transplanted on to the antero-inferior aspect of the glenoid margins. The attached tendons of biceps (short head) and coracobrachialis act as a muscle sling with the bony block (coracoid process) to prevent anterior dislocation.
2. The *Putti–Platt procedure* (*Fig. 4.8b*) utilizes dividing and overlapping the stretched subscapularis and anterior capsule. Recurrence is nine times more common than with the Bristow technique.
3. The *Bankart operation* (*Fig. 4.8c*) repairs the damaged capsule and reattaches the labrum to the margins of the glenoid cavity. This operation is often carried out with the Putti–Platt or other procedures. Recently early active mobilization (2–3 days) has been reported as giving excellent results after this procedure.
4. The *Magnusson–Stack operation* (*Fig. 4.8d*) transfers the subscapularis in the arm to a more lateral position (i.e. to the outer aspect of the biceps sulcus). After surgery the arm is bandaged to the side for 4–6 weeks. It is a simple operation with a low recurrence and may be especially suitable in the non-active or elderly.

 • *All procedures involve tightening the anterior structures to prevent the dislocating external rotation and abduction forces.* The Bristow procedure is especially effective in sportspeople and allows almost a full range of movements. (As a final point: the Romans achieved a similar ideal by applying a red hot iron to the shoulder anteriorly).

Recurrent Posterior Dislocation
This is uncommon and accounts for less than 5% of recurrent shoulder problems. Characteristically it can occur during the push-up position in gymnastics. The capsule is tightened through a posterior approach and the infraspinatus muscle is transferred laterally for stability, or a posterior wedge osteotomy of the neck of the scapula can be performed.

82 An outline of fractures and dislocations

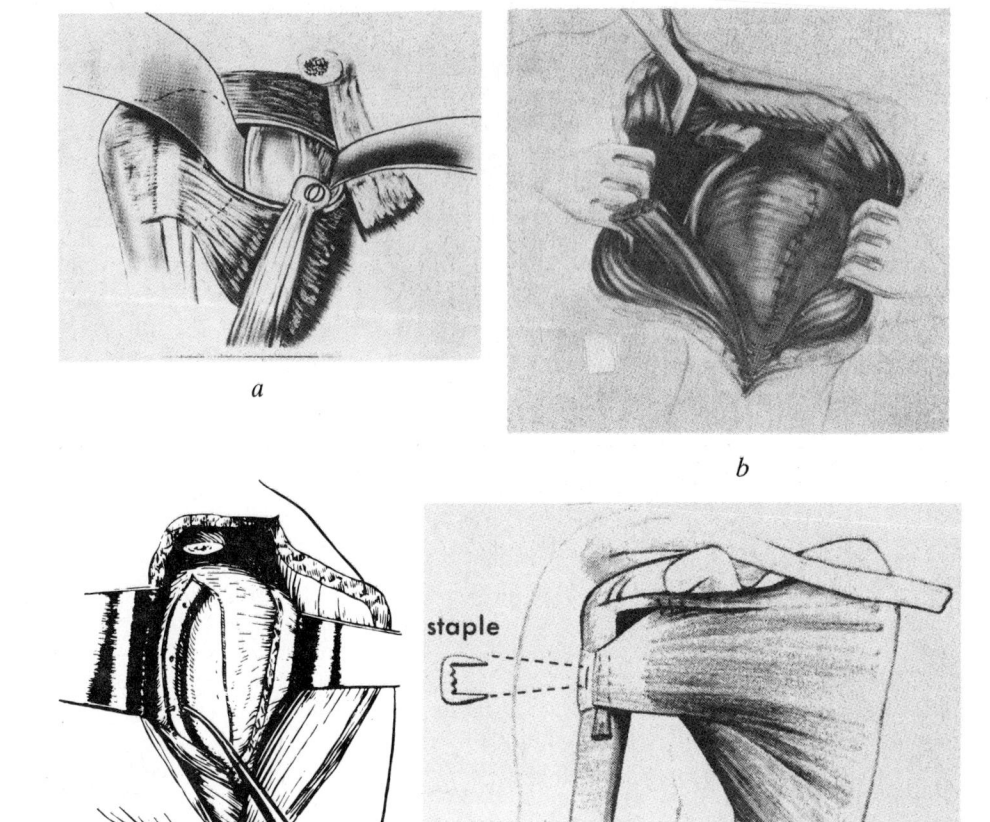

Fig. 4.8. *a*, The Bristow procedure. *b*, The Putti–Platt procedure. *c*, The Bankart procedure. *d*, The Magnusson–Stack procedure.

- **Tears of the Rotator Cuff**

    The intimate relationship of the rotator cuff makes it vulnerable to tearing during shoulder dislocation, especially the supraspinatus muscle (*Fig.* 4.9).

Diagnosis
Usually the action of supraspinatus is lost and the patient is unable to initiate abduction of the shoulder unless the arm is supported through the first 30° of movement. There is tenderness over the shoulder capsule and often a subdeltoid bursitis.

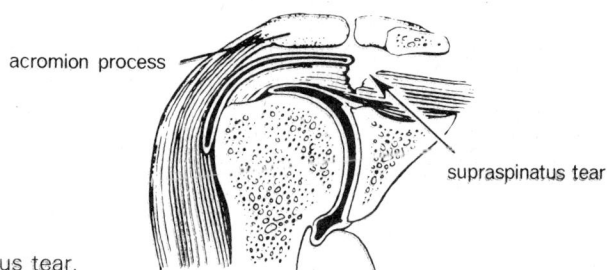

Fig. 4.9. Supraspinatus tear.

Treatment
In young or active patients the cuff is repaired; in older people the shoulder is mobilized with physiotherapy.

- **Fractures of the Humerus**
  These occur at three levels:
1. Upper humerus (shoulder region).
2. Shaft.
3. Lower humerus (including elbow).

Upper Humerus (*Fig.* 4.10)
1. Anatomical neck.
2. Greater tuberosity.
3. Surgical neck (often impacted).
4. Avulsion by supraspinatus tendon.
5. Epiphyseal.
- *As with Colles fractures and femoral neck fractures such injuries are usually the prerogative of the aged with osteoporosis.*

Diagnosis
There is local pain and restricted shoulder mobility. Eventually bruising appears in the upper arm.

Treatment
Undisplaced fractures require a sling or a collar and cuff. Occasionally widely *displaced* fractures need internal fixation. In each case the sling or cuff is worn for 6 weeks.

Complications
1. The *biceps tendon* may be trapped in the fracture.
2. The humeral head rarely develops *avascular necrosis* and osteoarthrosis supervenes (*Fig.* 4.10d).
3. An *associated dislocation*.
4. When there is an *overlap of the shaft* on the humeral head a hanging cast is applied, sometimes open reduction and fixation are required.
5. In children epiphyseal injuries may cause some *loss of growth*. Fracture separation of the proximal epiphysis may be unstable.

84 An outline of fractures and dislocations

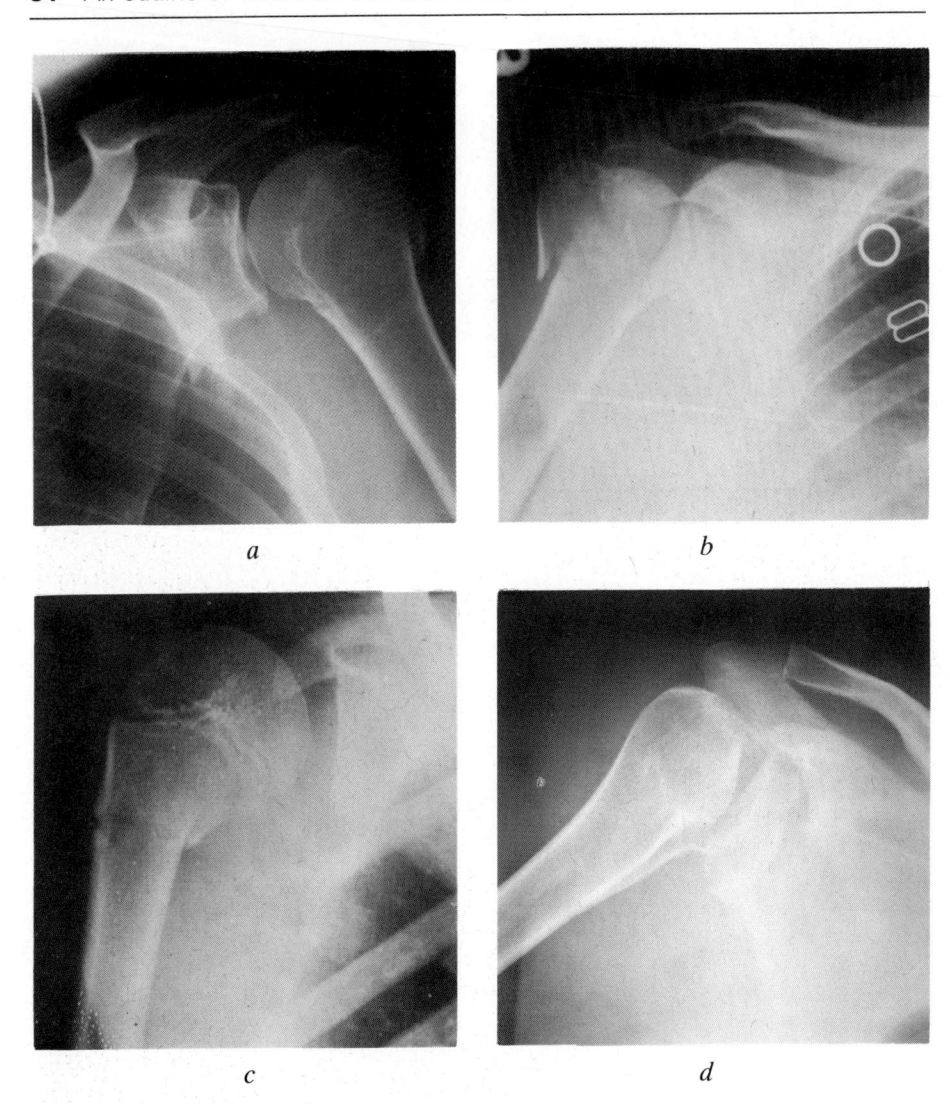

Fig. 4.10. Upper humeral fractures. *a*, Fractures of the L greater tuberosity with extension across the surgical neck. *b*, Impacted surgical neck (in a 54-year-old patient with a Colles fracture). *c*, Transverse upper humerus (surgical neck) in a 10-year-old boy. *d*, A rare complication—avascular necrosis following a fracture of the anatomical neck (note the head within a head) in a 30-year-old man.

Shaft of the Humerus

● *The most important feature of these injuries is radial nerve damage which occurs in almost 15% of cases* (*Fig.* 4.11). Sometimes there is nerve bruising (neuropraxia) which settles in 6–8 weeks but with compound, comminuted or widely displaced fractures nerve severance is found and demands urgent surgical repair.

85 Injuries to the shoulder, arm and elbow

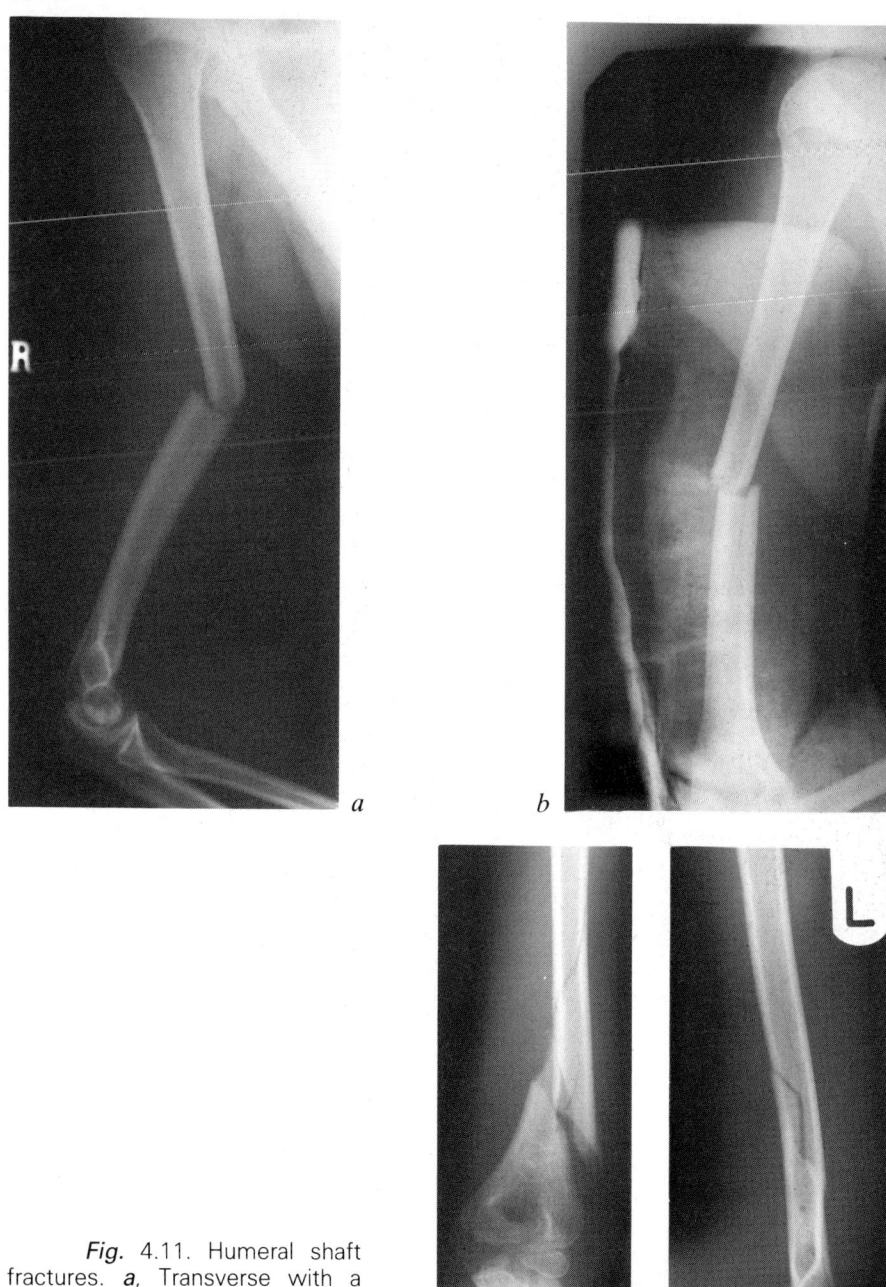

Fig. 4.11. Humeral shaft fractures. *a*, Transverse with a radial nerve neuropraxia. *b*, In a hanging cast, recovery took place in 4 weeks. *c*, A spiral fracture in an 8-year-old girl which clinically resembled a supracondylar fracture, due to the local haematoma.

When neuropraxia is suspected nerve conduction studies can be performed and if they indicate severance then exploration is undertaken. If immediate surgery is carried out the fracture is stabilized before nerve suture; defects in the nerve can be overcome by shortening the humerus (usually when comminuted, by 2·5 cm or so) or by nerve grafts (e.g. using the sural nerve). A lively splint is worn to support the wrist and hand and to encourage movement.

Diagnosis
This is easily established both clinically and radiologically but the function of the radial nerve must be tested. X-ray may show a spiral, transverse or oblique fracture; comminution occurs in high speed accidents.

Treatment
A cotton wool pad is placed in the axilla and a body bandage or sling given; with angulation or overlap a plaster cast is applied as a U-slab extending from the tip of the shoulder under the elbow to the inner arm. Then a collar and cuff is worn for 6–8 weeks. Alternatively, a functional cast brace can be used. It is made from plaster or polypropylene and extends from the axilla to the medial epicondyle and is adjusted by velcro straps. Mobilization occurs at 6–8 weeks. Internal fixation with plates or intra-medullary nails can be used when reduction is poor due to soft-tissue interposition.

Complications
Shortening and angulation cause little trouble unless severe but rotational deformities lead to problems of forearm movements. Such problems may occur because the sling is positioned with the forearm across the chest wall, i.e. in marked internal rotation. If *rotational* deformity is suspected it is better to apply a cast brace and by elbow movements realign the fragments.

Non-union. This is uncommon but when it occurs it is very refractory to treatment. Thus comminuted or markedly displaced humeral fractures are best treated by internal fixation, either by intra-medullary methods such as a Rush or Küntscher nail, or by a compression plate. With established non-union a bone graft is added to the fixation (a cortico-cancellous iliac crest graft can be used).

Radial nerve injury (*see above*).

Humeral Injuries around the Elbow
- *This is an important area for two reasons:*
1. Supracondylar fractures are often associated with vascular injury.
2. The natural variations of the elbow's epiphyses can cause confusion unless a comparative X-ray is taken with the uninjured elbow.

Supracondylar Fracture of the Humerus (*Fig.* 4.12)

There are 4 types:
1. *Undisplaced* (30% of all supracondylar fractures).
2. The *extension* injury with the lower fragment *displaced posteriorly* (95% of displaced fractures).
3. The *flexion* injury with the lower fragment *displaced anteriorly* (5% of displaced fractures).

87 Injuries to the shoulder, arm and elbow

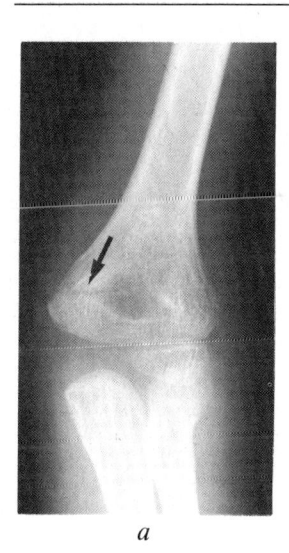

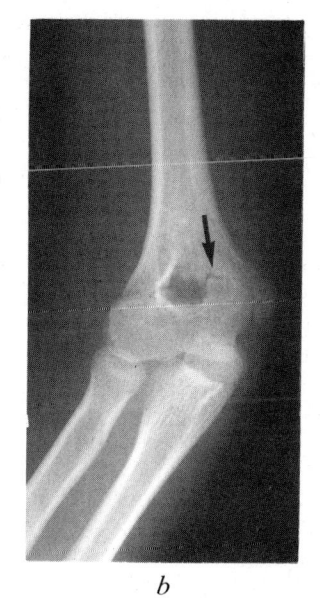

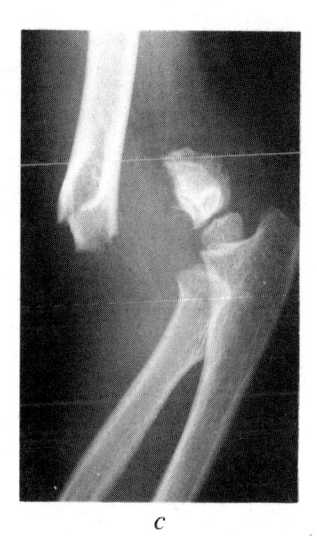

Fig. 4.12. Supracondylar fractures. *a*, Crack medial cortex. *b*, Transverse (undisplaced). *c*, The common posterior displacement. *d*, Anterior.

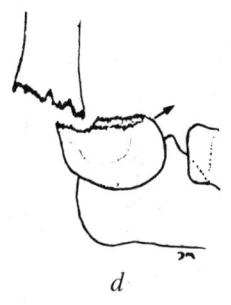

4. A *T-shaped* or *Y-shaped* extension into the intercondylar region (often in adults).

● **Very common in children, with boys three times more frequently affected than girls.**

Diagnosis
The immediate pain and deformity are obvious, the forearm may be cold and showing other signs of vascular impairment.

Treatment
Undisplaced fractures require a plaster backslab for 3 weeks. *Displaced* fractures need reduction—*urgent* when there are brachial artery problems (10% of cases).

Posterior Displacement
Under general anaesthesia longitudinal traction is applied to restore length to the limb and the posterior position of the lower fragment is corrected by flexing the elbow. However, the lateral or medial displacement must be corrected as well.

How should the limb be immobilized? As always, in the opposite position of the limb at the moment of fracture. Since the posterior displacement occurs with a fall on to the bent elbow and the limb is forced into extension, the reduced elbow is placed in flexion. When the hand is in *pronation* at the moment of impact the lower fragment is forced *laterally* (outwards); thus *supination* is required after reduction. When the hand is in *supination* at the moment of impact the lower fragment is pushed medially (inwards) and the forearm is placed in *pronation* after reduction. A simple rule!

Although it is often taught to immobilize the reduced posterior fracture with a collar-and-cuff, a plaster is much more comfortable and protective—it is worn for 3–4 weeks.

- *After flexion of the elbow to 90–100° the radial pulse must be checked along with the capillary circulation in the fingers (usually the nail bed). If the radial pulse is absent or diminished reduce the amount of flexion until it returns.* When the pulse is only present with an extended elbow then *Dunlop traction* (skin traction with crêpe and wool) is applied or *balanced suspended traction* with a Kirschner wire through the olecranon.
- *The circulation must be checked for at least 24–48 h.*

With *anterior displacement* of the lower fragment the limb is held in extension (since this is a forced flexion injury) after reduction. A plaster backslab is used for 3–4 weeks; the circulation is checked for 24 h but rarely impaired. In adults a *Y- or T-shaped fracture* may occur and if displaced require internal fixation, with plaster for 4 weeks.

Some centres favour open reduction or the closed insertion of percutaneous pins, especially when a supracondylar fracture feels unstable. A plaster is used for 3–4 weeks and the pins removed.

Complications
1. Injury to the *brachial artery*. A failure of the radial pulse to return after complete reduction, especially with elbow extension, demands an arteriogram and urgent exploration.
2. Injury to the *median, ulnar or radial nerves* may occur. There is usually a neuropraxia but exploration may be required if severance is suspected (*see* humeral shaft/radial nerve injury).
3. *Volkmann's ischaemic contracture* (*see* Chapter 3).
4. *Alteration in carrying angle* due to either malunion (most commonly) or loss of growth at the epiphysis. Some alteration occurs in almost 50% of cases. In cubitus varus the angle is decreased; in cubitus valgus the angle is increased. The normal carrying angle in the child is 6° (range 0–12°).
5. *Elbow stiffness.*
6. *Myositis ossificans.*
7. *Progressive ulnar nerve palsy* due to cubitus valgus (increased carrying angle causing traction on the nerve behind the medial epicondyle).
8. *Instability of the elbow.*

Injuries to the shoulder, arm and elbow

Fractures of the Condyles of the Humerus

The *lateral* condyle fracture is found in children and a great part of the detached fragment may be cartilaginous (*Fig.* 4.13a,b) and thus appears much smaller on X-rays than at surgery. Because the fracture is intra-articular correct realignment is essential. Medial condylar fracture is uncommon.

Diagnosis
The elbow is swollen and painful, and on X-ray the fat pad in the olecranon fossa is elevated with a translucent line beneath (the 'fat pad' sign).

Treatment
A plaster is used for 3 weeks; displaced fragments need open reduction and internal fixation with a small screw or pins (*Fig.* 4.13c).

Complications
1. *Non-union* due to the intra-articular nature.
2. *Rotation of the capitellum* (may be rotated through 90°).
3. *Malalignment of the forearm* due to displacement of condylar fragment or loss of growth in the epiphysis.
4. *Osteoarthritis* may develop from joint incongruity.

Fractures of the Epicondyle of the Humerus

Whereas most condylar fractures (*Fig.* 4.13a) occur laterally, *epicondylar* fractures are commonly found on the *medial* aspect (*Fig.* 4.13d). They occur at all ages and are usually an avulsion injury.

Diagnosis
Tenderness on palpation of the prominent epicondyle, which is often displaced.

Treatment
Plaster to relieve pain for 3 weeks. However, if the medial fragment becomes trapped within the elbow joint or there is injury to the ulnar nerve, surgery with fixation is carried out.

Complications
1. *Fragment trapped* in the joint.
2. *Ulnar nerve damage*.
3. *Elbow stiffness*.

Unusual Elbow Injuries

Epiphyseal injury: a fracture-separation of the distal humeral epiphysis is uncommon.

Shear fracture of the capitellum or trochlea.

Little league elbow: a baseball-induced avulsion of the medial epicondyle and a compression fracture of the capitellum (or an osteochondritis dissecans of the capitellum).

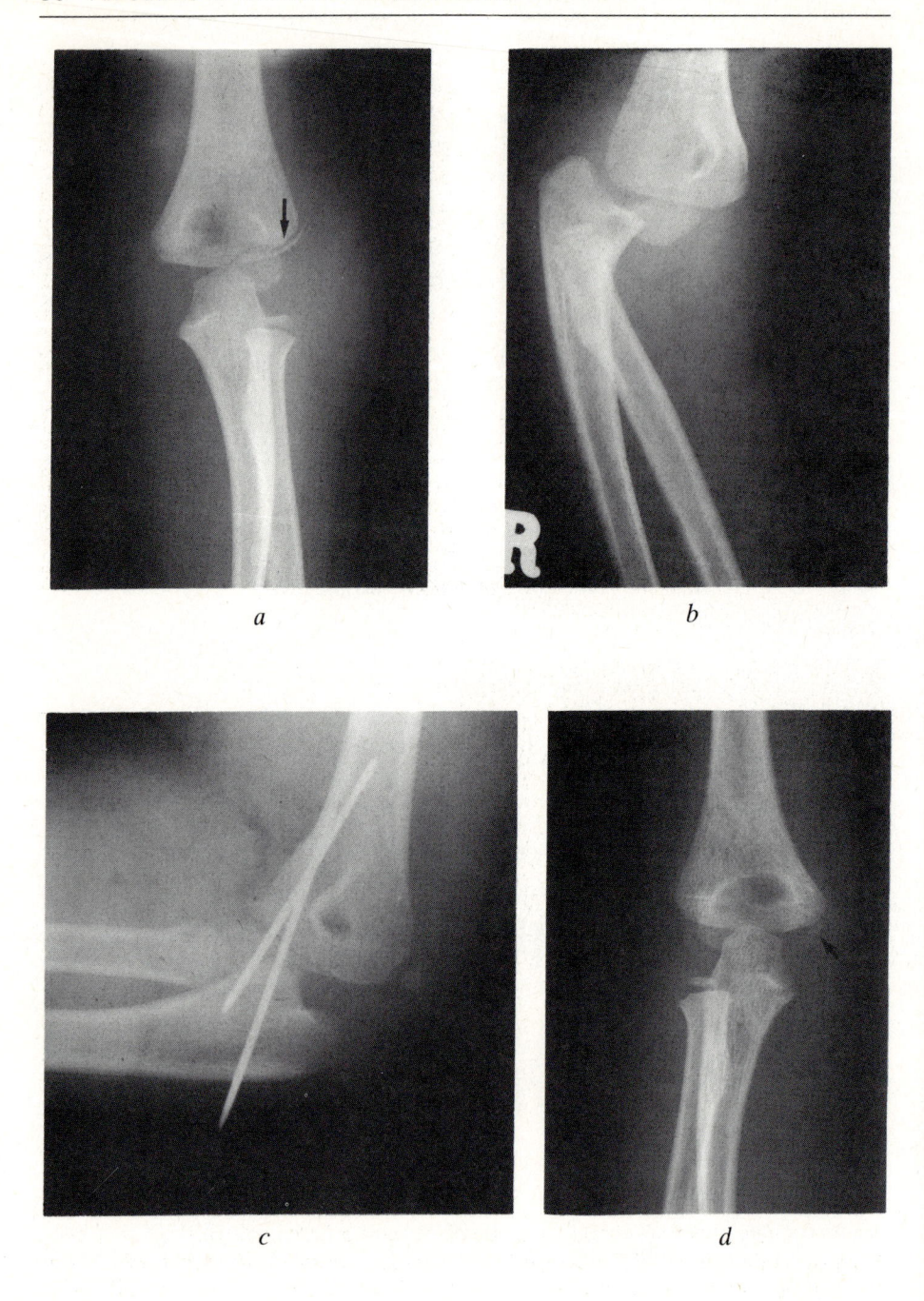

Fig. 4.13. *a*, Undisplaced lateral condyle of the humerus. *b*, Displaced (with a posterior dislocation of the elbow). *c*, Fixed with a Kirschner wire. *d*, Undisplaced fracture, medial epicondyle (denoted by soft-tissue swelling and local tenderness).

91 Injuries to the shoulder, arm and elbow

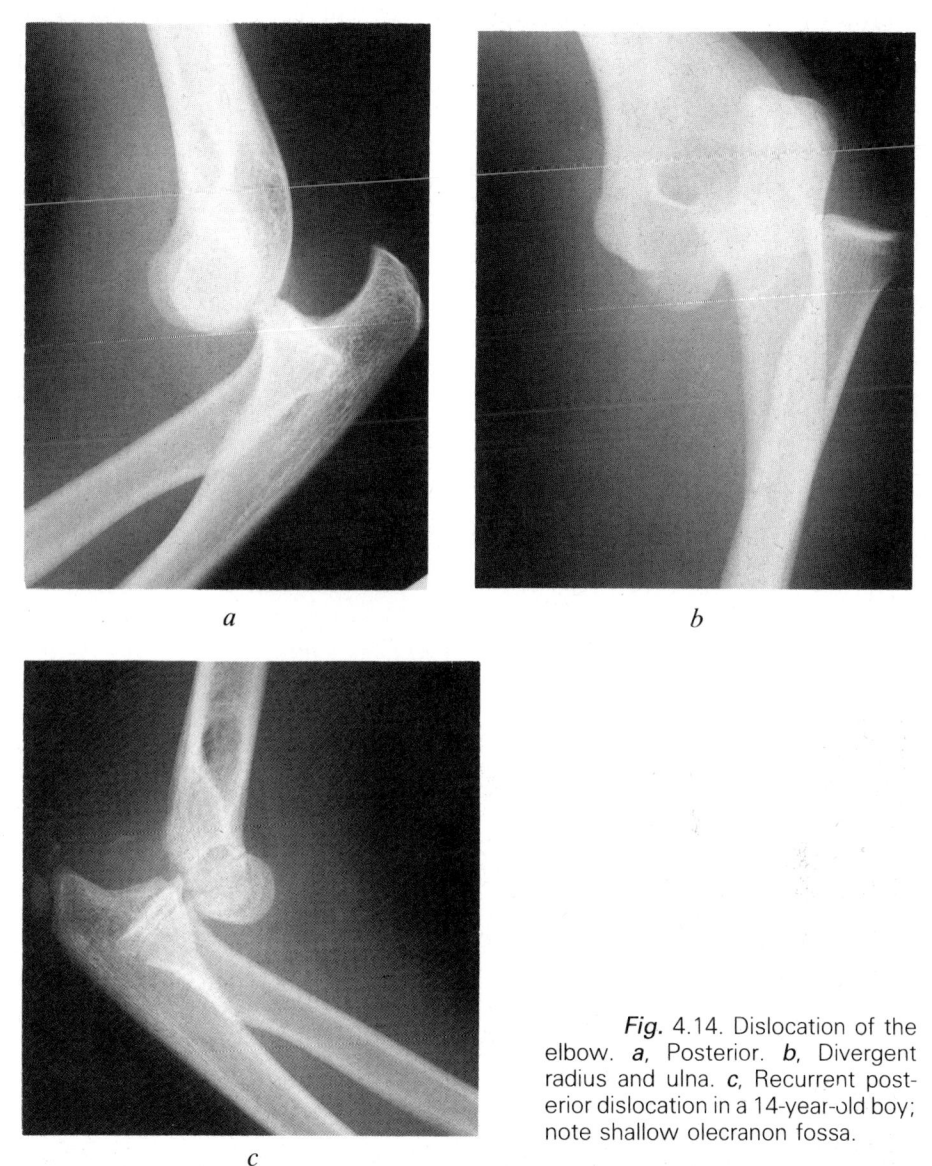

Fig. 4.14. Dislocation of the elbow. *a*, Posterior. *b*, Divergent radius and ulna. *c*, Recurrent posterior dislocation in a 14-year-old boy; note shallow olecranon fossa.

Dislocation of the Elbow Joint

Nearly always *posterior*, i.e. the olecranon points backwards (*Fig.* 4.14*a*). Very occasionally may be either *anterior*, *medial*, *lateral* or *divergent* (*Fig.* 4.14*b*) (the bones may be split apart in a *V-shaped* manner or lie parallel—the *transverse separation*).

Diagnosis
Obvious both clinically and radiologically.

Treatment
A *posterior dislocation* reduces very easily with traction (either under sedation or general anaesthesia). The reduced elbow is flexed and a plaster backslab is worn for 1–2 weeks; some centres advocate even more rapid mobilization within 5 days, a collar-and-cuff being used. Thereafter mobilization must be gentle or myositis ossificans may be induced by forced movements.

Anterior dislocation needs immobilization in extension for 2–3 weeks but the other varieties may need open reduction and repair.

Complications
1. The *ulnar nerve* can be stretched or torn.
2. The *median nerve* is sometimes trapped.
3. The *brachial vessels* may be injured.
4. *Joint stiffness* due to capsular tearing; when severe this can be treated by a turnbuckle splint which has a hinge that can be slowly extended by a screw every day. Physiotherapy can use resistance exercises and ice facilitation. Progress is often slow but steady. In refractory cases a manipulation under general anaesthesia may be required at 4–6 weeks.
5. *Myositis ossificans*. When this condition appears on the X-ray the limb is rested completely in a plaster for 2 weeks. Calcification can occur in the capsule and ligaments.
6. *Irreducible dislocation* due to trapping of bony fragment e.g. medial epicondyle.
7. *An associated fracture* of the lower humerus, lateral condyle, radial head, olecranon or coronoid process.
8. *Recurrent dislocation* which occurs in 2% of cases, especially when there is an anatomical defect in a child such as a shallow olecranon fossa (*Fig.* 4.14c).
9. An *unreduced dislocation* can be reduced by surgery and the results are often encouraging but the same basic problems of stiffness and osteoarthrosis are found as in the shoulder.
10. *Osteoarthrosis*: this may demand excision arthroplasty or a joint replacement.

Recurrent Dislocation of the Elbow
In the young the olecranon fossa is often deficient (*Fig.* 4.14c) due to poor growth. In the adult the soft tissues are usually lax.

Diagnosis
There is a clear history of elbow dislocation, sometimes relatively painless; the ulnar nerve may be irritated.

Treatment
The posterior lax capsule and related structures are tightened. A plaster is worn in flexion for 4 weeks. Then gentle mobilization begins.

5

Fractures of the forearm, wrist and hand

- **Fractures of the Olecranon Process**
    These may be *displaced* or *undisplaced*; usually the fracture is intra-articular, i.e. in the middle of the trochlear notch (*Fig. 5.1a*).

Diagnosis
With an undisplaced fracture there is localized bony tenderness; with displaced fractures the subcutaneous gap is palpable.

Treatment
With an *undisplaced fracture* or in the *very elderly* (with displacement) a plaster is worn for 3–6 weeks; in the *active patient* with a *displaced* fracture internal fixation is performed using either a screw (*Fig. 5.1b*) or a figure-of-eight tension band wire (*Fig. 2.15*). Elbow mobilization can begin almost immediately the soft-tissue discomfort and swelling have subsided. With a *comminuted* fracture the fragments are excised and the triceps attached to the distal part of the olecranon. Separation of the *olecranon epiphysis* is treated like an undisplaced fracture.

Complications
Non-union This is uncommon and can be accepted in the aged, but excision of the scar tissue and screw fixation are usually needed in active patients.
    Osteoarthritis develops when the articular surface is irregular.

- **Anterior Dislocation**
    Anterior dislocation of the radius and ulna may occur with fracturing of the lower humerus and upper ulna (sidesweep injury—when the elbow points invitingly out of the car window). Surgery is required with open reduction and internal fixation.

94   An outline of fractures and dislocations

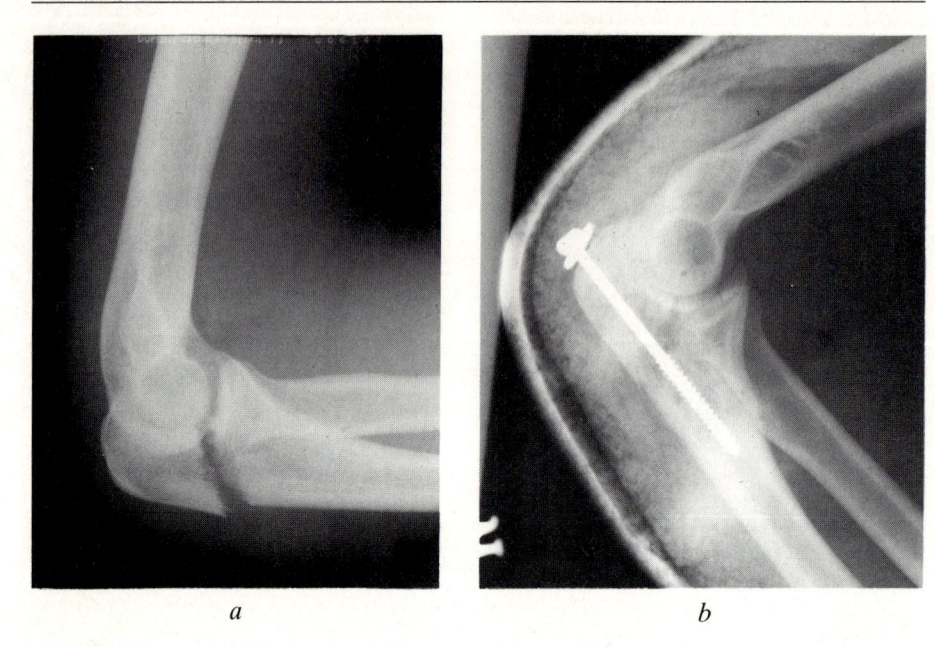

a   *b*

Fig. 5.1. *a,* Transverse fracture of the olecranon. *b,* Fixed by a bone screw.

- **Fractures of the Coronoid Process**
    Seldom fractured except with dislocation of the elbow; attention is directed to the dislocation.

- **Fractures of the Head of the Radius**
    Often indirectly caused by a fall on to the outstretched hand with an extended elbow and supinated forearm. The radial head knocks against the capitellum, causing damage to both joint surfaces. The head may fracture or the radial neck; in the child the epiphysis fails. Sometimes a direct blow to the outer elbow is the cause.

Diagnosis
Frequently missed on X-ray unless several oblique views are taken; there is local tenderness over the radial head with pain on full extension and supination.
    The types of fracture are (*Fig.* 5.2):
1.   *Undisplaced*
                    linear cracks
                    fissure fractures (T-shaped)
                    fractures of the neck of radius (transverse)

95 Fractures of the forearm, wrist and hand

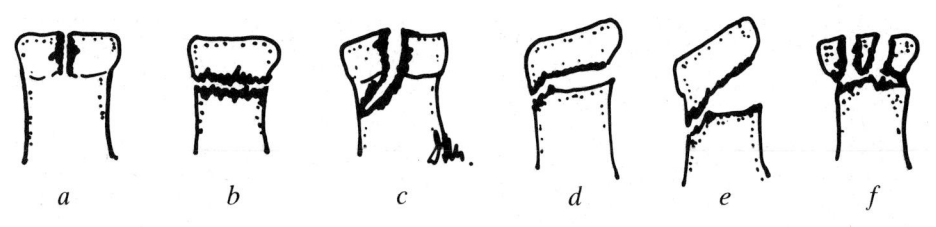

Fig. 5.2. Radial head fractures. *a*, Linear. *b*, Transverse. *c*, Oblique. *d*, Angulated, less than 20°. *e*, More than 20°. *f*, Comminuted.

2. *Displaced*
   lateral margin
   angulation of the radial head (less than 20°)
   (tilting greater than 20°)
   severe comminution

Treatment
Undisplaced fractures need a collar-and-cuff for 3 weeks.
   Displaced fractures can be reduced by traction on the limb in extension while pressure over the radial head affects reduction. However, surgery may be required and in the case of comminuted fractures the fragments are excised, sometimes being replaced by a synthetic component of plastic or carbon.
   If there is only a margin fracture it can be treated with a small lag screw. Tilting of less than 20° can be left; above this figure it must be corrected, often by open reduction, and a plaster is worn for 4 weeks.

Complications
1. *Localized osteoarthrosis* from capitellum damage, irregularity of the head or excessive tilting.
2. *Joint stiffness*, with limitation of extension and supination.
(*Note*: A radial head fracture may be associated with an elbow dislocation.)

- **Dislocation of the Radial Head**
   In a child (2–4 years) wrenched or lifted by his upper limb, the radial head may sublux in the annular ligament—the *pulled elbow*.

Diagnosis
The child is usually reluctant to move the elbow.

Treatment
The subluxation is reduced by pushing the forearm upwards with gentle rotatory movements.

Anterior Dislocation (*Fig.* 5.3)
Forced pronation can cause the head to be displaced forwards and it is reduced by pressure over the radial head with supination. A plaster is worn with the elbow in flexion for 6 weeks.
- *An isolated dislocation of the radial head is very rare and more commonly the ulnar shaft is fractured (a Monteggia fracture-dislocation).* The function of the radial nerve must be checked.

(*Special note*: Rarely the head of the radius is congenitally dislocated but the head shows a rounded appearance without the usual concavity on the upper surface.)

- **Fractures of the Shaft of the Radius and Ulna**
These bones are closely linked by the interosseous membrane and the gap between the forearm bones is widest in the neutral position and least at the extremes of pronation and supination. The main checks on such rotatory movements are the interosseous membrane and tightening of the forearm muscles, especially the impingement of the flexor pollicis longus on the flexor digitorum profundus. However, the normal 9° curve of the radial shaft lessens such impingement until the full range is reached. Thus with forearm fracture this radial arch is lost and the muscle and interosseous membrane check becomes distorted, especially if the bones are allowed to unite in an angulated or rotated position. Shoulder movements can accommodate up to 40° loss of pronation/supination.

Isolated Fractures of the Ulna
These occur from a direct blow or a fall on to the outstretched hand. They may be *undisplaced* or *displaced* (*Fig.* 5.4).
1. Greenstick fracture (child).
2. Transverse or oblique mid-shaft in an adult.
3. Comminuted fracture.
4. Angular fracture.
- *Always X-ray the elbow to exclude a Monteggia lesion.*

Diagnosis
The subcutaneous border easily localizes the fracture area.

Treatment
Special note: This is one fracture that may be better treated *without rigid immobilization*. Plaster can lead to non-union. Functional cast bracing is accepted as the treatment of choice at present, because a number of fractures treated by plating fail to unite. The brace is used for 6–12 weeks.

Complications
1. *Non-union*.
2. *Dislocation* or fracture of the *radial head* (*Figs.* 5.5, 5.6).

97 Fractures of the forearm, wrist and hand

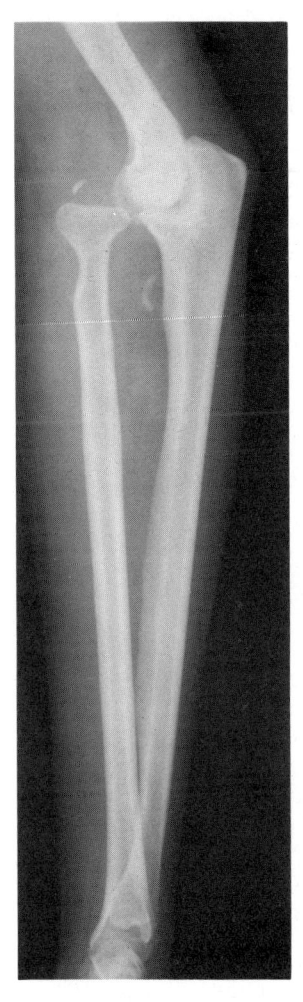

Fig. 5.3. Anterior dislocation of the radial head—a rare injury.

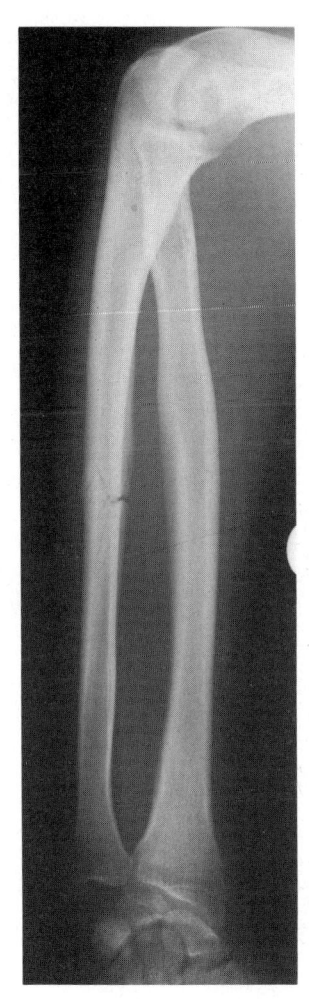

Fig. 5.4. An isolated fracture of the ulna—also uncommon.

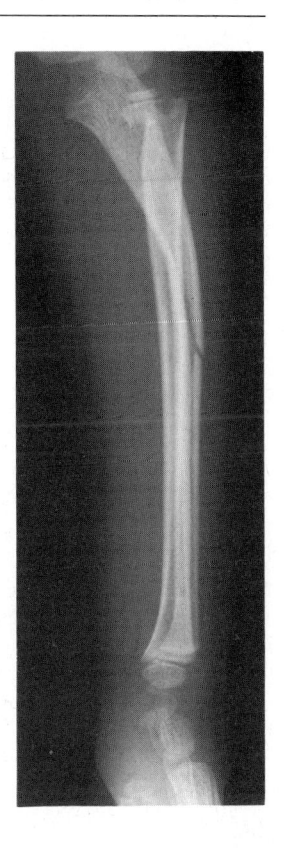

Fig. 5.5. An unusual fracture of the ulnar shaft and radial head in a child (a type of Monteggia lesion).

3. Occasionally the *inferior radio-ulnar joint* subluxes.
4. *Angulation* or *rotational* deformity.

Monteggia Fracture-dislocation
    Usually the radial head is displaced anteriorly (*Fig.* 5.6).
    Rarely posterior dislocation occurs. *Such displacements happen because the ulnar shaft fractures* and the parallel alignment is lost.

Diagnosis
Severe pain and swelling; the deformity is obvious.

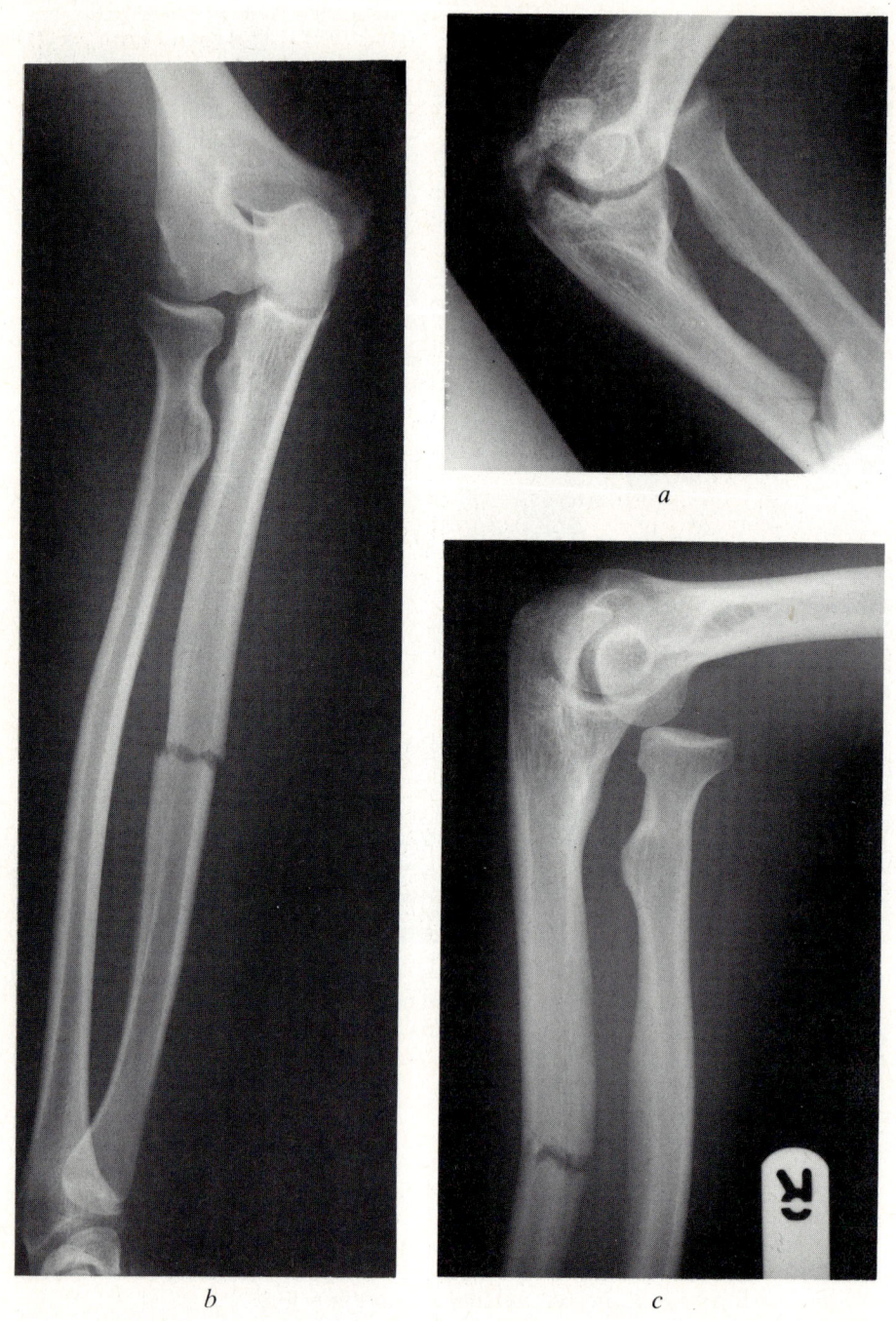

Fig. 5.6. *a,* A fracture of the olecranon with anterior dislocation of the radial head and an ulnar shaft fracture (a complex Monteggia lesion). *b, c,* The typical Monteggia fracture.

Treatment
Accurate reduction is essential and is usually only achieved by surgery. *Closed reduction* is effective in children. Since the injuring force is one of a fall or blow with forced pronation the ulna is reduced in supination with the elbow flexed at 90° to contain the reduced radial head. An above-elbow plaster is retained for 6–8 weeks. *Surgery*: Often the ulnar fracture is secured either with an intramedullary nail inserted through the olecranon, or a plate. The annular ligament may be repaired at the same time. After surgery a plaster is worn for 6 weeks to contain the radial head, then intensive mobilization exercises begin.

Complications
1. *Loss of elbow movement and forearm rotation.*
2. Failure to recognize the *radial head dislocation.*
3. *Non-union of the ulna.*
4. *Interposition* of capsule or annular ligament.
5. *Radial nerve injury* (15% of cases).
6. *Damage to the radial epiphysis* in children.
7. *Late osteoarthrosis* of the radio-ulnar and radiohumeral joint.
8. *Synostosis* between radius and ulna.

With *posterior* Monteggia dislocations the elbow is placed in extension and the forearm in the neutral position.

Surgery may not be needed but if the head is unstable the annular ligament must be repaired.

Fractures of the Radial Shaft
• **Check the inferior radio-ulnar joint for ulnar subluxation or dislocation.**
May be *undisplaced* or *displaced*.

Diagnosis
Local tenderness and restriction of forearm movement are easily detected.

Treatment
Closed manipulation usually reduces this fracture when displaced but alignment must be checked and the normal curve of the shaft maintained. Sometimes plating is required.

A plaster is used for 6 weeks.

Galeazzi Fracture-dislocation
This is a fracture of the shaft of the radius (usually lower third) with dislocation of the inferior radio-ulnar joint (i.e. at the wrist) (*Fig.* 5.7). The head of the ulna may pass either medially, anteriorly or posteriorly. This is a very unstable lesion. Also in children separation of the distal ulnar epiphysis may occur or a fracture of the distal 1 in of ulna.

Diagnosis
An X-ray must include the wrist joint in all cases of isolated radial shaft fractures.

100 An outline of fractures and dislocations

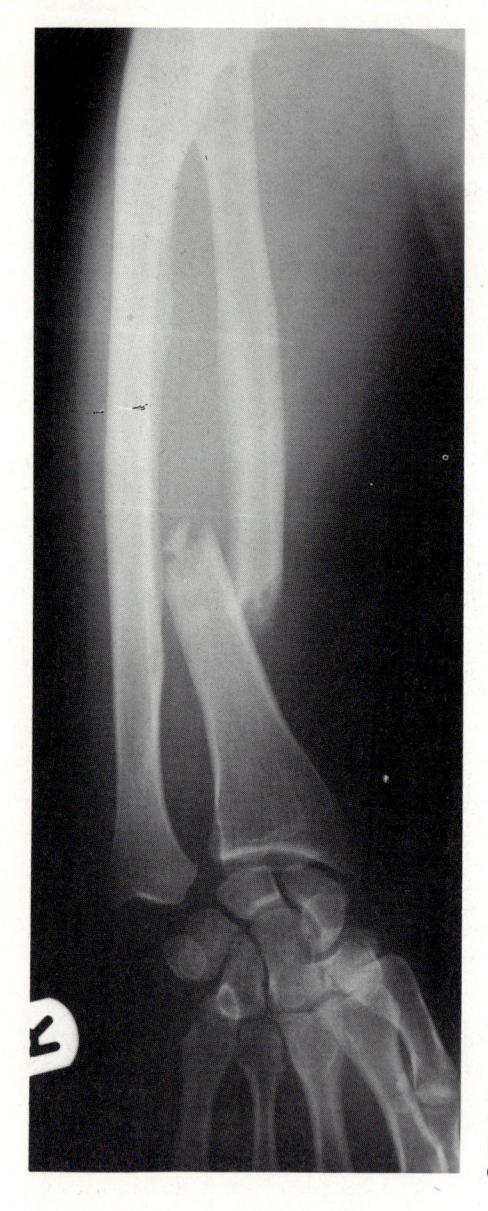

Fig. 5.7. A fracture of the radius (shaft) with a dislocation of the inferior radio-ulnar joint (Galeazzi fracture-dislocation).

Treatment
Perfect reduction is essential for full restoration of function. The fragments are usually held in supination. The best results occur when the radius is plated and the joint is fixed with a fine Kirschner wire. Plaster is worn for 6–8 weeks, then intensive mobilization exercises begin after wire removal.

Fracture of Both Forearm Bones

Commonly both bones are fractured, either due to a direct blow or indirectly through a fall onto the hand. They may be *undisplaced* (usually a greenstick fracture) (*Fig.* 5.8*d*) or *displaced* (*Fig.* 5.8*e*). Displaced fractures can occur in the adult with marked angulation. *Fracturing* may be found in the *upper, middle* or *lower* thirds (*Fig.* 5.8*a,b,c*).

Diagnosis
In children these fractures are more difficult to diagnose because swelling and pain can be slight; in adults there is usually marked swelling and deformity.

Treatment
For *undisplaced* fractures a plaster is worn for 3–6 weeks.

With *displaced fractures* the forearm is manipulated and an above-elbow plaster used. However, the position of the forearm is crucial for reduction and unfortunately this positioning often causes a great deal of confusion.
- *Simply remember the level of radial shaft fracture* (recall US:MN:LP).

With an *upper third* fracture (*Fig.* 5.8*a*), the upper part is pulled into supination, thus the forearm is placed in *supination* to match (US).

With a fracture in the *middle third* the break lies below the supinators and the pronator teres (*Fig.* 5.8*b*); thus the upper fragment lies in *neutral rotation*—the forearm is placed in neutral rotation (MN) to match.

With a fracture of the *lower third* (*Fig.* 5.8*c*) of the radius the pronator quadratus acts pulling this bone into *pronation*—the position the forearm assumes after reduction (LP).

After all reductions it is best to relieve the full pronation/supination by derotating the forearm a few degrees, thus slightly widening the interosseous membrane; also in full pronation the weight of the hand displaces the distal pieces downwards.

Any angulation will also narrow the interosseous space and lead to diminished mobility.
- *Because of instability and difficulty in apposing the narrow bone ends fractures of the radius and ulna often need internal fixation with compression plates* (*see Figs.* 2.13*a* and 5.8*h*).

With closed reduction a plaster (for 6 weeks) is applied above the elbow and must be snugly fitting; thus after reduction limb elevation and observation of the finger circulation are essential. After internal fixation a crêpe-and-wool support or plaster backslab is required for 2–3 weeks.

With comminuted fractures or when there are skin problems (a wound or skin loss) external fixation can be used for 6–8 weeks (*see Fig.* 2.17) or a Sarmiento plaster with a hinge brace at the wrist can also be used to allow early mobilization.

Special note: With *fractures* of the *lower forearm* (*Fig.* 5.8*f*), especially in *children* (*Fig.* 5.8*g*), the small chunky fragments are often difficult to reduce and later float apart in the swelling. To reduce, the wrist is placed in pronation and hyperextended with traction on the lower fragment. The bone ends are hooked together and the distal fragment is flexed to about 30°.

N.B. Correct any lateral displacement. Always use a full-arm plaster because brachioradialis will act as a displacing force and can cause volar angulation. The plaster is moulded with three-point fixation and worn for 4 weeks.

102 An outline of fractures and dislocations

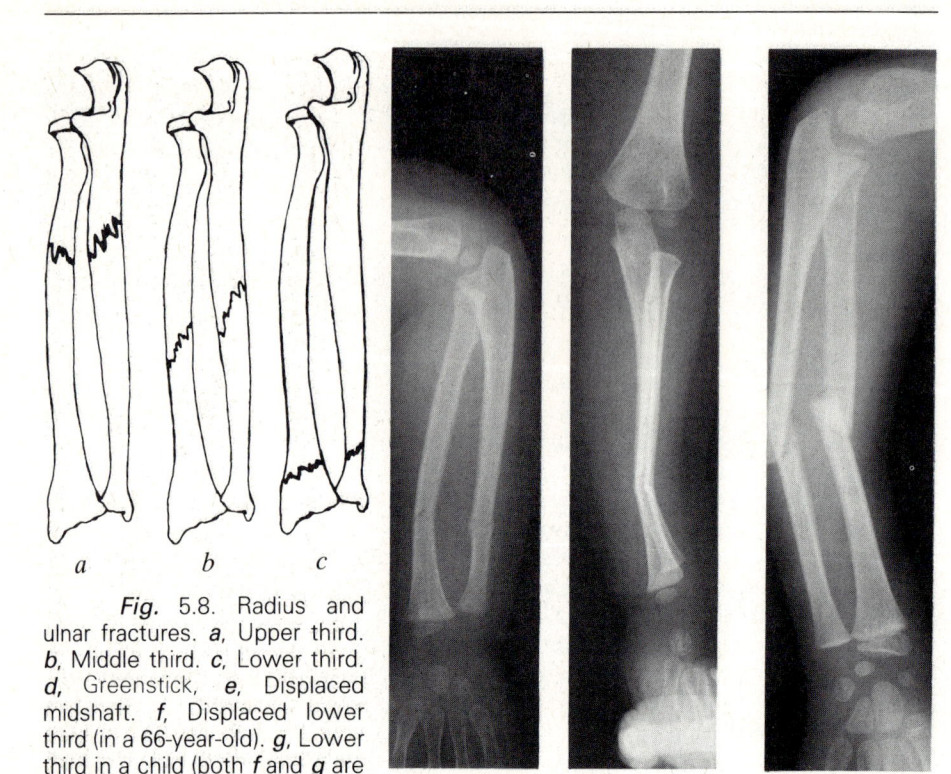

Fig. 5.8. Radius and ulnar fractures. *a*, Upper third. *b*, Middle third. *c*, Lower third. *d*, Greenstick. *e*, Displaced midshaft. *f*, Displaced lower third (in a 66-year-old). *g*, Lower third in a child (both *f* and *g* are difficult to reduce). *h*, AO compression plating forearm fractures.

Complications
1. These fractures *commonly displace* and forearm X-rays must be taken at weekly intervals, if necessary, for the first 3 weeks of immobilization, although slipping is uncommon after 2 weeks. When the position cannot be maintained by plaster, compression plating may be required (*Fig.* 5.8*h*).
2. *Ischaemic necrosis* of the forearm muscles (Volkmann's), thus the circulation must be watched for 24–48 h.
3. *Rotation and angulation* leading to marked restriction of pronation/supination. Angulation will usually spontaneously cancel in children below 8 years, even if greater than 20°. However, there may be an occasional increased angulation which proves unsightly, requiring an osteotomy.
4. *Injury to the anterior interosseous nerve* especially as it emerges from the pronator teres.
5. *Non-union* with comminuted fracture or when there has been segmental loss; fixation with a compression plate and bone-grafting is used.

f   *g*   *h*

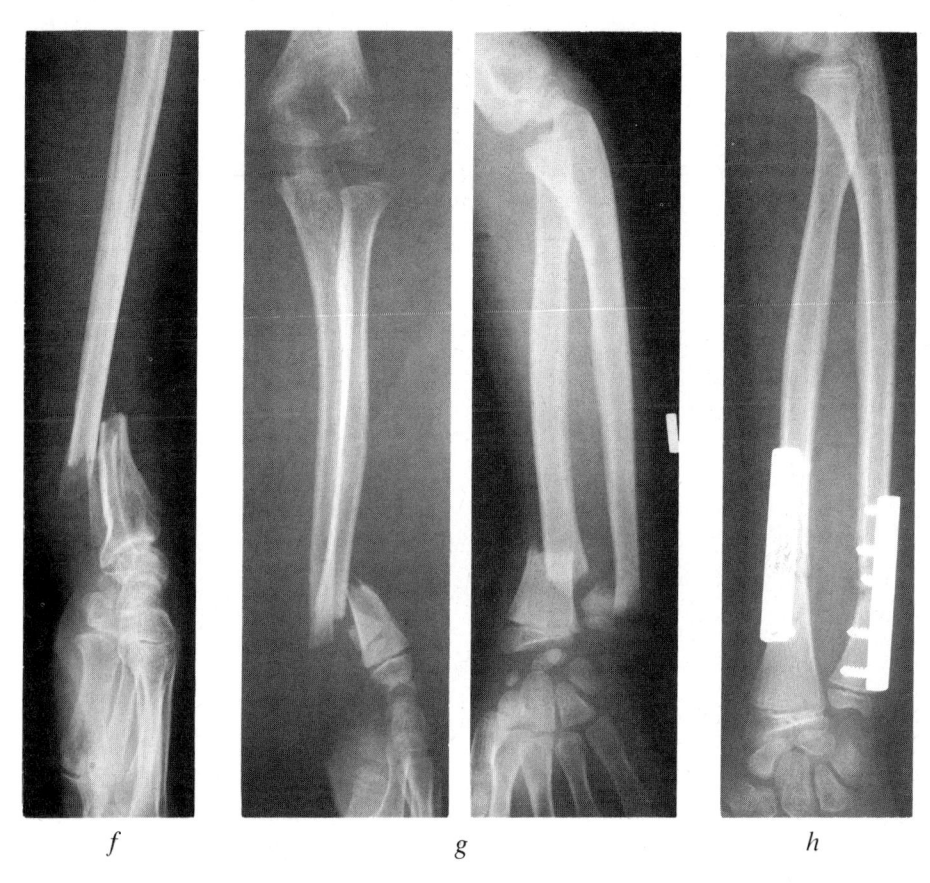

Fig. 5.8. (*cont.*)

Fractures of the Lower Radius (Children)
    This fracture may occur with a chip fracture of the tip of the ulnar styloid process. Commonly it is a greenstick fracture (*Fig.* 5.9*a*) or undisplaced (*Fig.* 5.9*b*) but when displaced it occurs through the lower radial epiphysis (*radial slipped epiphysis*) (*Fig.* 5.9*c*). The lower fragment is usually pushed backwards.

Diagnosis
There is usually marked tenderness over the radial epiphysis with a dorsal bump on the wrist. Check the hand circulation when displacement is marked.

Treatment
Reduction under anaesthesia is often easy unless there is full displacement, when open reduction and gentle leverage of the epiphysis back into position are needed. A forearm plaster is worn for 4 weeks.

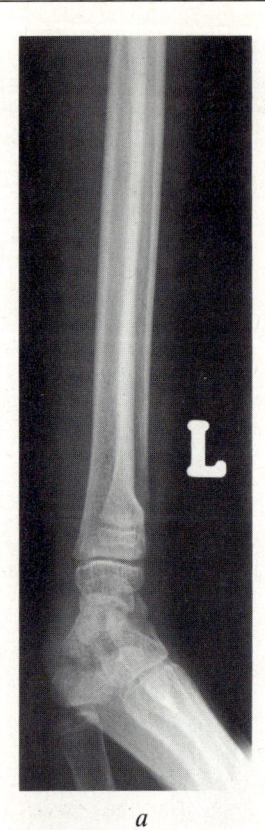

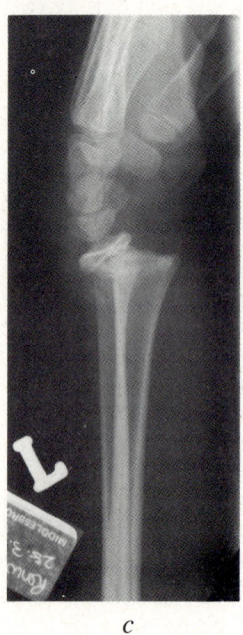

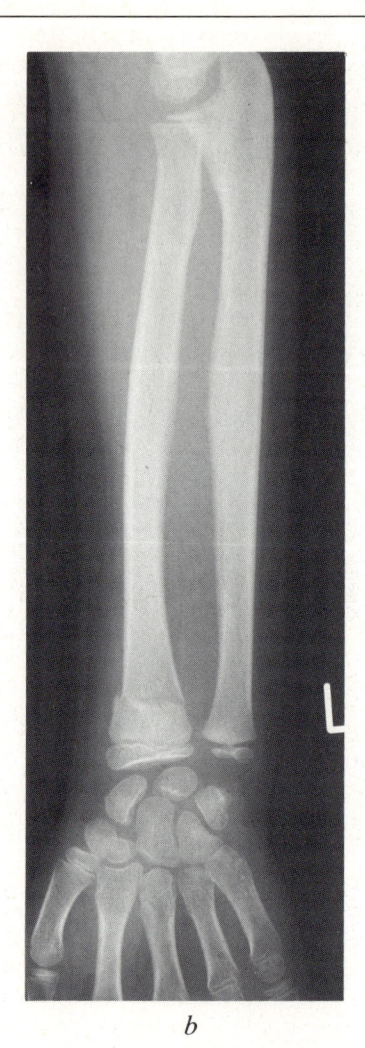

Fig. 5.9. Lower radial fractures in children. *a*, The typical, often missed, greenstick fracture of the radius (lateral view) in a 10-year-old boy. *b*, Transverse, undisplaced in an 8-year-old girl. *c*, Displaced radial epiphysis in a 12-year-old boy.

Complications
Loss of growth, more common after crushing injuries (Type IV), rarely may cause Madelung's deformity when the ulnar styloid becomes more prominent and the hand deviates radially. (For other complications see next section.)

Fractures of the Lower Radius (Adults)
The eponymic fractures: Colles, Smith's and Barton's fractures.

Colles Fractures
This fracture with its dinner fork deformity (*Fig.* 5.10*a*) is amongst the most ubiquitous of all orthopaedic emergencies. A fall onto the dorsiflexed hand forcibly supinates the forearm, breaking the radius just above the wrist. There are *three* components: radial shortening, radial deviation and dorsal angulation.

Colles fracture is typically an injury of osteoporotic bones in elderly women (70%). The same hyperextension injury from a fall in a young adult produces a scaphoid fracture, or in a child a slipped epiphysis.

The radius may fracture in isolation or more commonly with the ulnar styloid process or lower ulnar shaft.

The radial fracture may be: *transverse* (*Fig.* 5.10*b*), an inch or so above the wrist; comminuted (*Fig.* 5.10*c,d*) or T-shaped into the joint (*Fig.* 5.10*e*).

Diagnosis
The classic dinner fork deformity is obvious.

Treatment
Apart from undisplaced cracks in the lower radius the true Colles fracture needs reduction by grasping the wrist above the fracture and applying traction to the hand via the lower fragment to unlock the pieces. The wrist is flexed and pronated and the distal fragment is pushed forwards and downwards with the palm of the hand. A high forearm plaster is worn for 1 month. During the first week a plaster back-slab allows the swelling to subside without compression of the soft tissues. It is completed on the 7th day and a check X-ray is taken. Then mobilization begins at 1 month to achieve dorsiflexion, essential for a good power grip.

The treatment of the comminuted fracture depends upon the degree of joint involvement; if there is depression of the articular surface or if the joint is unstable then open reduction with stabilization through a thick Steinmann pin is required, or an external fixation device is applied. A plaster is used for 4 weeks. N.B. When active mobilization begins the patient is warned that bony union takes approximately 12 weeks and some discomfort may be experienced during this 4–12 week interval. However, prolonged plaster immobilization (to 6 weeks) increases the risk of joint stiffness. Contrast bathing (hot to cold water for 10–20 min three times daily) with exercises to regain full dorsiflexion and supination are required.

Special note: The commonly taught forced flexion, pronation and ulnar deviation is a rotten position for the wrist. Should stiffness supervene then the power grip is lost, while the pull of brachioradialis accentuates the deformity and median nerve compression can result. Thus the forearm is placed just short of full pronation and the wrist rests in only 20° of flexion.

106 An outline of fractures and dislocations

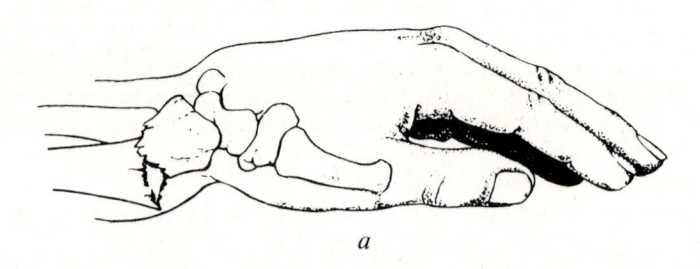

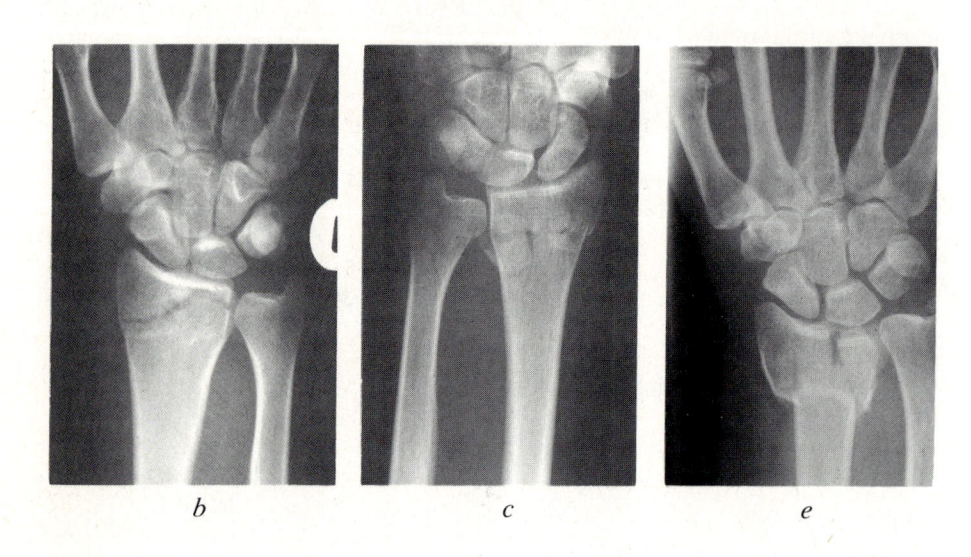

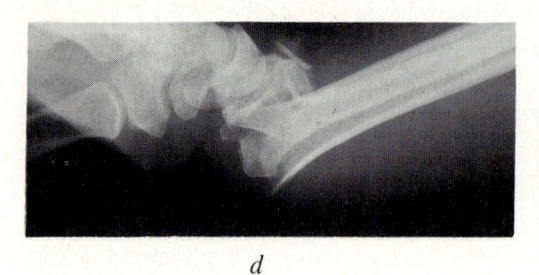

Fig. 5.10. Colles fracture. *a*, The 'dinner-fork' deformity. *b*, Transverse (extra-articular, but close to the joint). *c*, Comminuted (extra-articular). *d*, Comminuted, displaced and intra-articular. *e*, T-shaped, intra-articular. *f*, Radial styloid, intra-articular, with ulnar styloid.

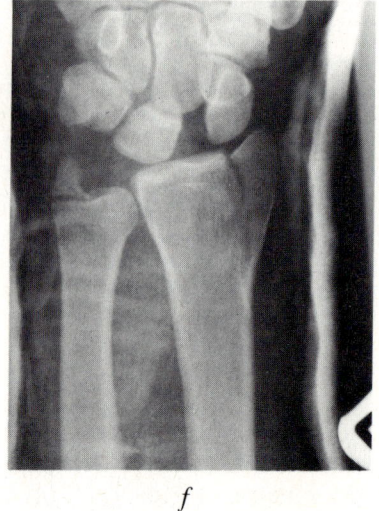

Complications
1. Poor grip strength and *finger stiffness*.
2. *Shoulder-hand syndrome*—pain, weakness and restricted movements are especially common in the shoulder and hand. Emphasis is given to early exercises with limited use of a sling (up to 7 days).
3. *Sudeck's atrophy*.
4. *Median nerve compression* (*acute*) or *late* (carpal tunnel syndrome) (3%). Sometimes an *ulnar* neuropathy occurs at the wrist.
5. *Rupture of the extensor pollicis longus* by spiculation at the fracture site. *Tenosynovitis* may occur, especially of the wrist flexors in the carpal tunnel.
6. *Malunion*. This is common and when severe may require an osteotomy to correct the angulation. *Prominence of the ulnar styloid* often leads to an ugly deformity and local discomfort. Excision of the prominent area may be carried out.
7. *Disruption of the radio-ulnar joint*.
8. Osteoarthrosis after comminuted injuries.
9. *A fracture of the scaphoid* (or other carpal bones) is found in 5% of Colles fractures. Under these circumstances the wrist is held in 25° of extension and radial deviation and the plaster includes the thumb and elbow. *Radial head* fractures and finger and thumb injuries occasionally coexist.
10. Volkmann's ischaemic contracture.

Smith's Fracture
This is the reverse of Colles' fracture (*Fig.* 5.11*a*), the lower fragment and the wrist displace in a volar direction. The cause is a heavy fall on a supinated wrist, often from a motor cycle.

Diagnosis
A concavity is noticed on the dorsum of the wrist with marked pain and restricted movements.

Treatment
This is a very unstable fracture. The hand is placed in supination and neutral flexion and kept in plaster for 4–6 weeks. With instability or comminution a small angled or T-shaped plate (*Fig.* 5.11*c*) is fixed to the volar surface of the radius after open reduction, or an external fixation device is used.

Complications
As for Colles fracture but damage to the median nerve and circulatory problems in the hand from swelling are more common. Redisplacement may follow conservative management.

Barton's Fracture
This is in reality a *fracture-dislocation* (*Fig.* 5.11*b*) with the wrist usually displaced forwards (volar) and a shear fracture through the articular margin of

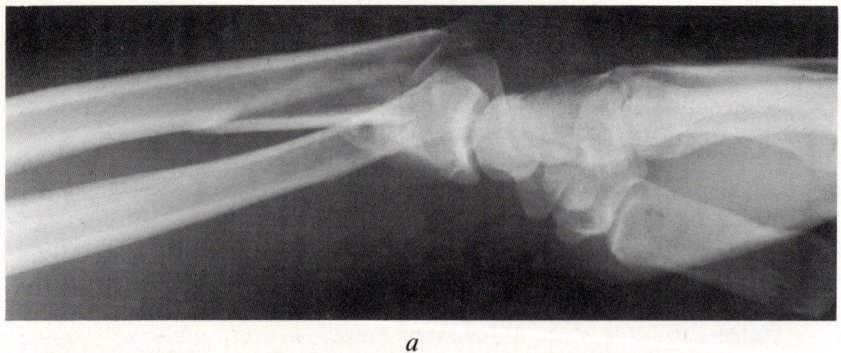

108 An outline of fractures and dislocations

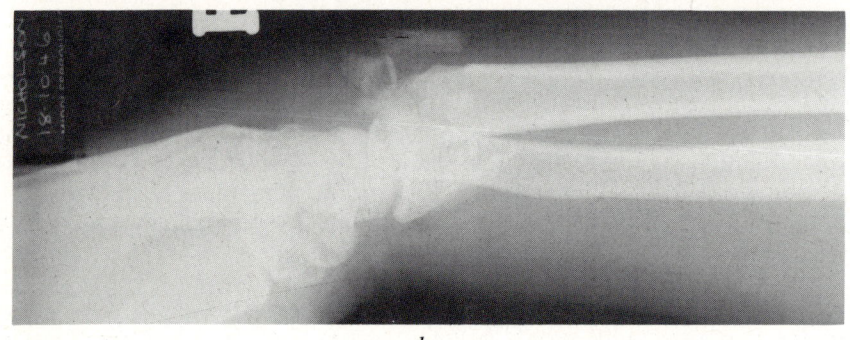

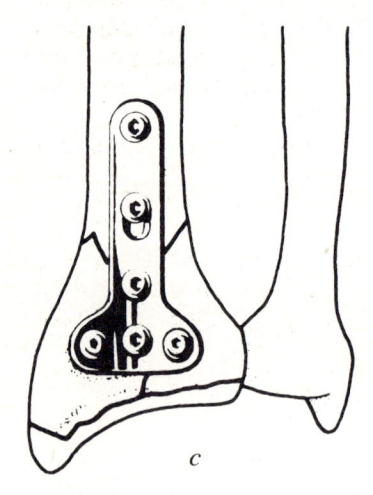

Fig. 5.11. *a*, Smith's fracture (L). *b*, Barton's fracture (R)—in the same patient. *c*, Buttress plate.

the radius—an *anterior marginal fracture*. (Sometimes the fracture is *comminuted* or there is *posterior marginal fracture*, resembling a Colles fracture; occasionally a radial styloid fracture coexists.)

Diagnosis
The common anterior fracture may be confused with Smith's fracture but the break is within the wrist joint and not proximal to it (as in the latter).

109 Fractures of the forearm, wrist and hand

Treatment
So unstable is this injury that open reduction is nearly always required with fixation by a buttress plate (the radial styloid can be held with a Kirschner wire). A plaster is used for 4 weeks and the wire removed then. An external fixation device can also be used for 6–12 weeks.

Fracture of the Radial Styloid
An undisplaced crack is treated with a light plaster for 3 weeks but the displaced fracture is important because it involves the radial articular surface (*see Fig. 5.10f*). Thus if there is imperfect reduction screw fixation may be needed after perfect alignment has been restored by surgery.
- *This fracture may occur with carpal injuries such as a perilunate dislocation. Always have adequate views of the carpal bones.*

Fracture of the Ulnar Styloid
Commonly found with lower radial fractures, it may occur in isolation as an avulsion injury due to the pull of the ulnar collateral ligament. Usually a light plaster is worn for 2–3 weeks.

Subluxation or Dislocation of the Distal Ulna
Subluxation or dislocation can occur *on its own* or with a *fracture of the radius* (Galeazzi) or *ulna*.

Diagnosis
The more serious dislocation is usually clearly visible on the *dorsal* or *volar* surface (depending on the direction of the dislocation). However, subluxation is commonly missed. Since there is a wide variation in X-ray appearance of the normal wrist the beam should be centred over the wrist, the elbow flexed and the forearm pronated giving lateral shift of the ulnar styloid.

In a child subluxation cannot be seen on X-ray and the condition is treated on clinical suspicion (*see* pulled elbow).

Treatment
With *dorsal dislocation* or subluxation the ulnar head is reduced by firm pressure and the limb immobilized for 4 weeks in *supination*. *Volar dislocation* needs *pronation* after reduction. The plaster must be above the elbow to prevent rotatory movement.

- **Fractures and Dislocations of the Carpal Bones**
The eight carpal bones (two rows of four) possess an almost global range of motion; the proximal row forming a smooth arch on the radius and articular disc (note that the ulna does not articulate with the carpus), while the distal row glides freely on the proximal. The 2nd and 3rd carpometacarpal joints remain practically immobile as a fixed keystone of the arched hand.
- *The scaphoid spans both rows and acting as a link rod is in a vulnerable position.*

110 An outline of fractures and dislocations

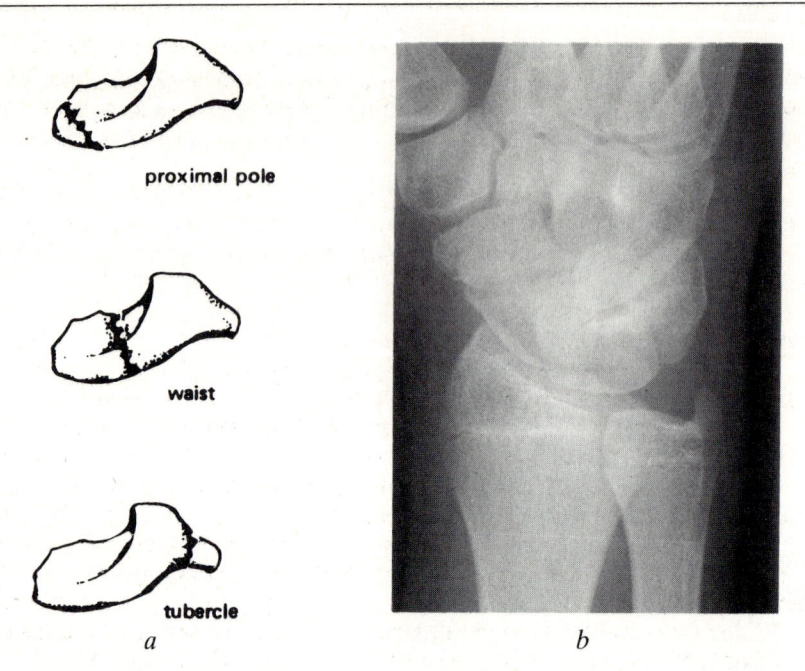

Fig. 5.12. *a*, Fractures of the scaphoid. *b*, An uncommon fracture involving both the waist and the tubercle.

N.B. Approximately 60% of extension occurs between radius and carpus. But with flexion the situation is reversed, i.e. 40% of flexion occurs at the radiocarpal joint.
 • *X-ray diagnosis requires* **four** *views of the wrist, with supplementary oblique views, if needed.*

Fractures of the Scaphoid
This bone is the most frequently fractured of all the carpal bones (*Fig.* 5.12): usually forced dorsiflexion breaking the mid-scaphoid (waist) region, i.e. the place that straddles the mid-carpal joint.

Ninety Per Cent Rule
 Approximately 90% of scaphoid fractures occur in the middle third (waist), are isolated injuries and unite with plaster immobilization.
 Fractures can be *undisplaced* mid-third (waist)
 distal third
 tubercle
 or *displaced* horizontal
 mid-third (waist)
 oblique
 proximal third

- *The principal vascular supply to the scaphoid is through the distal portion and this arrangement means that both displaced fractures and injuries of the proximal third and waist risk avascular necrosis of the proximal fragment.*

Diagnosis
- *Any painful wrist (usually labelled a 'sprain') demands good X-rays (several views).* The patient may grip the scaphoid area with his index finger and thumb when describing the pain, and palpation of the anatomical snuff box hurts.

Treatment
- *If no fracture is seen apply a scaphoid plaster for 2 weeks and re-X-ray (out of plaster).* If still negative exclude a scapholunate subluxation.

If X-rays are positive initially (or at 2 weeks) but the fracture is *undisplaced* a scaphoid plaster is used for 6–12 weeks. The thumb is placed in the grasp postion with the wrist in slight extension and radial deviation. The plaster extends dorsally from the metacarpal heads to the upper forearm and to the palmar crease ventrally. At 6 weeks the fracture is tested clinically; if *non-tender* it is mobilized; if *tender* the plaster is reapplied for a further 4–6 weeks. If the fracture persists after 12 weeks the wrist must be mobilized to avoid stiffness.

With *displacement* the fracture is reduced and fixed with a percutaneous wire; sometimes open reduction and a small lag screw are required.

- *Fractures of the* **tubercle** *can be treated with wrist strapping for 2–3 weeks.*

Complications
This fracture causes more problems than its size warrants (the 'mighty mouse' of fractures). However, the prognosis is more optimistic (90%) than most books suggest.
1. *Avascular necrosis of the proximal fragment (Fig.* 5.13a). 5–10% develop this complication which is most frequent with proximal third fractures (also with horizontal, displaced, oblique fractures and carpal dislocations). The avascular area is clearly visible on X-ray. A technetium bone scan can be used to assess bone viability at 3–6 months. (For treatment *see* non-union, *below.*)
2. *Non-union.* 5–10% develop non-union (*Fig.* 5.13b) which may exist without symptoms. Cystic change, fibrous union and collapse of the proximal fragment occur, usually at 6–12 months. Without symptoms no treatment is needed; with pain and restricted wrist power a bone graft is required with screw or wire fixation.

Alternatively, the small dead fragment can be excised and replaced with a silicone rubber implant.
3. *Associated fracture.* 10% have Colles, transcapitate or other fractures.
4. *Associated dislocation.* There may be other carpal dislocations including trans-scaphoid dislocation (*Fig.* 5.13c) or a scapholunate subluxation.
5. *Missed fracture.* Over 90% of fractures discovered within a month will heal with plaster immobilization—even a delay of several months will not affect union in 70% of cases.

The plaster is worn for 6–12 weeks.

112 An outline of fractures and dislocations

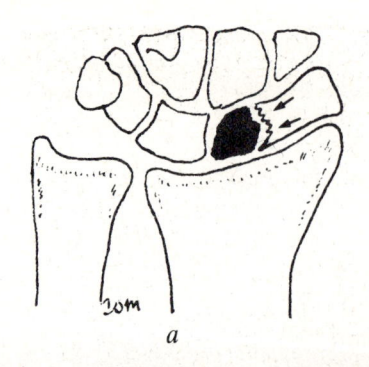

Fig. 5.13. *a*, Avascular necrosis of the proximal fragment. *b*, Non-union and cystic changes. *c*, Trans-scaphoid fracture with displacement of the proximal fragment due to lunate subluxation.

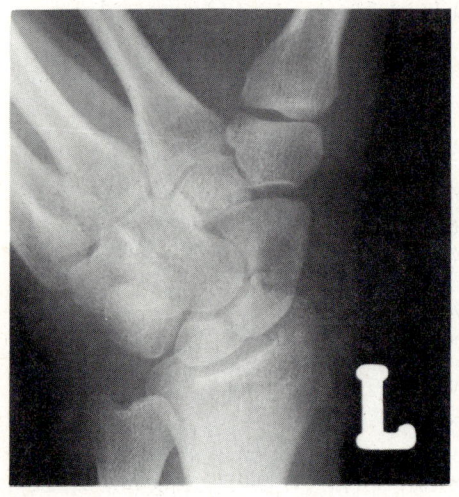

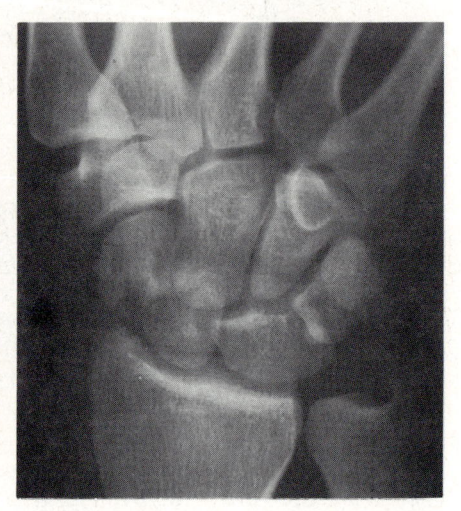

- **Even if the fracture line is visible when the plaster is removed after 12 weeks,** it **frequently becomes obliterated** *within 6–12 months.*

6. *Osteoarthritis.* This develops at the radioscaphoid junction and symptoms may respond to a wrist support (leather or polyethylene), to excision of the radial styloid, or to a carbon pad implant into the osteoarthritic area. Rarely, arthrodesis or wrist arthroplasty is necessary.

7. *Median nerve compression* occurs with associated major carpal dislocation.

8. *Finger stiffness and Sudeck's atrophy*

Note: Congenital bipartite scaphoid is rarely found. It has a clear, smooth joint line and is usually present in both wrists.

Scaphoid Fracture with Lunate Dislocation

The same dorsiflexion force that fractures the scaphoid can cause lunate dislocation or subluxation (*Fig.* 5.13c), carrying with it the proximal half of the scaphoid. Treatment consists of lunate reduction and, if unstable, fixation of the scaphoid fracture with a screw. The plaster is applied and maintained as for a scaphoid fracture.

113 Fractures of the forearm, wrist and hand

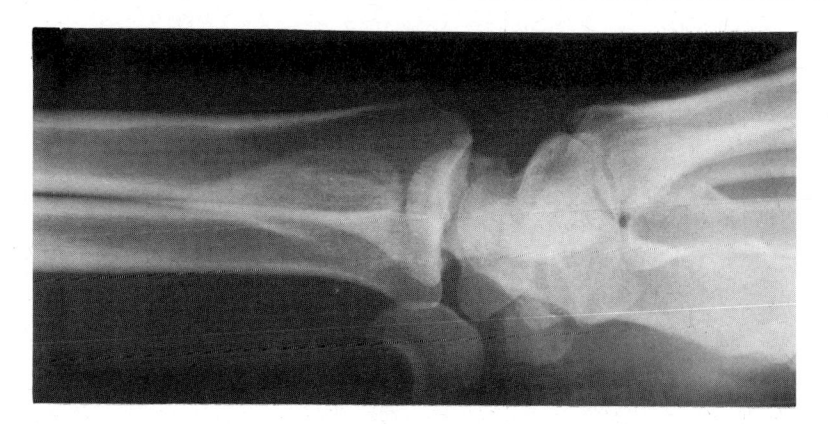

Fig. 5.14. Volar dislocation of the lunate.

Volar Dislocation of the Lunate
    This is one of the common uncommon carpal injuries (*Fig.* 5.14); a fall onto the extended hand squeezes the snugly placed lunate like a pip into the volar aspect of the wrist, tearing its dorsal ligament.

Diagnosis
The lunate can be palpated on the front of the wrist and X-ray shows the articular surface to be tilted forwards. There may be compression on the median nerve.

Treatment
The wrist is dorsiflexed with strong traction to open up the space and the thumb presses on the lunate, which 'pops' backwards. The wrist is flexed to 45° and a plaster worn for 6 weeks.

Complications
1.   *Missed dislocation.* May need surgery to replace lunate.
2.   *Avascular necrosis* (Kienböck's disease). May need excision and replacement with silicone rubber prosthesis.
3.   *Median nerve compression.*
4.   *Associated fracture* especially scaphoid waist (*see above*).
5.   *Osteoarthrosis* (if avascular fragment is not excised or a dislocation is missed).
6.   *Persistent subluxation of the scapholunate* joint. (*See* Other wrist injuries.)

Perilunate Dislocation of the Carpus
    In this condition the lunate stays in place (*Fig.* 5.15) and the remaining carpal bones (with the hand) dislocate dorsally, giving a 'desert fork' deformity (smaller and lower than the Colles fracture). This fracture reduces with pressure over the dorsum of the wrist. *Note:* so far as the relationship between the lunate and the remaining carpus is concerned there is no relative difference between this injury and a lunate dislocation. Indeed reduction might convert one injury

114   An outline of fractures and dislocations

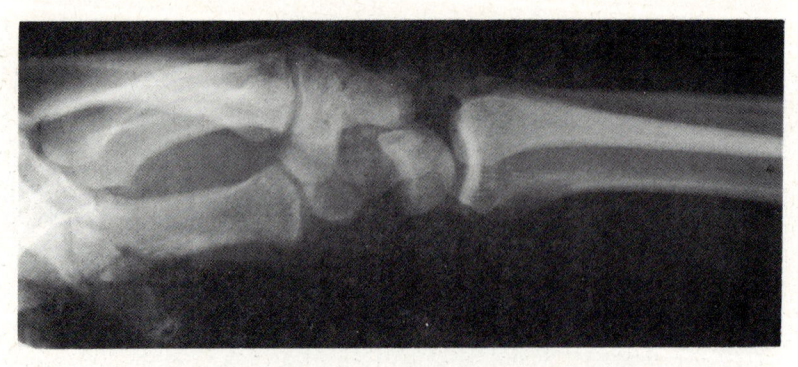

Fig. 5.15. Perilunate dislocation of the carpus.

into the other, thus immediate check X-rays are required before the plaster is applied for 6 weeks. (*See* Lunate dislocation.)

- **Other Wrist Injuries**
1. *Scaphoid subluxation (rotatory)*. This may occur after an incomplete carpal dislocation, or independently in people who use their wrists in a rotatory manner, e.g. joiners. There is pain over the scaphoid, a click on extension of the wrist and a weak grip. X-ray shows a gap over 2 mm between scaphoid and lunate on the anteroposterior view, while there is malalignment of the lunate, capitate and scaphoid on the lateral film. This is a condition which is *frequently missed*, being considered clinically as a scaphoid fracture initially and then dismissed after two negative X-rays for fracture. Since the small ligaments are difficult to repair the reduced carpus is held by two Kirschner wires passed through the scaphoid, one into the lunate and the other in the capitate. The plaster and wires are removed at 6 weeks.
2. *Dorsal carpal dislocation* around the lunate and scaphoid (reduction as for 'perilunate dislocations').
3. *Dislocation of the lunate and scaphoid* anteriorly (reduction as for 'lunate dislocation').
4. *Dislocation of the metacarpals*—may be an anterior dislocation and the carpus is displaced dorsally. The ulnar nerve is commonly damaged. Pressure over the base of the displaced carpal bones with the wrist dorsiflexed reduces this injury. The wrist is held in palmar flexion for 4–6 weeks.

With the *dorsal* dislocation (*Fig.* 5.16a) the reverse manoeuvre is applied. This injury is more common in motorcyclists who grip the handlebars during impact. If the dislocation is unstable wire fixation (using a small external fixation device) may be required.

5. *Subluxation of the capitate-hamate* leads to malrotation of the second and third fingers and a finger fracture is often suspected. Surgery is required to decompress the ulnar nerve while the torn transverse ligament is repaired or stabilized with a wire. A plaster is used for 4 weeks.

115　Fractures of the forearm, wrist and hand

a

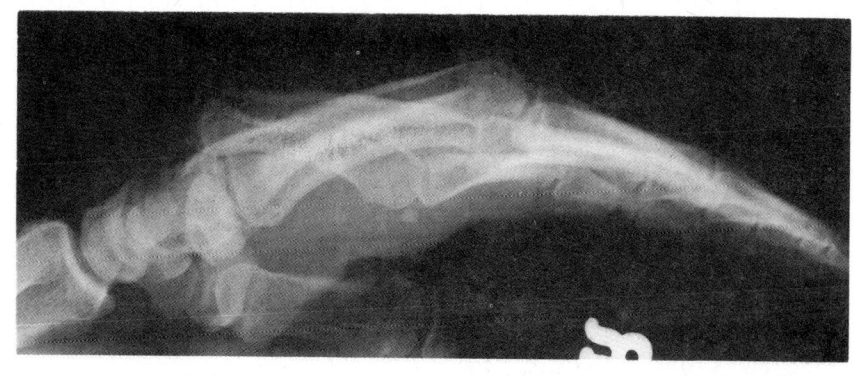

b

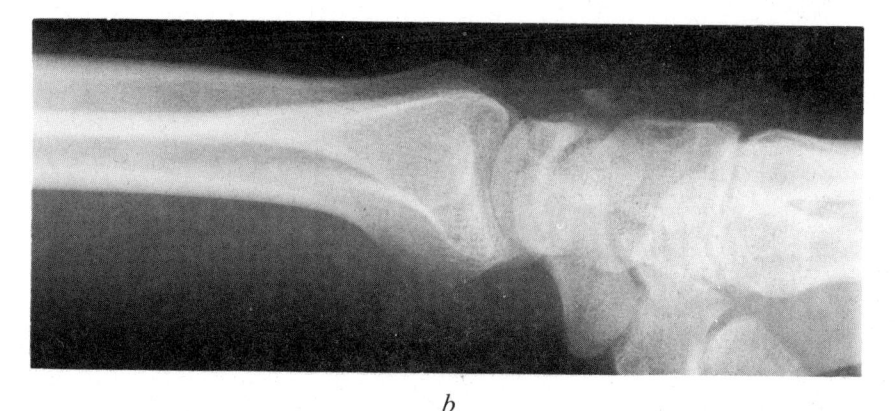

Fig. 5.16. *a*, Dorsal metacarpal dislocation. *b*, Flake fracture of the triquetrum.

6.　*Fractures of the capitate, flake fracture of triquetrum (Fig.* 5.16*b*), *pisiform and hook of hamate* are usually due to direct trauma and require a plaster for 3–4 weeks. If troublesome, tender un-united fragments can be excised.

- **Fractures of the Metacarpals and Phalanges**
  - *There is great versatility in the hand from precision pinch to power grip and thus fractures in this area demand careful attention.*

    There are *five longitudinal* arches—carpals, metacarpals and fingers (or thumb) and *two transverse* (the rigid base of the metacarpals and the distal carpal bones being one; while the second is the heads of the metacarpals and their transverse ligaments).
  - *These arches must be maintained during plaster immobilization.*
  - *Each metacarpophalangeal joint is made so that during flexion the fingers do not overlap.* This arrangement does not allow for angulation or rotation of metacarpal or phalangeal fractures (*see Fig.* 5.20*b*).

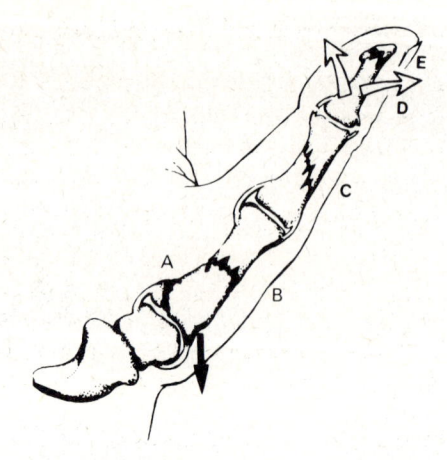

Fig. 5.17. Fracture of the thumb. A, Bennett's, B, Transverse mid-shaft, C, Oblique proximal phalanx, D, Dislocation (often with avulsion of a flake of bone), E, Fracture of the terminal phalanx.

- *The metacarpophalangeal joint of the thumb must be stable for pinch grip and thus has the functions of an interphalangeal joint of the finger (indeed the first metacarpal ossifies like the proximal phalanx).* Loss of thumb function is equivalent to loss of half the hand.

Fractures of the Thumb Metacarpal
Fractures of the first metacarpal may be *stable* or *unstable* (*Fig.* 5.17)
Stable   Transverse/shaft (Boxer's thumb)
         Greenstick
Unstable Oblique/shaft
         Comminuted
         Base/Oblique (Bennett's fracture)

Stable fractures are maintained in plaster for 3–4 weeks with the thumb abducted and in the apposed position. The terminal joint is free from plaster which extends to the upper forearm.

Unstable fractures often require internal fixation with screws or wires after reduction (a small external fixation device can be used) (*see* Bennett's fracture).

Fracture-dislocation of the Carpometacarpal Joint of the Thumb (Bennett's Fracture)
This is an oblique fracture through the base of the first metacarpal with dislocation of the radial part of the thumb (*Fig.* 5.17A).

Diagnosis
Painful movements of the thumb with palpable angulation.

Treatment
An attempt can be made to realign the fragments by extension/abduction at the carpometacarpal joint and, if successful, a plaster applied for 4 weeks. Check

X-rays are taken after 1 week if internal fixation is not used since the fracture may displace.

Generally, closed reduction gives imperfect results.

The thumb is abducted to realign the shaft to the small medial fragment and fixed under image-intensifier X-ray control with a wire (through the large fragment and into the trapezium) or a small screw across both fragments. A plaster is worn for 3–4 weeks.

Complications
1. The fracture is immobilized in an unreduced state; or *slips* because the wire is placed into the tiny medial fragment; or the thumb is incorrectly immobilized (with flexion/adduction at the carpometacarpal joint).
2. *Osteoarthrosis* This may lead to arthrodesis, arthroplasty or excision of the trapezium.
3. *Angulation, rotation* and *shortening* may require osteotomy.

Other Metacarpal Fractures (2–5)

These occur through: the base, the shaft, the neck (with metacarpal head angulation) (*Fig.* 5.18A,B).

In the great majority the displacement is slight because of the strong soft-tissue connections (interossei muscles and transverse ligaments). A crêpe support with immediate finger movements are encouraged with *undisplaced* fractures; sometimes a dorsal plaster slab is used for 7–10 days.

With *displaced* fractures the angulation, rotation or overlap must be corrected. Many can be reduced by gentle manipulation but the length of the injured metacarpal must be maintained to preserve the palmar arch; if necessary a transverse wire (*Fig.* 5.18c) can be passed across the adjoining metacarpal heads to stabilize the fracture. The wire and plaster are removed after 3 weeks. With neck fractures often the finger is flexed over a rolled bandage in the palm for 7–10 days. Sometimes open reduction and screw fixation are needed.

- **Dislocation of the Thumb**

The carpometacarpal joint may be dislocated in motorcycle accidents (or as part of a Bennett's fracture); however, subluxation is more usual. Dislocation of the thumb phalanges (*see Fig.* 5.17D) (often at the metacarpophalangeal joint) is fairly common and easily reduced. A thumb spica strapping or a moulded plaster can be used for 1–2 weeks, the latter being preferred with frank carpometacarpal dislocations.

Abduction of the thumb during a fall at skiing or during soccer can cause a sprain of disruption of the *ulnar collateral ligament* usually at the metacarpal head origin (gamekeeper's thumb). With a sprain a plaster is applied with the metacarpophalangeal joint slightly flexed to relax the collateral ligaments. This is worn for 2–3 weeks. An arthogram may show complete rupture and the ligaments are repaired with plaster for 3 weeks.

118 An outline of fractures and dislocations

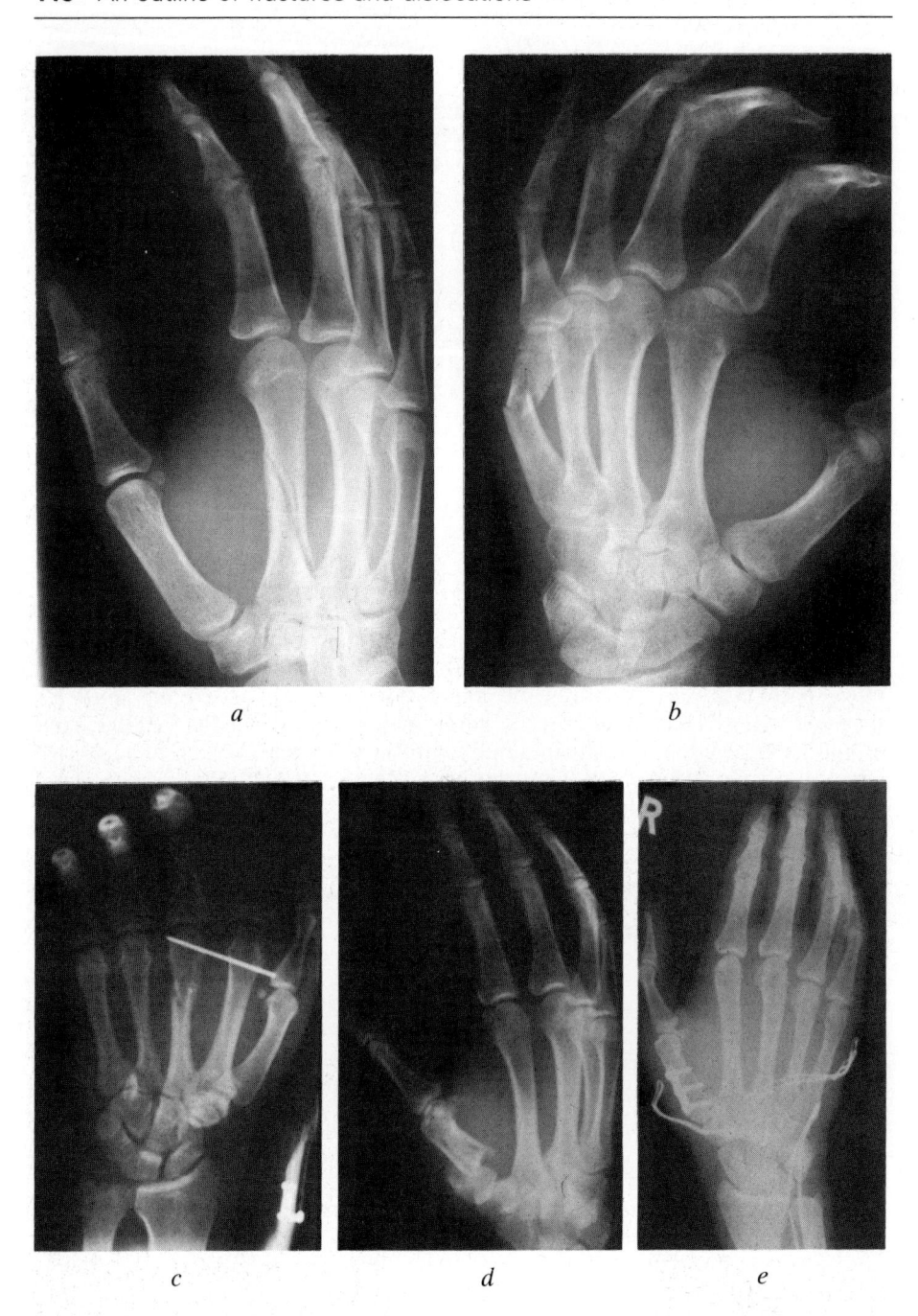

Fig. 5.18. *a*, Spiral fracture 2nd metacarpal. *b*, Fractured neck of 5th metacarpal. *c*, Metacarpal transverse arch maintained with a transverse wire. *d*, Displaced 1st metacarpal fracture. *e*, Held by a small plate and screws.

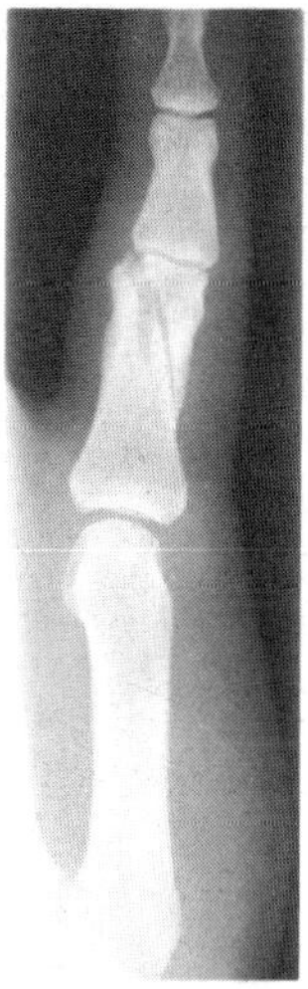

119 Fractures of the forearm, wrist and hand

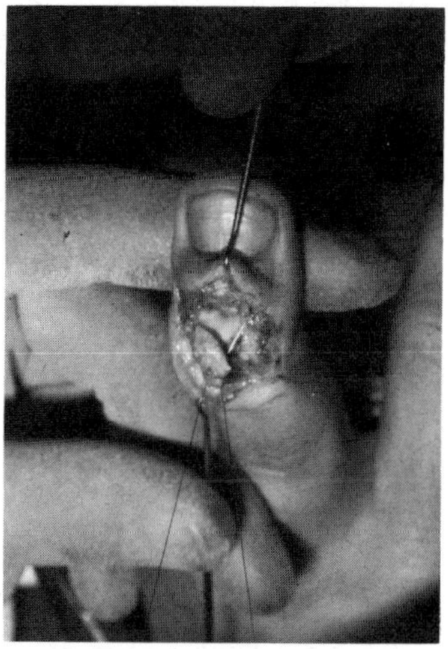

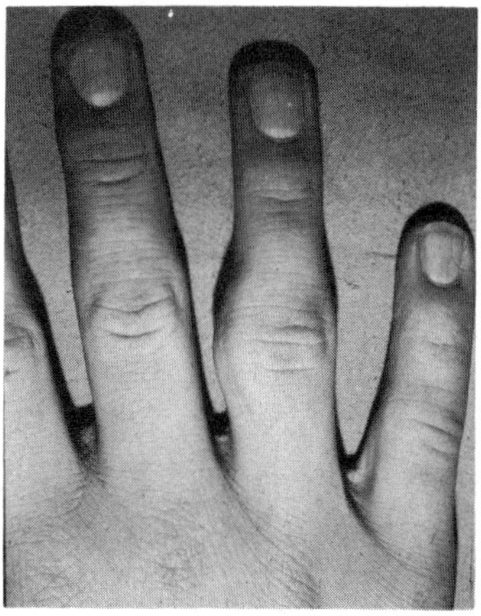

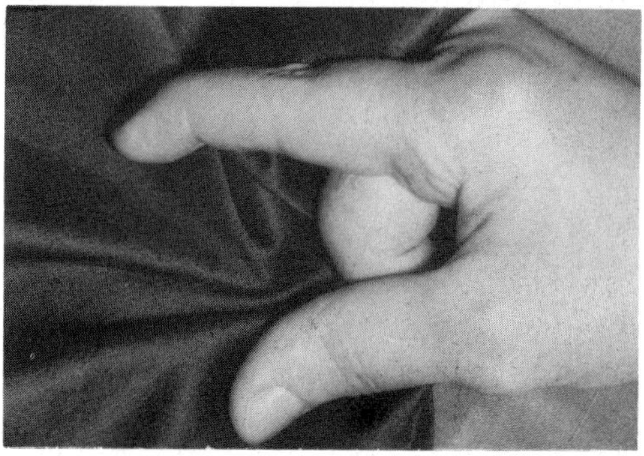

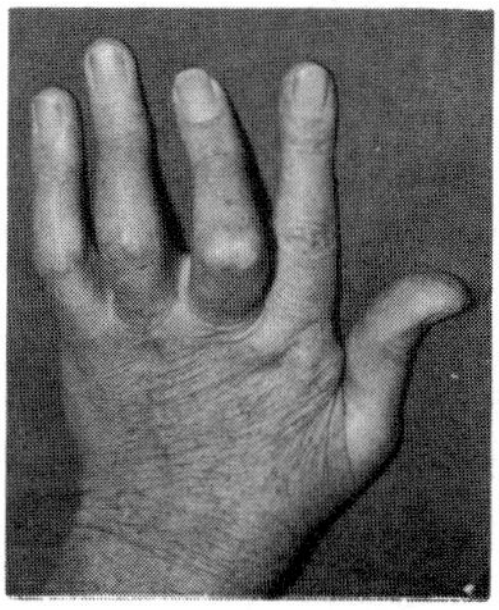

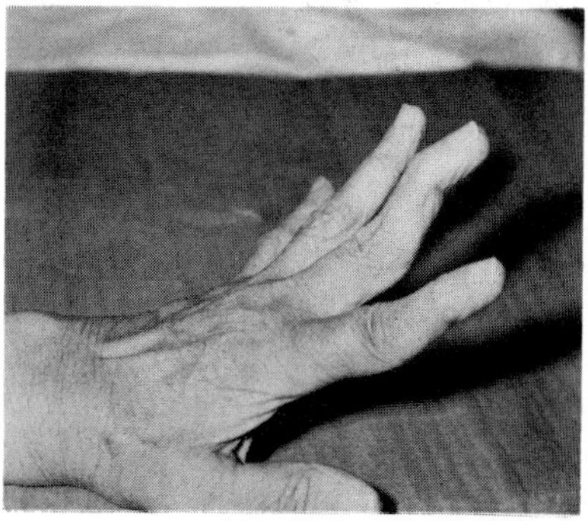

Fig. 5.19. *a*, Fractured proximal phalanx. *b*, Avulsion injury terminal phalanx. *c*, Previous haemarthrosis proximal interphalangeal joint and chronic thickening. *d*, Mallet finger. *e*, Boutonnière deformity. *f*, Swan-neck deformity.

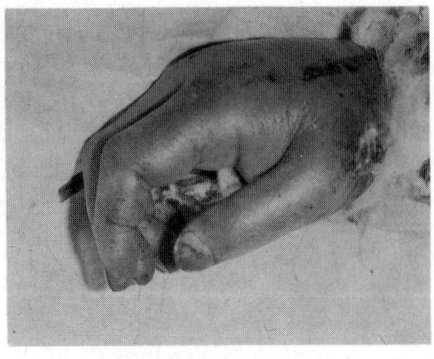

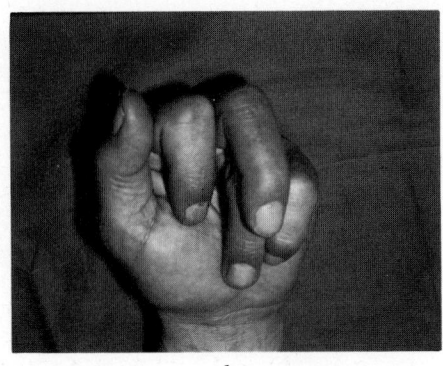

Fig. 5.20. Two common complications of hand injuries: *a*, Gross oedema. *b*, Malrotation of the fingers.

- **Fractures and Dislocations of the Phalanges**

Fractures of the phalanges may be *undisplaced* or *displaced* (*Fig.* 5.19). An intra-articular fracture may cause marked stiffness (only a few millilitres of blood fill these joints!) and all finger injuries demand mobilization as quickly as possible. A simple method is to bind the injured finger to the adjacent normal one, often with a finger garter or strapping. With comminuted terminal fractures the nail bed may be avulsed but can be retained as a natural splint if only torn.

Unstable fractures (usually oblique) can be fixed with small compression screws or wires, the fracture can be reduced by an external compression clamp and the wires passed percutaneously.

Dislocations are easily reduced under local anaesthesia and should be immobilized for 10–14 days by strapping to adjacent fingers.

Special Associated Tendon Injuries are:
1. *Avulsion of the extensor tendon* (*Fig.* 5.19b) from the dorsum of the terminal phalanx (mallet finger or baseball finger). This is treated by a mallet splint which hyperextends the tip of the finger. Late cases can be treated by leaving well alone, if symptom-free; by tightening and repair of the extensor tendon; or by arthrodesis of the terminal interphalangeal joint.
2. *Avulsion of fragment* from *middle* phalanx or *proximal* phalanx by flexor profundus or sublimis tendons respectively.
3. *Boutonnière deformity* (*Fig.* 5.19e) is due to a rupture of the central slip of the extensor tendon over the middle phalanx. The lateral slips pass to the volar axis of the proximal interphalangeal joint and hyperextension of the distal interphalangeal joint occurs with flexion of the middle joint.
4. *Pseudo-Boutonnière deformity*. A hyperextension injury to the proximal interphalangeal joint disrupts the volar capsule and plate and the joint subluxes inferiorly leading eventually to a fixed flexion contracture of the proximal interphalangeal joint.

5. *Swan-neck deformity* (*Fig.* 5.19*f*). (This is the reverse of 3), the hyperextension of the proximal interphalangeal joint damaging the volar capsule and plate (or fracturing the middle phalanx) and the flexor profundus pulls the distal phalanx into flexion.

Lateral instability of the proximal interphalangeal joint usually results from a radial collateral ligament tear after a lateral dislocation.

The treatment of these injuries usually requires surgical intervention and repair by a surgeon specializing in hand injuries.

- *After all upper limb injuries, and especially injuries of the hand, oedema (Fig. 5.20) is controlled by limb elevation for at least 24 hours. Joint stiffness (especially in the fingers) needs intensive but graduated physiotherapy—once these joints become stiff then recovery is greatly delayed.*

It is also worth emphasizing that in an injured limb mobilization of all uninjured areas is imperative.

6

Spinal injuries

Spinal injuries are commonly found in road traffic accidents and approximately 30% develop neurological changes.
- **With head and facial injuries always examine the cervical spine.**

- **Fractures and Dislocations of the Cervical Spine**

The cervical spine has developed extreme flexibility at the expense of stability in order to facilitate the special senses located in the head. Stability especially depends upon the ligamentous supports and articulations. Severe injuries that displace the vertebral bodies usually involve the disc.

The atlanto-occipital joint allows side to side motion but there is little flexion/extension and no rotation. At the atlanto-axial joint there is 45° of rotation but minimal flexion and extension. From C2 to C7 there is flexion and extension of approximately 9° at each level.

- *Fractures are either* **stable** *or* **unstable.** *In* **unstable** *fractures the cord may have been damaged or, if it has escaped, it may be subsequently injured. Thus it is important to reach a firm diagnosis regarding stability. If the posterior ligaments are intact the spine is* **stable.** *If they are torn, it is* **unstable.** Flexion and extension films and tomography are required in all suspected cases of spinal instability, even after a simple 'whiplash' injury, should symptoms be severe or fail to remit.

Fractures and Dislocations of the Atlas and Axis (Upper Cervical Spine)

Dislocations of the *occiput* on the *axis* are extremely uncommon and usually fatal.

Severe trauma causing hyperflexion produces a forward shift of the *atlas on the axis* with rupture of the transverse ligament (*Fig.* 6.1*a*). (This condition can be found in patients with rheumatoid arthritis involving the C1–2 articulation. Radiologically there may also be a congenitally absent odontoid process or abnormalities of the C1–2 articulation.)

A fracture of the arch of the atlas (*Fig.* 6.1*b,c*) is usually due to a heavy object falling on to the top of the head with the spine straight or a diving accident. The condyles of the occiput split the ring and spread the lateral masses. Generally no neurological deficit results because the spinal canal is widened.

The odontoid process (C2) (*Fig.* 6.1*d,e*) can be fractured (often with a mandibular injury). Occasionally it is displaced either anteriorly or posteriorly, with neurological problems.

A fracture of the neural arch of C2 (*Fig.* 6.1*f*) (Hangman's fracture) is due to a hypertension force producing a wide separation of the fragments and anterior displacement of the body of C2. Once again the neurological deficit may not be severe because of the large capacity of the spinal canal at this level. However, it may be associated with a cervical fracture-dislocation at a lower level.

Diagnosis
Fractures and fracture-dislocations of the upper cervical spine may be relatively painless but there will be associated muscle spasm and in severe cases nerve damage. It is important to have adequate X-rays, including an open mouth view, tomography and computerized tomography (CT scan).

Treatment
Undisplaced fractures require a firm collar for 6–12 weeks.

If there is any degree of *displacement* reduction can be achieved by gentle manipulation or skull traction. However, prolonged traction, especially in the case of an odontoid fracture, can lead to non-union. A halo-cast (*Fig.* 6.2) can be applied or a Minerva plaster. If there is instability in the upper cervical spine it is important to carry out fusion between C1 and C2 (or C2 and C3) depending on the fracture level. A bone graft and (often) wire fixation are used in combination linking the spinous processes or laminae. The patient rests in bed with a collar or brace for 2–4 weeks. Then a firm supportive collar is used until fusion is evident, usually at 12–16 weeks.

Unilateral or Bilateral Dislocation of a Cervical Vertebra (C3–C7)

Unilateral dislocation (*Fig.* 6.3*a*) is usually produced by a lateral and rotatory force with rupture of the interspinous ligament and joint capsule on that side. As a rule the cord is not involved, but in 30% of cases there may be impingement on a nerve root. A lateral X-ray of these injuries characteristically shows *anterior displacement of approximately 25%* of the width of the vertebral body.

Bilateral dislocation (*Fig.* 6.3*b*) is quite rare without a fracture. There is severe disruption of all posterior structures and also the posterior longitudinal ligament and disc. The displacement is approximately 50% on the adjoining vertebral body and usually the cord is severely damaged. Reduction can be achieved under X-ray control by gentle traction through skull *tongs* (*Fig.* 6.4). Approximately 15 lb (6·8 kg) of traction is applied with increments of 5 lb (2·3 kg) every 15 min, up to 35 lb (15·9 kg).

A constant check is made for any neurological changes. Once disengagement has occurred, traction is reduced to a minimum load of 15–20 lb (6·8–9·1 kg).

• *It is important to avoid over-distraction of dislocations in the cervical spine, especially bilateral dislocations, because cord damage is a sequel.*

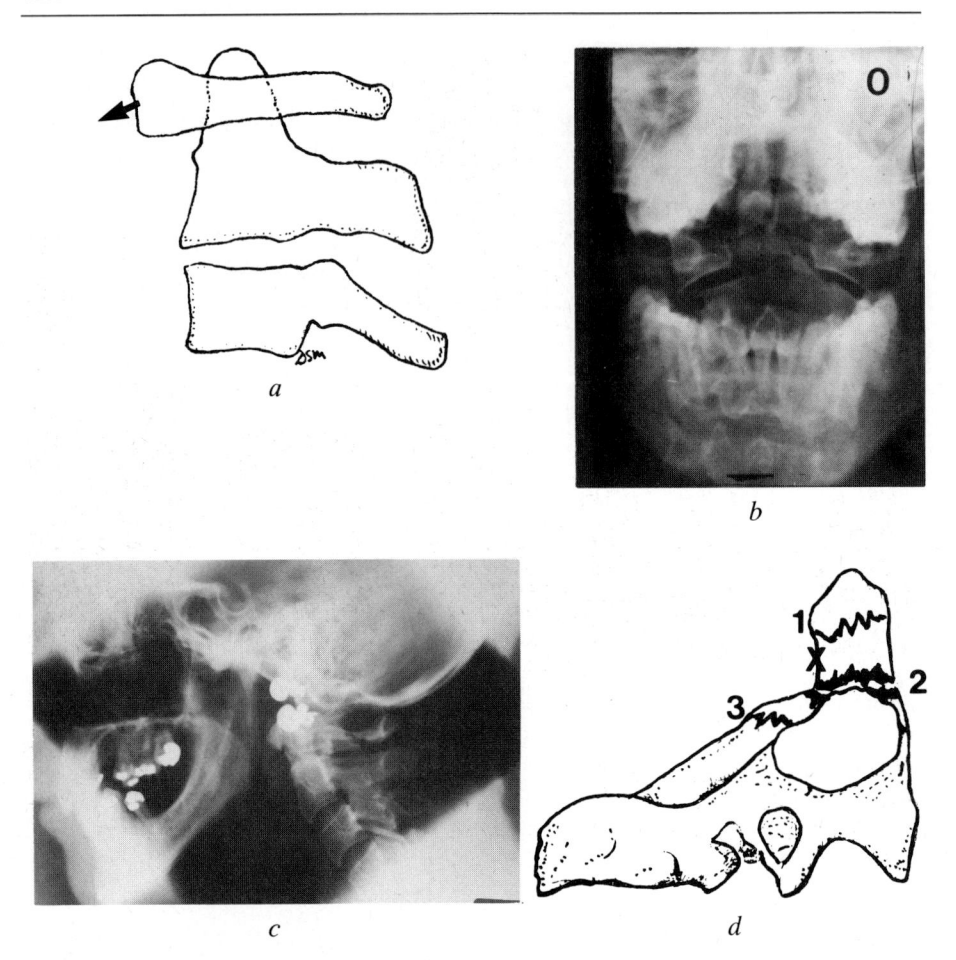

Treatment
After reduction patients with a stable *unilateral* dislocation can be given a firm cervical collar for 6–12 weeks.

Patients with a *bilateral* dislocation will require surgery, as will patients with an irreducible or unstable unilateral dislocation. After reduction spinal fusion is carried out involving one vertebra below and usually one above the involved level. Postoperatively, skull traction is maintained for 3 weeks until the soft tissues have healed, with a weight of 8–10 lb (3·6–4·5 kg). A collar or brace is employed for a further 12–24 months.

Fractures and Fracture-dislocations of the C3–C7 Vertebrae

Simple Compression Fractures
These are stable fractures due to vertical loading in the neck with slight flexion. There is usually compression of C5. Although the discs may be damaged the ligamentous structures are intact and generally no neurological damage occurs because the posterior part of the vertebral body remains intact.

125 Spinal injuries

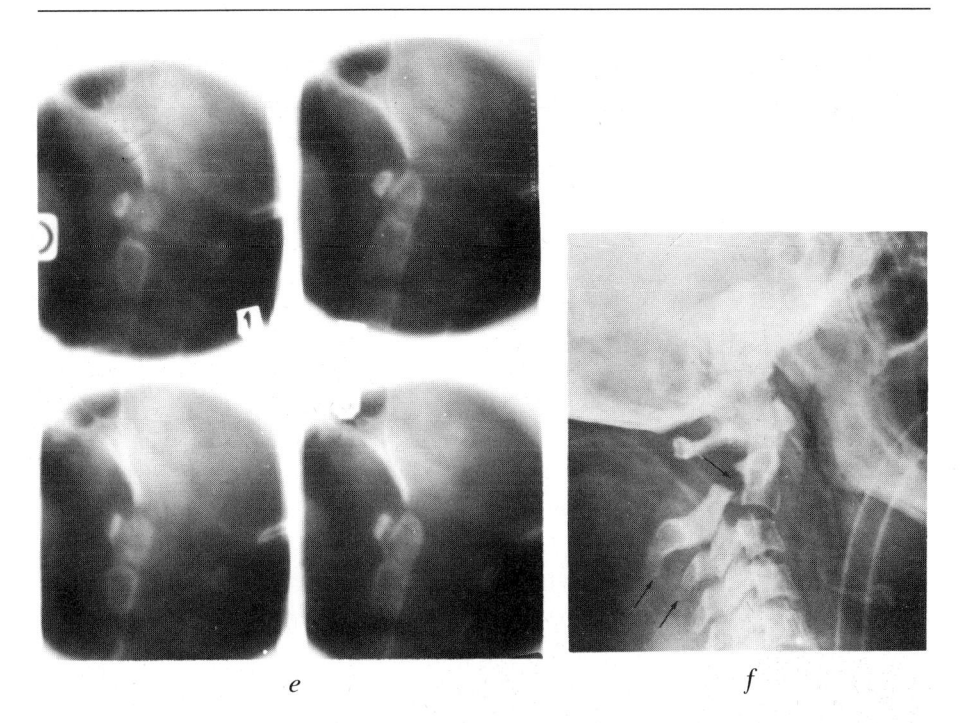

Fig. 6.1. Injuries to the upper cervical spine (C1 and C2). *a*, Atlanto-axial subluxation. *b*, Fractured arch of atlas (C1) in an open mouth view. *c*, Atlas arch fracture extending towards spinous process. *d*, Common C2 (axis) fractures 1=tip, and 2=base of odontoid, 3=arch. *e*, An odontoid fracture outlined on a tomogram. *f*, Hangman's fracture.

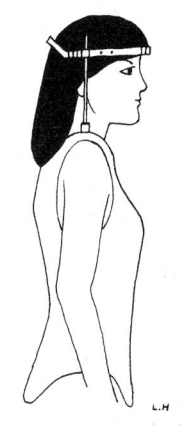

Fig. 6.2. A halo-cast.

126 An outline of fractures and dislocations

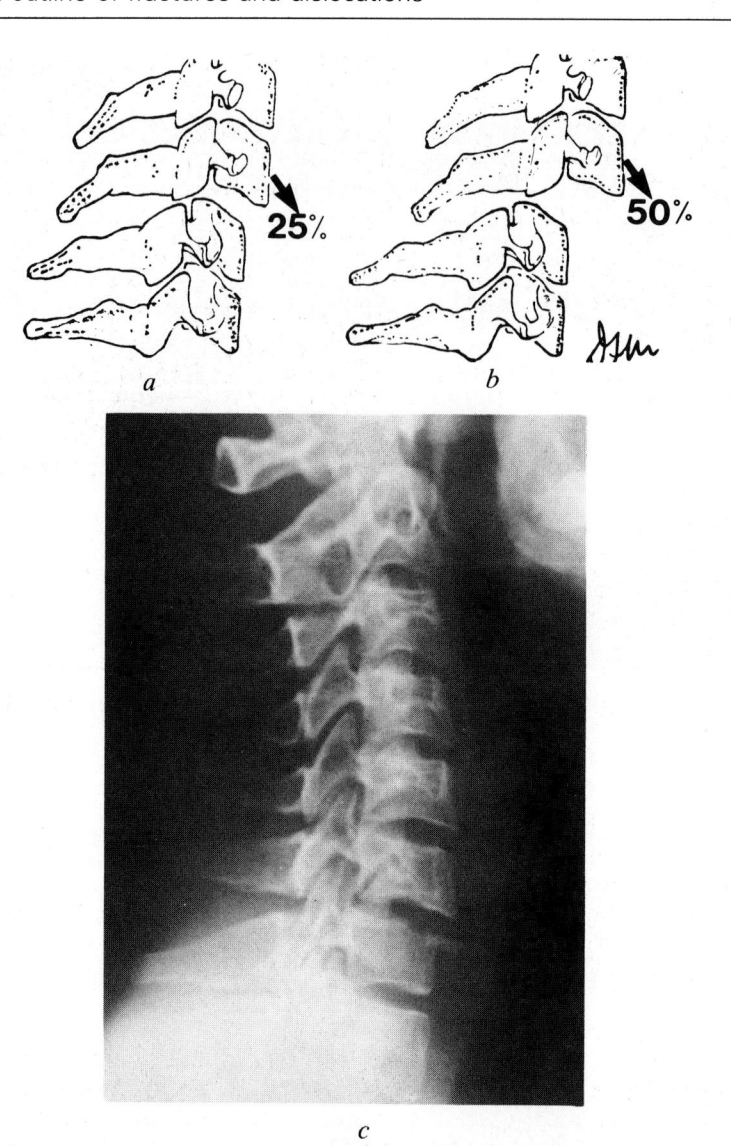

Fig. 6.3. *a*, Unilateral dislocation in the cervical spine (less than 25% shift on the lateral film). *b*, Bilateral dislocation. *c*, Unilateral posterior joint dislocation with flake fracture.

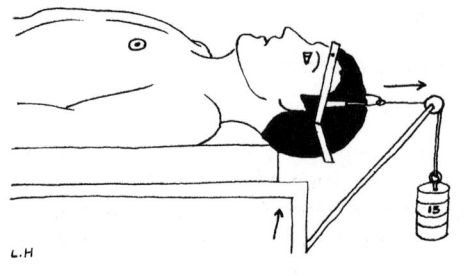

Fig. 6.4. Traction to the cervical spine through skull tongs.

127 Spinal injuries

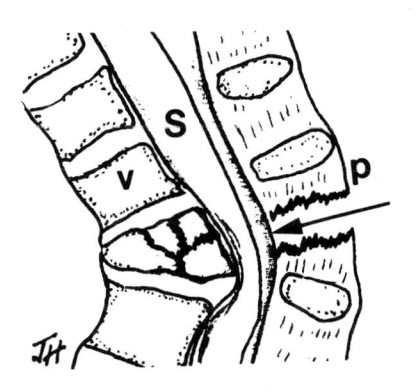

Fig. 6.5. Marked hyperflexion leading to unstable fracture due to posterior ligament tearing (p) (V, vertebral body; S, spinal cord).

Fig. 6.6. Burst fracture C5 (unstable).

Diagnosis
There is a history of a blow to the head in slight flexion with immediate neck pain and spasm. X-rays reveal the wedge-shaped fracture.

Treatment
A collar is worn for 3–4 months.

Fracture of the Spinous Process
This often occurs at C7 (clay-shoveller's fracture) and is stable. A collar is required for 3–6 weeks. Other associated more serious injuries must be excluded, such as fracture-dislocation of C7 on T1.

Fracture-dislocation of the Cervical Spine (C3–C7)
There is marked hyperflexion in a fracture-dislocation (*Fig.* 6.5) and neurological complications may vary from transient paralysis to complete quadriplegia. The associated fractures are crushing of one or more vertebral bodies, fracture of the pedicles, articular processes and often one or more spinous processes and laminae. Such injuries commonly occur between C4 and C6.

Diagnosis
There is severe pain, usually with neurological changes.

Treatment
Traction is applied by tongs (Crutchfield's). Later, when the condition of the patient permits, spinal fusion is carried out once reduction has become complete. A bone graft with wiring of the spinous process, or an anterior plating of the vertebral bodies, can be used. A collar is worn for 6–12 months.

Laminectomy results in a high mortality rate and loss of motor function—any decompression should be via an anterior route.

Burst Fractures of the Cervical Vertebrae (teardrop fracture)
This is commonly due to a fall on to the head with slight hyperflexion and marked comminution occurring in the vertebral body (*Fig.* 6.6), often with a fracture of the associated lamina.

Diagnosis
As above for fracture-dislocation.

Treatment
Anterior decompression and a fusion can be carried out (as above); or halo-pelvic traction can be used for 3–4 months, usually after 4–6 weeks of bed traction using skull tongs to maintain alignment.

Hyperextension Injury with Anterior Chip Fracture
A force in hyperextension can rupture the anterior longitudinal ligament with avulsion of bone from the anterior superior margin of the body. The disc is usually torn and the cervical cord damaged.

Diagnosis
As above.

Treatment
If there is no neurological change a halo-cast is used. With paralysis anterior decompression and fusion are carried out (as above).

Fracture-dislocation produced by Hyperextension and Compression
These injuries produce severe disruption of the posterior bony element. The anterior longitudinal ligament ruptures, avulsing a chip from the anterior margins of the lower vertebra (as above), while the lamina (and spinous process below) are fractured, with a fracture-dislocation of the articular process.

Treatment
The spine is reduced into normal alignment with skull traction. Later a spinal fusion may be carried out using bone graft and internal fixation device (*Fig.* 6.7a-c). Traction is maintained for 4–6 weeks, and a firm cervical collar for 12–24 months.

Complications
All cervical fractures may suffer from the following complications:
1. *Disc involvement.* Herniation or rupture of the disc can cause impingement on the dura. Pain radiates to the neck and over the trapezius region. Occasionally it passes to the occipital and intrascapular areas. In severe cases it radiates down the arms. Such problems are treated by traction, physiotherapy and cervical support.

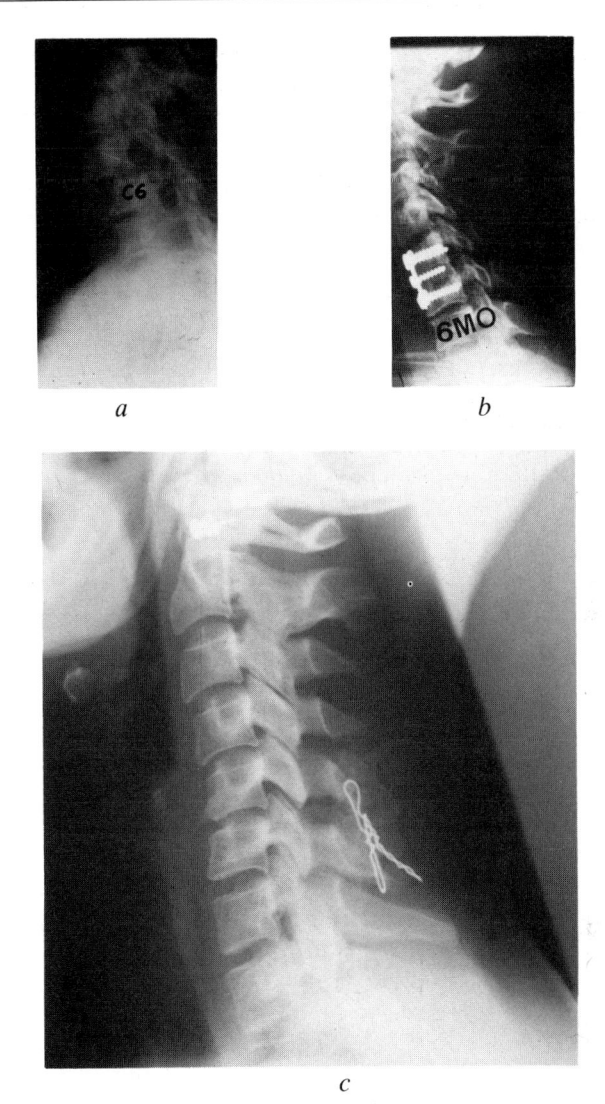

Fig. 6.7. a, Unstable dislocation C5/C6. *b*, Treated by anterior fixation (result at 6 months). *c*, The more commonly used posterior spinal fusion with a bone graft and wire (also a C5/C6 dislocation in a young nurse) at 6 months.

2. *Osteoarthrosis of the facet joints.* This can occur directly from injury or later through malalignment of the cervical vertebrae. Treatment is as for cervical disc.
3. *Nerve root involvement.* This may consist of partial or complete severance of the nerve root or several roots. When the *5th and 6th* roots are involved there is a decrease or absence of the biceps reflex with diminished muscle power in the arm and shoulder, especially in the biceps. There is paraesthesia in the thumb. With the *7th* nerve root

involvement the triceps power and reflex are diminished and the paraesthesia extends to the index and middle finger. With *8th* nerve root involvement there is paraesthesia on the ulnar aspect of the hand and little finger with diminished muscle power in all fingers. There are no reflex changes. During the phase of nerve recovery passive and active exercises are carried out. Appropriate splintage (wrist or elbow supports or a lively splint for fingers) is used to encourage rehabilitation.

4. *Cord damage.* Quadriplegia is paralysis in all four limbs. With *cord concussion* recovery begins within 8–24 hours, motor power, sensation and visceral recovery occurring simultaneously. With *cord transection* the neurones below the damaged area begin to show independent activity after 24 hours or more; the plantar response becomes extensor and reflexes return and muscles become increasingly spastic—showing clonus and increased reflex responses. The use of steroids may not enhance recovery.

During the initial phases of skull traction the patient is turned approximately every 2 hours. A turning frame may be used. Intermittent positive-pressure respiration, gastric intubation, indwelling urethral catheterization and a bowel control programme should be instituted. Light padded splints can be used to hold the limbs in a functional position.

The level of the nerve root involvement makes a significant difference to later muscle control and function. Involvement from C5 down leaves only neck muscle control. Thus the patient will have to use an electrically-powered wheelchair and externally powered hand splints for limited self-care. With involvement from C6 level down the patient will have control of his shoulder muscles and elbow flexors, thus permitting self-transfer with an overhead sling and the use of a propelled wheelchair. With involvement from C7 down the patient will have wrist extension and supination, thus permitting more independence for transfer, self-care and driving a car with hand controls. With involvement of C8 downwards the patient is handicapped by weak hand grip and some loss of elbow extension but is more able to look after himself.

5. Injuries at C1/C2 may be associated with intermittent symptoms of motor paralysis or *drop attacks*, due either to impingement of the cord or, more likely, to alteration in blood flow in the vertebral arteries.

6. Chronic instability. With non-operative measures 42% of cervical fracture-dislocations may develop instability and require fusion.
N.B. Pseudarthrosis and displacement of an anterior graft are uncommon but require re-fusion.

- *Remember head injuries and cervical spine injuries regularly coexist.*

- **Fractures and Fracture-dislocation in the Thoracic Spine**

The thoracic spine is very stable. Fractures of the thoracic vertebral bodies (*Fig.* 6.8) and transverse process, articular facets and laminae are quite rare, apart from penetrating injuries and osteoporotic collapse in the elderly.

Spinal injuries

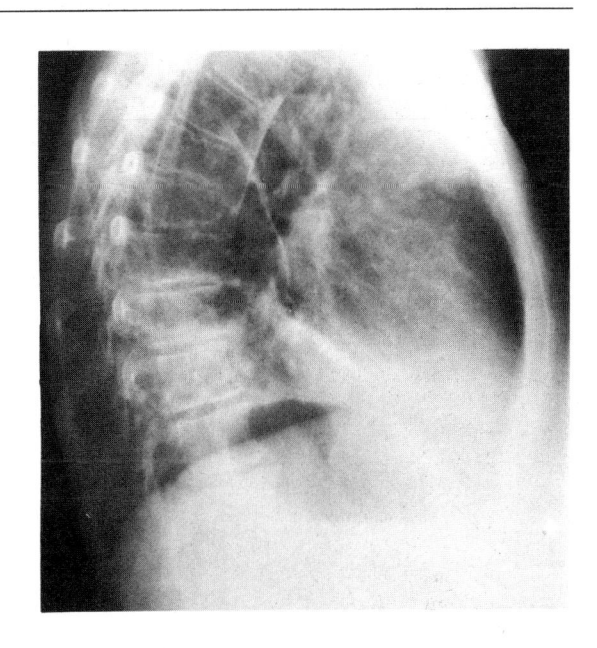

Fig. 6.8. Commonly seen compression fractures in the thoracic spine in the elderly with osteoporosis.

However, the abrupt transition from the thoracic kyphosis to the lumbar lordosis does lead to fracture-dislocations at the T12 to L2 level. These injuries will be considered with lumbar fracture-dislocations. It is important to remember that the cord ends at L1 and with slight variations the nerve roots generally occupy the canal below this level.

• Fractures and Fracture-dislocations of the Lumbar Vertebrae

Compression Fracture of the Lumbar Vertebrae
This is usually due to a vertically transmitted force with the spine in the neutral position or slight flexion.
It is common in patients with osteoporosis. There is collapse of the vertebral body (*Figs.* 6.9, 6.10). There are no neurological changes in most instances and the patient is treated with 1–2 weeks of bed rest and a well-fitting spinal support for 3–4 months.

Burst Fracture of the Lumbar Vertebrae
Here the vertical compression is more severe and the vertebral body shatters (*Fig.* 6.9) with the disc material displaced into the body. The displacement of the vertebral body can cause cord and nerve root damage.

Diagnosis
Discomfort localized to affected level with occasional nerve involvement.

132 An outline of fractures and dislocations

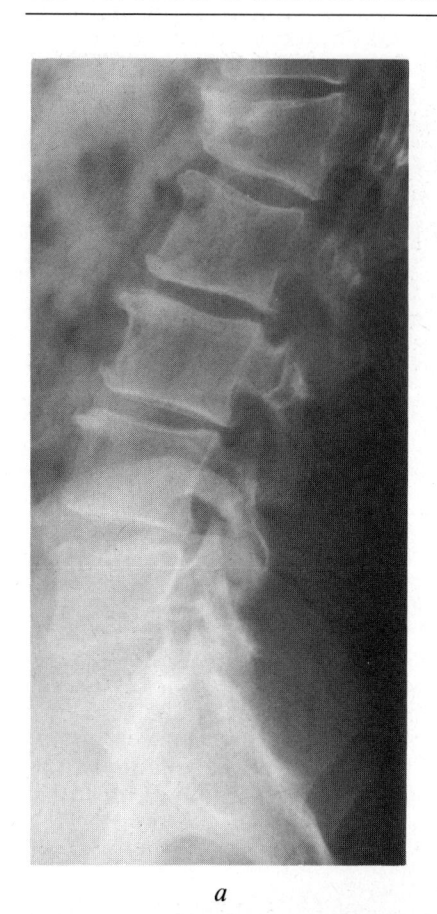

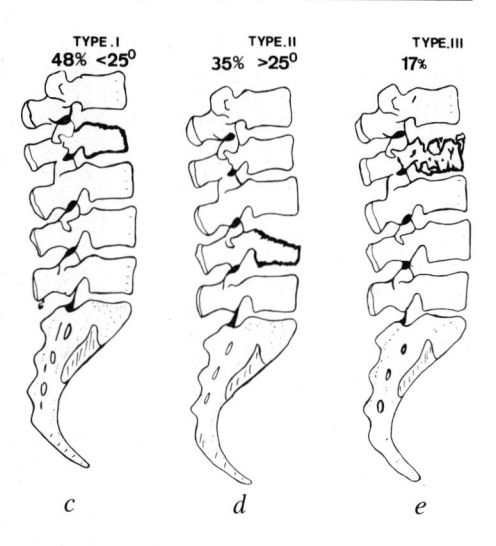

Fig. 6.9. *a*, Stable, lumbar compression fracture of L1. Three types identified are (*b*) Type I and (*c*) Type II (which are stable and differ according to the lateral angulation either below or above 25°; and (*d*) Type III which is often unstable due to comminution.

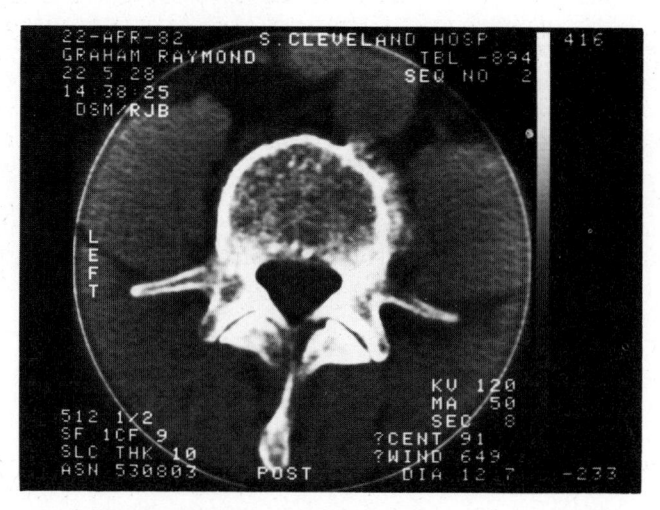

Fig. 6.10. A CT scan showing irregularity of the body of L2 following a fracture 9 months previously but no spinal stenosis.

133 Spinal injuries

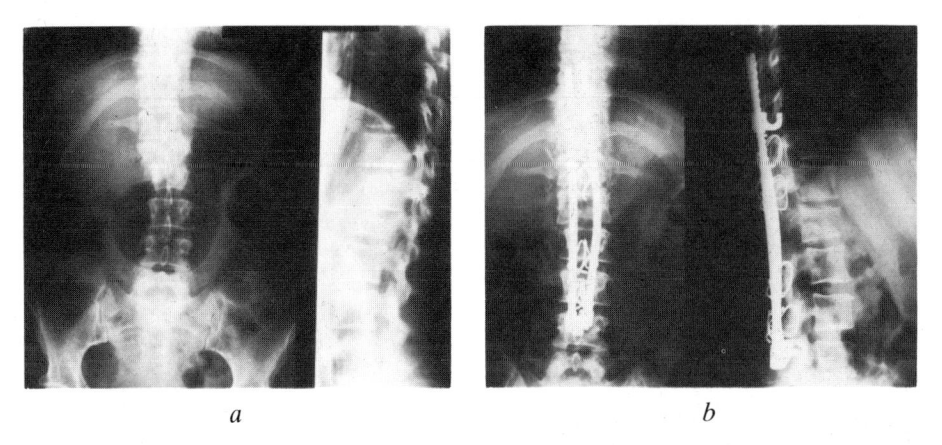

Fig. 6.11. *a*, A flexion/rotation fracture in the lumbar spine. *b*, Treated by Harrington rods and intersegmental wiring.

Treatment
Usually such fractures are stable (*see above*) but in the presence of marked (or progressive) neurological involvement it is advantageous to have a myelogram and bone scan (CT) and to consider decompression and internal fixation with plates (attached to the spinous processes) or spinal (Harrington) rods (between laminae) to effect distraction and stability.

- **Fracture-dislocation of the Lumbar Vertebrae**

    This is usually due to a flexion/rotation mechanism (*Fig.* 6.11) as when the passenger is thrown around in a motor vehicle or in the past when a miner was struck on the back while kneeling. There is a slice fracture of the superior aspect of the vertebral body and a horizontal displacement of the entire vertebra. This injury commonly occurs at the thoracolumbar junction and produces paraplegia, both from cord and nerve root damage. The articular processes and posterior ligaments are also injured, causing forward displacement of one vertebra on another. Occasionally a hyperextension shear mechanism, such as occurs when a victim is hit from behind by a motor vehicle, causes hyperextension and anterior displacement of the lower lumbar vertebrae, slice fracture of the vertebral body and disruption of the articular process.

Diagnosis
There is severe pain and leg paralysis, sensation is lost below the fracture level.

Treatment
It is often worthwhile treating such unstable injuries with open reduction and internal fixation (*Fig.* 6.11) (but not laminectomy which adds to the instability).

After rod or plate fixation the patient is mobilized at 2–3 weeks in a cast for 20 weeks, unless nerve damage dictates otherwise.

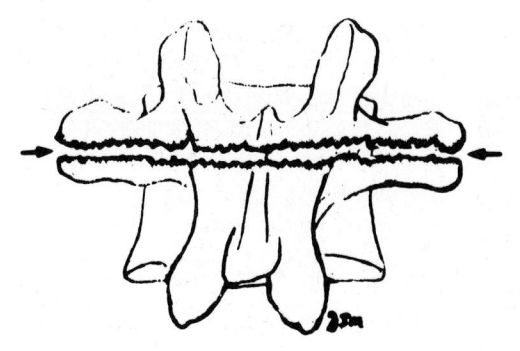

Fig. 6.12. Chance (seat-belt) fracture.

Some centres simply use conservative measures, believing that surgery adds to the spinal trauma. A special spinal bed with a turning frame is required for 2–3 months, depending on the severity of bone, soft tissue and neurological damage. An intensive rehabilitation programme is instituted depending on the level and degree of nerve injury (*see below*).

Seat-belt Fracture (Chance Fracture)
Distraction loading of the lumbar spine produced by the lap seat belt has become a recent addition to thoracolumbar injuries. Hyperflexion over the seat-belt produces spinal distraction and fracture through either the disc or the vertebral bodies (*Fig.* 6.12) and across the remaining supporting structures. It is important to remember that the abdominal viscera may be injured at the same time. If there is only bony injury a plaster cast in extension for 12 weeks is sufficient immobilization. However, if there appears to be instability, fusion with internal fixation using plates, Harrington rods or compression instrumentation may be necessary.

Other Stable Lumbar Fractures
Isolated fractures of the lumbar transverse and spinous processes cause little difficulty, even when displaced (*Fig.* 6.13)
- *It is always important to remember that the kidneys can be damaged. Isolated fractures of the lamina and spinous process may require lumbosacral support for 6–12 weeks.*

Complications
1. *Persistent back discomfort.* After stable crush fractures of the lumbar vertebrae there may be persistent back discomfort in 40% of cases. This is due to either osteoarthrosis at the level of the fracture or later to osteoarthritic changes developing in the lower facet joints of the lumbar spine consequent upon abnormal stresses due to altered spinal mechanics. There may be a localized kyphosis.
2. *Damage to the spinal cord or nerve roots.* It is important always to test completely for any sensory or motor function present below the injury level. *Good prognostic signs* are the preservation of any voluntary movement including toe motion or voluntary anal sphincter contraction.

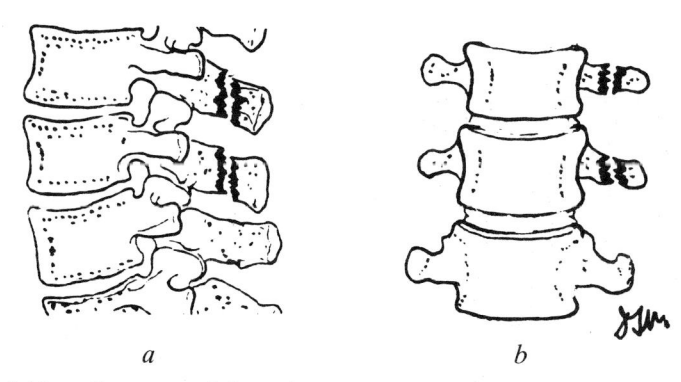

Fig. 6.13. *a*, Fractures of the spinous processes. *b*, Fractures of the transverse processes—in the lumbar region.

The preservation of any perianal sensation is also a good sign. A *poor prognostic* sign is flaccid weakness which lasts more than 24 hours and the return of any superficial reflex. Such reflexes as the bulbocavernosus reflex, anal reflex (when pinching the perineum causes contraction of the rectal sphincter), slow toe flexion and extension reflex (positive Babinski signs) and priapism.

The same post-injury problems regarding bladder, bowel, etc. apply as for cervical injuries. With involvement from *T1–T8* levels the patient will have normal hand muscles permitting independent hygiene and some limited standing with lower limb splints.

With involvement of *T9–T12* trunk stability is achieved which allows some ambulation with the use of bilateral long leg braces.

With involvement of *L1–L5* there is pelvic stability which allows the patient to walk with long leg braces or crutches.

With involvement of *S1–S2* level the patient has knee extension and hip flexion which permits effective ambulation with short leg braces, crutches or sticks.

- **Fracture of the Sacrum**

This uncommon injury is caused by a fall or direct blow to the sacral area. Usually there is an undisplaced crack. Occasionally there is displacement with risk of injury to the cauda equina. Bed rest is prescribed for 2–4 weeks.

- **Fracture of the Coccyx**

This is produced by a fall. There is immediate pain which occasionally can become refractory and requires excision of the coccyx. Both fractures of the sacrum and coccyx can be treated by analgesics and the use of a soft rubber ring for several weeks to allow sitting.

- **Fractures of the Ribs**

Most fractures of the ribs are caused by direct injury. The fracture usually occurs near the angle of the rib and there is seldom displacement. Multiple rib fractures may occur in road traffic accidents and produce a haemothorax or haemopneumothorax.

Clinical Diagnosis
There is localized pain over the fractured ribs, aggravated by deep breathing. Palpation reveals localized tenderness.

Treatment
Most rib fractures unite spontaneously and only simple analgesics are given. For multiple rib fractures long-acting anaesthetics can be injected or the flail segment is controlled by intermittent positive-pressure respiration. Rarely, internal fixation with wires or pins is required.

- **Fractures of the Sternum**

Fractures of the sternum may be caused by a direct blow or from compression of the thoracic cage. The sternal fragment can be displaced posteriorly, producing airway impairment.

Undisplaced fractures need no special treatment other than analgesics.

If there is *displacement* it may have to be reduced by open method and wire or plate fixation.

- *It is important to remember that fractures of the sternum are often associated with thoracic visceral injuries and spinal fracture-dislocations.*

7

Fractures of the pelvis, thigh and knee

- **Fractures of the Pelvis**
    - *30% of all pelvic fractures are complicated by other severe injuries and major blood loss* (since they are caused by high speed accidents) with a mortality rate of 10%. The pelvis, sacrum and sacro-iliac joints form a ring which can be indented or prised apart (*Fig. 7.1*).

    Minor fractures: single pubic ramus
    wing of ilium
    ischium
    avulsion fractures
    Major fractures: ilium (body)
    unilateral or bilateral pubic rami
    bilateral ischial rami
    separation of the symphysis pubis
    subluxation of the sacro-iliac joint
    fracture-dislocation of the hemipelvis
    acetabular fractures

Minor Fractures of the Pelvis

Diagnosis
There is localized pain from a direct blow to the pelvis and the fracture is usually visible on X-rays although a single pubic ramus fracture may be difficult to see in osteoporotic bones.

Treatment
This is symptomatic with bed rest for 2 weeks in the elderly and more rapid mobilization with crutches, if necessary, in the young adult. Avulsion injuries (anterior superior, anterior inferior iliac spine, ischial tuberosity) in teenage athletes usually mean a cessation of sport for 3–4 weeks.

Major Fractures of the Pelvis
Fractures of the body of the *ilium* may be associated with brisk bleeding and thus require a careful assessment of the circulatory volume (e.g. blood pressure and pulse).

138 An outline of fractures and dislocations

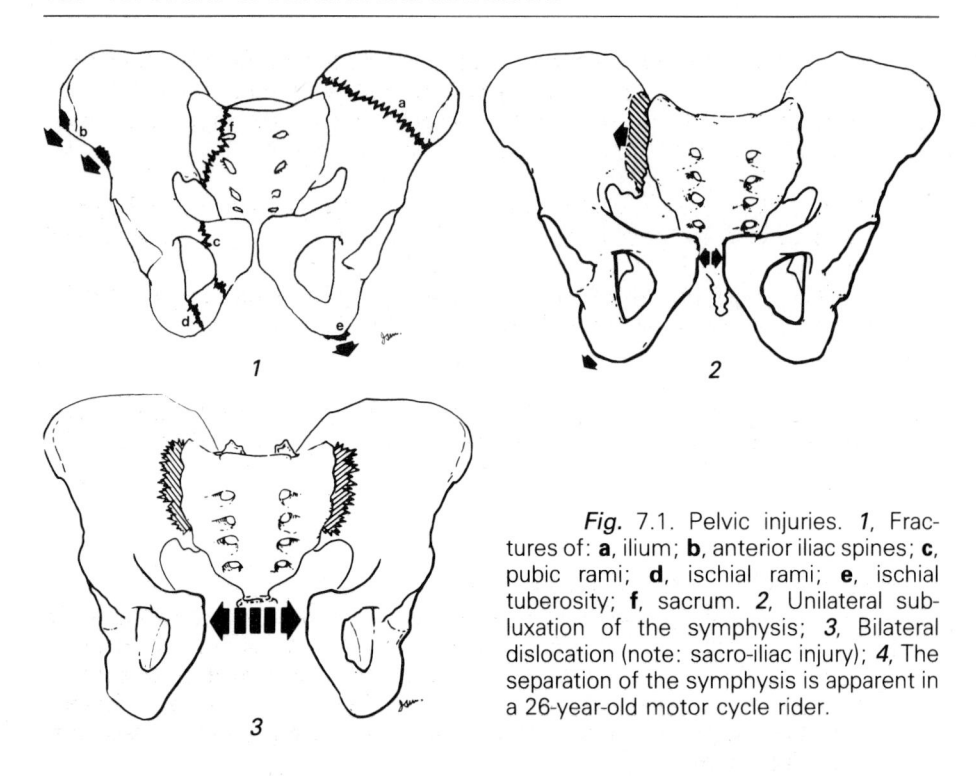

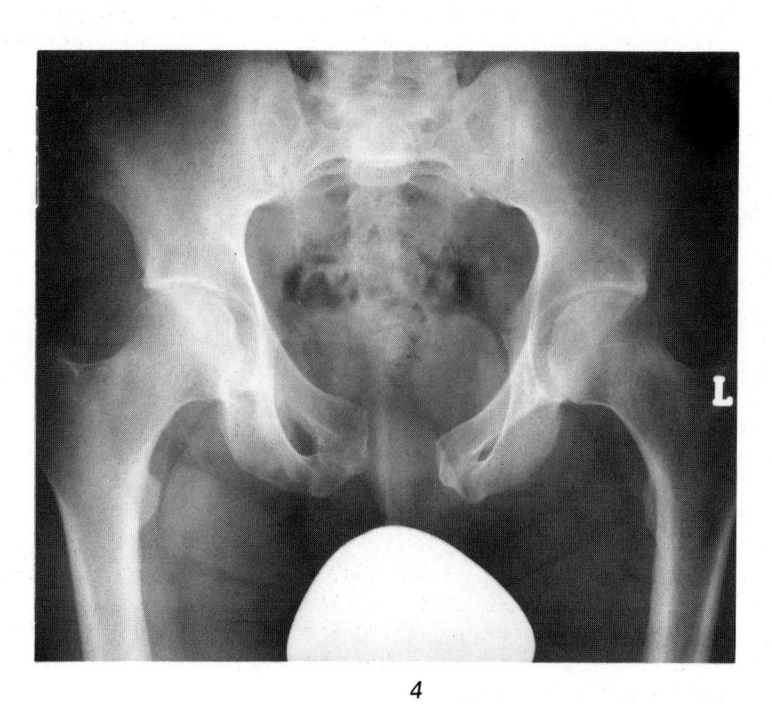

Fig. 7.1. Pelvic injuries. *1*, Fractures of: **a**, ilium; **b**, anterior iliac spines; **c**, pubic rami; **d**, ischial rami; **e**, ischial tuberosity; **f**, sacrum. *2*, Unilateral subluxation of the symphysis; *3*, Bilateral dislocation (note: sacro-iliac injury); *4*, The separation of the symphysis is apparent in a 26-year-old motor cycle rider.

Unilateral pubic rami fractures (*Fig.* 7.1(1)*c*) (or ischial rami fractures) are common (40% of all pelvic injuries) and are usually uncomplicated; bilateral fractures (pubis or ischium) may have associated bleeding and an urethral injury. Bed rest may be needed for 3 weeks and mobilization usually requires crutches or a walking frame.

Subluxation of the symphysis pubis (*Fig.* 7.1(2)(4)) is treated by bed rest for 2–4 weeks, in a double pelvic sling if badly separated; or by compression of the pelvis under anaesthesia and a well fitting plaster spica for 4 weeks.

Subluxation of the sacro-iliac joint (*Fig.* 7.1(2)(3)) is rare and treated by manipulation under general anaesthesia and a spica for 4 weeks.

Diagnosis
The above injuries are usually readily apparent on X-rays and the patient must be carefully assessed for damage to the pelvic viscera, vessels and nerves.

Treatment
As above.

Fracture-dislocation of the Hemipelvis

1. Commonly one half of the ring of the pelvis is damaged simultaneously *anteriorly* and *posteriorly* (*Fig.* 7.1). The anterior disruption consists of a fracture of both pubic (or ischial) rami with the posterior disruption through the sacro-iliac joint. Thus one half of the pelvis becomes unstable. Sometimes the symphysis separates along with the ipsilateral sacro-iliac joint.
2. When the ring is damaged *anteriorly* only there is a bilateral fracture separation of both pubic (or ischial rami) leaving the front of the pelvis unstable.

Diagnosis
Severe trauma with a characteristic X-ray appearance. There must be an immediate check for major visceral, vessel or nerve injury.

Treatment
With the combined anterior and posterior dislocation the hemipelvis is reduced under general anaesthesia and maintained by either crossed pelvic slings or a hip spica for 6 weeks. When the general condition of the patient does not allow an anaesthetic conservative management with a sling is used. Shock is corrected and other visceral injuries may take priority.

Anterior pelvic ring injuries are treated by bed rest for 2–4 weeks with a crossed pelvic sling if necessary.

Complications
1. *Shock*. Blood loss may be 2–4 l. In severe cases either open surgery with vessel ligation or repair (usually internal iliac or branches) is required or selective arterial embolization with Gelfoam strips is carried out.
2. *Urethral damage*. Blood is seen at the external meatus with perineal swelling and bruising. The prostate feels high in the rectum. Urgent urological advice is needed.

140 An outline of fractures and dislocations

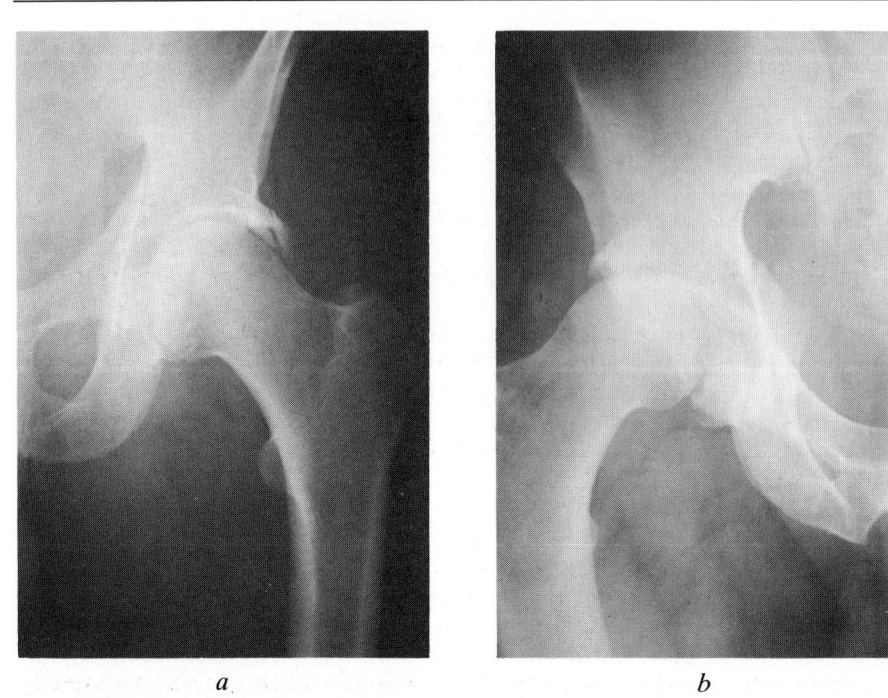

a   *b*

Fig.* 7.2. *a, Fracture of the acetabular margin following a posterior hip dislocation. ***b***, Comminuted acetabular fossa (R).

3. *Rectal and vaginal tears* need urgent repair. The *bladder* may be directly damaged and is sutured with catheter drainage.
4. *Damage to sciatic nerve and lumbosacral plexus.*
5. *Chronic sacro-iliac pain* from minor subluxation.
6. *Retroperitoneal abscess.*
7. *Chronic subluxation of the symphysis pubis.* May be asymptomatic or require bone grafting with wire or plate fixation.

Fractures of the Acetabulum

Isolated fractures (*Fig.* 7.2a) occur usually with posterior hip dislocations and may require fixation with screws (*see below*).

Comminuted fractures (*Fig.* 7.2b) occur when a lateral blow to the trochanteric region is transmitted via the femoral neck and head to the acetabulum—in severe cases a central dislocation results (*see below*).

- **Dislocations of the Hip**
  - *In contrast to the shoulder the hip is a very stable joint. Thus dislocations and fracture-dislocations in the adult require violent forces such as a road traffic accident.* However, in the mobile child's hip a less violent mechanism is needed. Many other structures can be damaged at the same time (*see later*). Incidentally,

141 Fractures of the pelvis, thigh and knee

the muscles attached to the greater trochanter act as a fulcrum and the head swings as a pendulum either forwards or backwards (*Fig. 7.3*).

Dislocations of the hip are: *Posterior* (85%)
Anterior (10%)
Central (5%)

Posterior Hip Dislocation

This is usually the result of a force driving the femur backwards (*Fig. 7.3a*) while the thigh is flexed and adducted (e.g. when the knee strikes the car dashboard).

The femoral head may assume a high (iliac) (*Fig. 7.3c*) or low (ischial) position depending upon the degree of hip flexion at the moment of impact.

Diagnosis

The hip is flexed, adducted and internally rotated, with the knee of the affected side resting on the opposite thigh. There is severe pain and the limb cannot lie flat on the bed.

As well as routine X-rays, oblique views should be taken to exclude associated hip fractures (femoral head and acetabulum).

Treatment

General anaesthesia with good muscle relaxation is required. The patient can be placed on a low trolley (or floor). An assistant steadies the iliac spines by downward pressure, and traction is applied to the affected limb. Then the hip is flexed to 90° with gentle rotatory movements to disengage the head from the external rotators. The thigh is pulled forwards and reduces. The limb is rested on a Thomas' splint with extension and slight abduction and skin traction is maintained for 3–6 weeks. Younger patients can begin non-weight-bearing with crutches earlier at 2 weeks for 6 weeks. The initial resting measures are designed to allow soft-tissue healing. Open reduction is used when closed methods fail, or when other complicating factors are present (such as a large acetabular fracture) which need internal fixation.

Complications

1. *Irreducible or incomplete reduction.* Approximately 10% of closed reductions fail due to button-holing of the femoral head through the capsule, or to obstruction by either piriformis, a bony fragment from the head or acetabulum, a detached piece of labrum or an osteocartilaginous loose body. X-rays show the femoral head is not concentric, that Shenton's line is broken and a wide gap exists between the head and the acetabulum. Surgery is needed to deal with the obstruction.
2. *Associated fracture of the posterior acetabular rim (see Fig. 7.2a).* A small fragment often reduces with the dislocation and stability is not affected. A large fragment requires screw fixation, with the limb rested for 4–6 weeks on a splint.
3. *Fracture of the femoral head.* Most fractures involve the inferior, non-weight-bearing third, and can be excised. With larger fragments (or when the ligamentum teres is attached) the fragment is retained and fixed with countersunk screws. After fragment removal the hip is mobilized at

142 An outline of fractures and dislocations

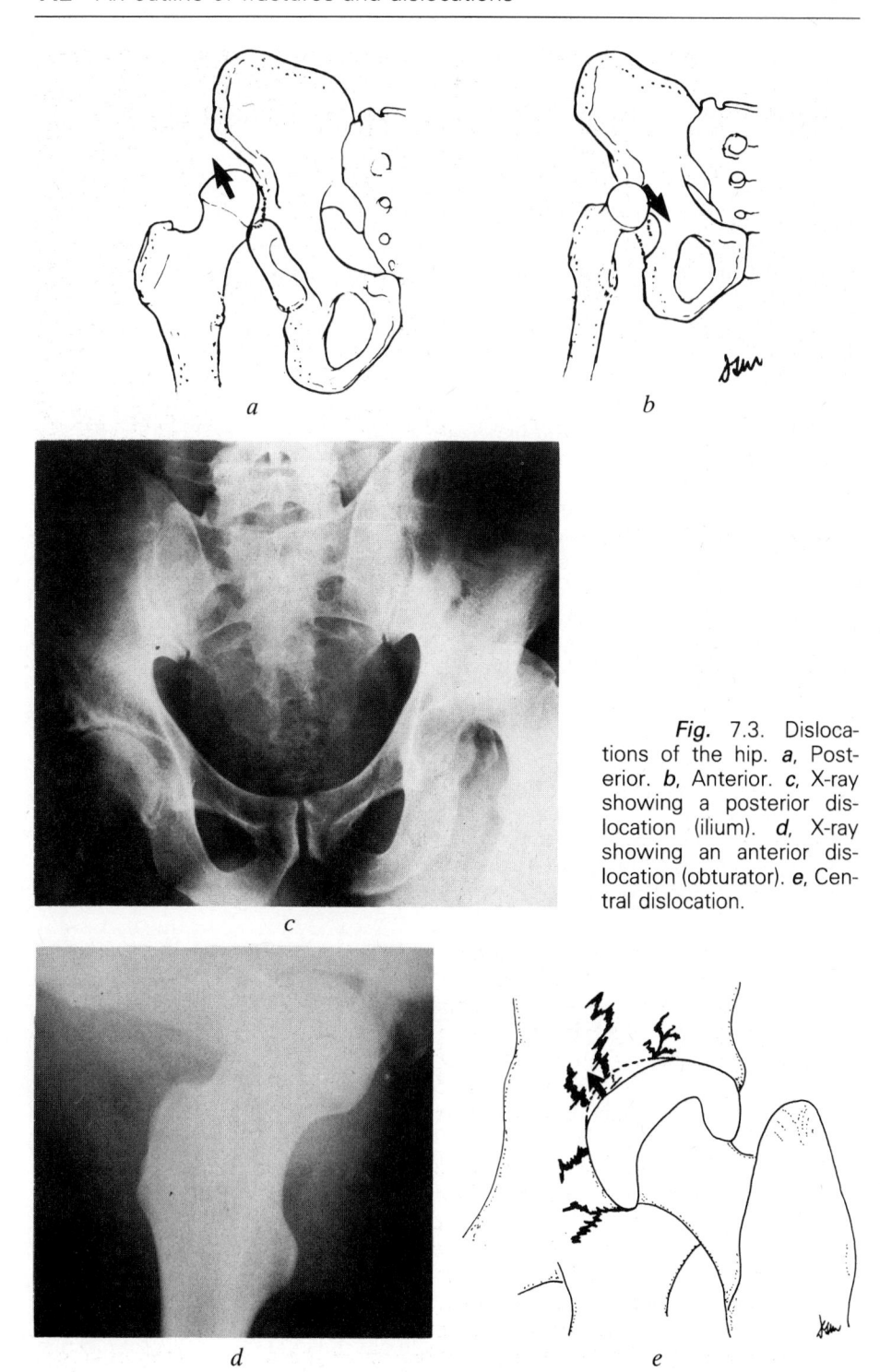

Fig. 7.3. Dislocations of the hip. *a*, Posterior. *b*, Anterior. *c*, X-ray showing a posterior dislocation (ilium). *d*, X-ray showing an anterior dislocation (obturator). *e*, Central dislocation.

143 Fractures of the pelvis, thigh and knee

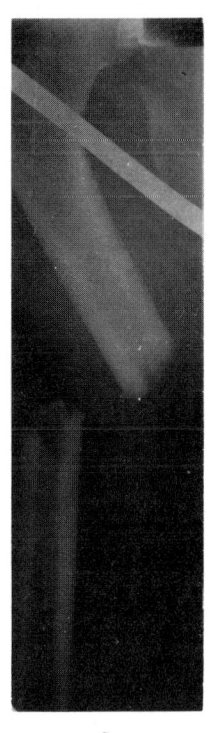

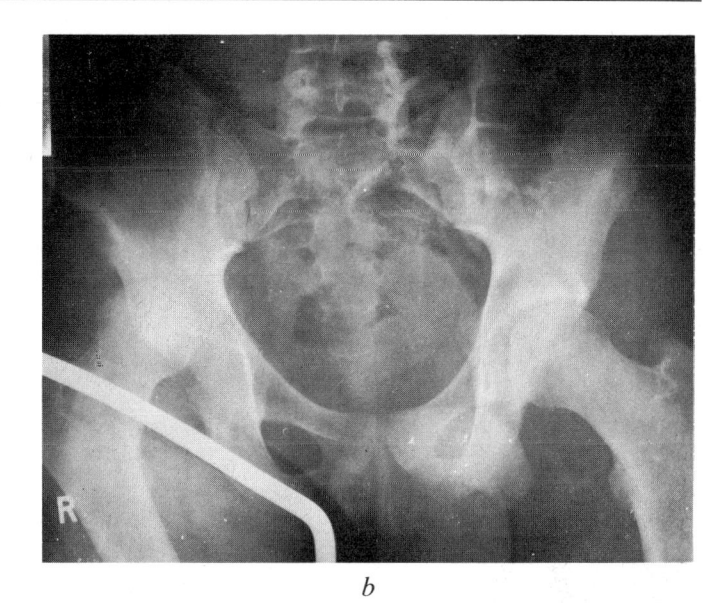

*Fig. 7.4. **a**, A suspicious femoral shaft fracture (note adduction of the shaft). **b**, The posterior dislocation of the femoral head.*

2–3 weeks, but with internal fixation the limb is rested on a splint for 6–8 weeks. Weight-bearing is delayed for 3–4 months.

4. *Fracture of the femoral neck.* This is treated by internal fixation with pins or a compression nail-plate; in the elderly a total hip arthroplasty is carried out.
5. *Fracture of the femoral shaft.* In 60% of cases the hip dislocation is missed (*Fig. 7.4*).
   - *In all cases of femoral shaft fracture the hip must be X-rayed.*

   With a fractured shaft the dislocation is reduced in the usual way but an assistant can help by applying direct pressure on the femoral head to effect reduction. Otherwise an intramedullary nail may be used to stabilize the fracture before reduction. The treatment is outlined in Fractures of the Femoral Shaft, *below*.
6. *Sciatic nerve injury.* This complication occurs in 15% of cases, especially if there is a fracture-dislocation.

   The lateral popliteal nerve is the most susceptible component.

   Occasionally the *nerve roots* may be avulsed in the lumbosacral region—myelography may show pouching and pseudomeningocele of L5 and S1 nerve roots. The commonest sciatic nerve injuries are neuropraxia (or stretching) but if recovery is delayed (over 6 weeks) or if there is evidence of a severe injury, then early exploration is carried out.
7. *Old unreduced dislocation.* This may occur when a femoral shaft fracture overshadows the hip injury or when there are multiple injuries. Open

reduction is carried out; however, hyaline cartilage necrosis may mean a total hip arthoplasty later.
8. *Avascular necrosis of the femoral head* (15%). This may demand arthrodesis or total hip arthroplasty.
9. *Recurrent posterior dislocation.* This is rare in the adult (1%) but may occur in childhood dislocations (6%). The posterior capsule has to be tightened to prevent dislocation.
10. *Osteoarthrosis* of the hip.
11. *Associated pelvic and spinal fractures.*
12. *Myositis ossificans.*

Anterior Hip Dislocation
This occurs in 10% of hip dislocations, the femoral head passing anteromedially (*see Fig. 7.3b*) to the *obturator foramen* (*see Fig. 7.3d*) or anterolaterally towards the *pubis*. The dislocating force is one of abduction, external rotation and extension. The pubic dislocation is often difficult to reduce.

Diagnosis
The hip is only slightly flexed, but the limb is externally rotated and abducted. (N.B. With pubic dislocation the hip is not abducted, just extended and externally rotated).
The X-ray shows the head is in the obturator foramen or on the pubic ramus anterior to the acetabulum.

Treatment
The patient is anaesthetized and placed on the floor in the supine position. An assistant presses on the iliac crests to brace the pelvis. With an *obturator* dislocation the knee and hip are flexed to a right angle with the limb in neutral rotation. Traction is applied and the femoral head is lifted posterolaterally into the acetabulum. The limb is gently lowered to the floor. With a *pubic* dislocation the limb is placed on the fracture table in a neutral rotation and traction is applied. The hip is hyperextended and posterior pressure is applied to the femoral head, so that it reduces backwards into the joint. The limb is rested on a splint with traction for 3–4 weeks and then partial to full weight-bearing begins over the ensuing month.

Complications
These are similar to those in posterior dislocation without sciatic damage, while a fracture of the femoral shaft and acetabular injuries (apart from slight margin fractures) are rare. However, the femoral vessels are at risk from an anterior dislocation, thus the circulation must be checked in the lower limb.

Central Hip Fracture-dislocation
The femoral head is driven through the medial acetabular wall (*see Fig. 7.3e*) and this injury occurs as a result of severe force, either to the knee or foot with the hip abducted, or directly against the lateral femur. The degree of displacement varies according to the force. Traction is applied through a screw passed into the greater trochanter, with the direction of pull downwards and

outwards for 4–6 weeks. If the hip is irreducible it can be left (almost as an arthrodesis) or open reduction can be performed.

Osteoarthrosis is inevitable and may demand an arthroplasty later.

Traumatic Dislocation of the Hip in Children
This condition is considerably less common in children than in adults and only a small percentage (15%) have an associated acetabular or femoral fracture. In children under 6 the hip may dislocate with minimal trauma; avascular necrosis is less frequent than in adults.

- ## Fractures of the Femoral Neck
  - *True fractures of the femoral neck (called subcapital or transcervical) are of special importance because the blood supply to the femoral head can be cut off and avascular necrosis result.*
  - *Fractures of the trochanteric region* (**inter-trochanteric, pertrochanteric, comminuted, subtrochanteric**) *behave as fractures of the femoral shaft (or any other long bone), i.e. they unite without complications on conservative treatment, although internal fixation is desirable for rapid mobilization and correct alignment.*

True Fractures of the Femoral Neck (Subcapital) (Intracapsular)
- *These may be UNDISPLACED (Grades I and II) (Garden classification) or DISPLACED (Grades III and IV).*
- *This injury is the unsolved fracture* (*Figs.* 7.5, 7.6), *a condition of the aged (average 70+ years) with osteoporosis or osteomalacia, while on medications for related medical problems that hamper the prognosis and treatment.* Women are affected four times more commonly than men.

Diagnosis
The classic triad of hip pain, limb shortening and external rotation is seen. X-ray shows the characteristic fracture line running obliquely from the lateral aspect of the femoral head to the distal medial cortex—produced by external torsion (*Figs.* 7.6, 7.7).

(N.B. Rarely the fracture crosses the lower neck—*transcervical* or *basal*).

Treatment
On admission the patient's medical condition should be fully evaluated and the limb maintained in neutral rotation by Russell traction.

With *undisplaced* (*impacted*) subcapital fractures (Grades I and II) the hip is fixed by percutaneous screws (either crossed or in parallel (*Fig.* 7.8)) or multiple pins. This relatively atraumatic procedure carries minimal blood loss, risk of infection and morbidity and is the procedure of choice in the very elderly or unfit, whose life expectancy is usually only in months or a few years. Younger patients (65 or less) may require a compression device for stability and rapid mobilization (*see below*).

With *displaced* subcapital fractures (Grades III and IV) the shaft is rotated outwards by the short external rotators opening up a gap anteriorly.

146   An outline of fractures and dislocations

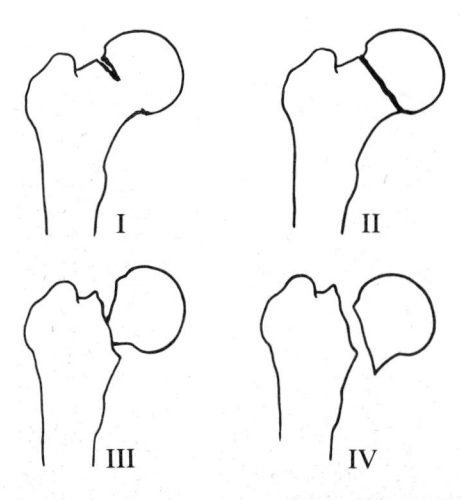

Fig. 7.5. Classification of subcapital femoral neck fractures: undisplaced (I and II), displaced (III and IV).

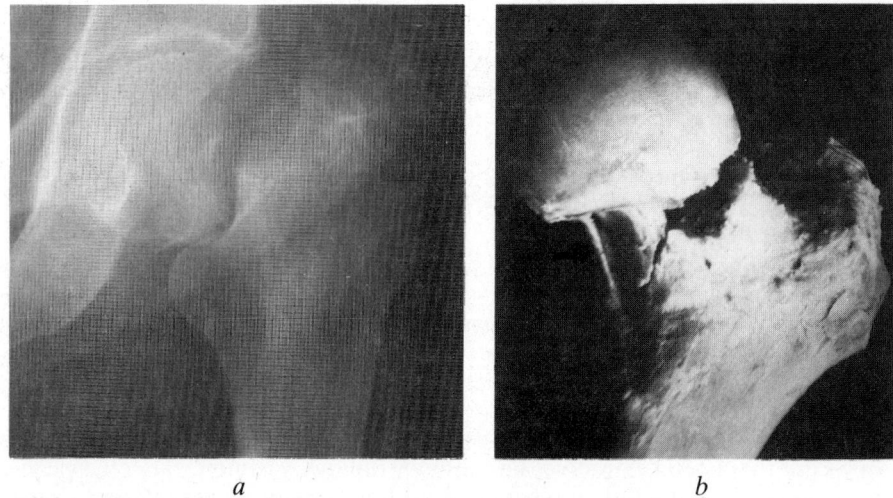

Fig. 7.6. *a*, The characteristic X-ray appearance of a subcapital fracture. *b*, The posterior cortex loss is apparent.

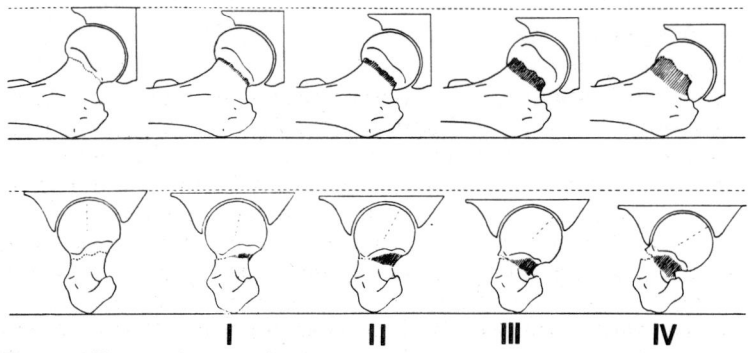

Fig. 7.7. The cortical loss is shown with each type of subcapital fracture.

147 Fractures of the pelvis, thigh and knee

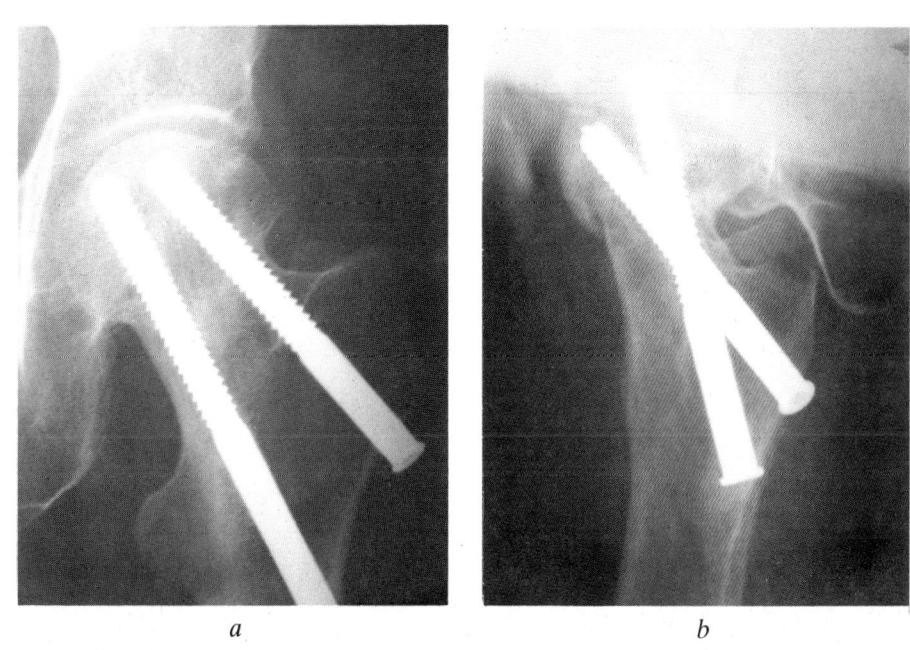

Fig. 7.8. *a*, A subcapital fracture at 2 years showing an excellent result with Garden screws (parallel). *b*, Often used crossed.

However, if the posterior cortex of the neck has collapsed (*see Figs.* 7.6, 7.7) the head springs back into its normal position in the acetabulum (and thus the trabeculae lie in correct alignment with those of the pelvis). The shaft displaces upwards (due to iliopsoas) and lies in front of the head. These fractures are reduced by traction on an orthopaedic table with minimal abduction (preferably neutral position since abduction opens the fracture site medially) and 45° or so of internal rotation. (However, Grade IV fractures are difficult to reduce perfectly because the defect in the posterior cortex renders it unstable).

With *younger (below 65 years), or fit elderly patients* subcapital fractures (III and IV) can be treated by internal fixation using:
1. A compression screw.
2. A nail-plate.
3. A sliding nail.
4. A pin and plate.

The compression device (*Fig.* 7.9) is the most popular at present but some centres believe that an additional posterior bone grafting is required if there is a cortical defect, especially in young (50+ years) patients. (The results in Grade IV cases are often poor due to avascular necrosis and some centres automatically proceed to a hip arthroplasty as a primary treatment (*see below*).

With very *elderly or unfit* patients a total hip replacement or a hemiarthroplasty is required in Grades III and IV fractures. Common forms of hemiarthroplasty are the Thompson's prosthesis, Moore's and Monk's prosthesis used with bone cement. The latter procedure (hemiarthroplasty) is only effective when there is no hyaline cartilage injury. It is worth noting that

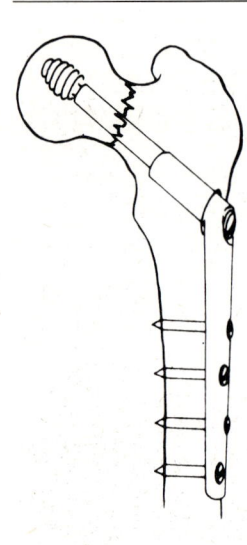

Fig. 7.9. Compression screw for subcapital fractures.

rarely do osteoarthrosis and femoral neck fractures coexist, considering the frequency of both conditions.

Mobilization is directly affected by the overall medical state of the patient; when there is good stability (I and II) or effective reduction (III) the patient can walk or hop with a walking frame after 2–4 days, a restriction on weight-bearing being enforced up to 4 months by use of the frame. With a Grade IV fracture, when there may be some posterior cortex instability, too early weight-bearing risks collapse and angulation. However, a delay in bed for several weeks risks postoperative complications such as bed sores or deep vein thrombosis (the devil–deep blue sea paradox). Unfit patients may manage with crutches or by hopping with a frame but these are the exceptions, sadly not the rule. Thus the hemiarthroplasty or hip replacement is preferred for rapid mobilization in the frail, unfit elderly.

Complications
1. In the first 3–6 months 15% *mortality* due to age and general ill-health.
2. *Avascular necrosis* (*Fig.* 7.10). This can be determined by technetium-99m uptake. Almost 30% of patients with displaced subcapital fractures suffer from either partial necrosis (*superior segmental collapse*) or *total femoral head necrosis* within 18 months. A hip arthroplasty may have to be performed in the fitter, mobile patient; the condition can be left alone in the feeble, bedridden patient unless there is marked pain. Incidentally, avascular necrosis occurs at any age—even children and young adults suffer this complication after subcapital fractures. Factors that affect the onset are: malreduction, ineffective stabilization, displacement, penetration by fixation device and over 3–4 days delay in surgery.
3. *Non-union* (*Fig.* 7.10). This occurs in approximately 30% of cases; the treatment is as for avascular necrosis. Younger patients can have a posterior pedicle bone graft (quadratus femoris plus bony attachment), although this procedure is not greatly successful in producing revascularization.

149 Fractures of the pelvis, thigh and knee

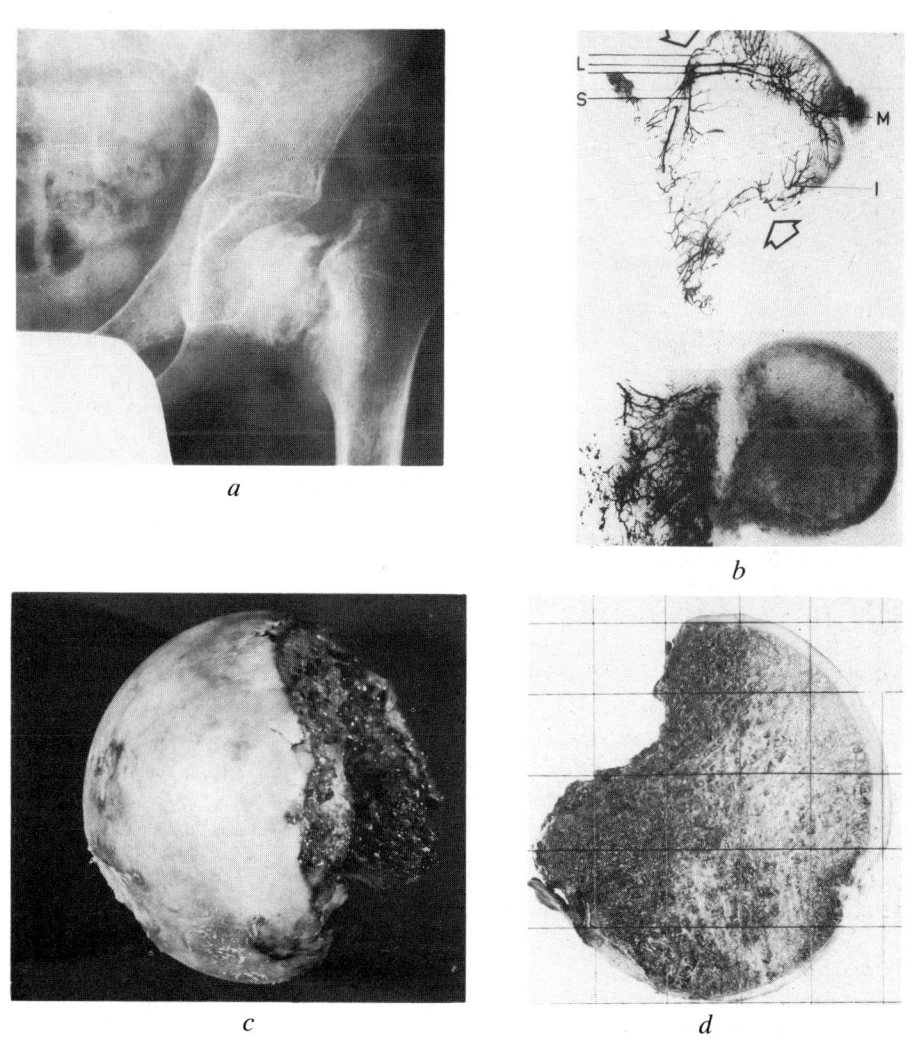

Fig. 7.10. Avascular changes following a subcapital fracture. *a*, X-ray appearance. *b*, Infarction of the femoral head shown on an angiogram (L, M = epiphyseal vessels; S, I = metaphyseal vessels). *c*, Hyaline cartilage injury seen on a femoral head removed after 4 days. *d*, Infarction is seen on cross-section.

4. *Failure of the metal implant.* Breakage of pins, nails, screws; penetration through the femoral head or shaft; failure of cement/bone or cement/metal interface may necessitate revision of the appliance or removal of the prosthesis.
5. *Associated with a dislocation of the hip, or femoral shaft fracture.*
6. *Coxa vara deformity.* The femoral neck/shaft angle may be reduced from 135° to 90°. A valgus angulation is achieved by a wedge osteotomy and nail-plate fixation of the upper femoral shaft.

150 An outline of fractures and dislocations

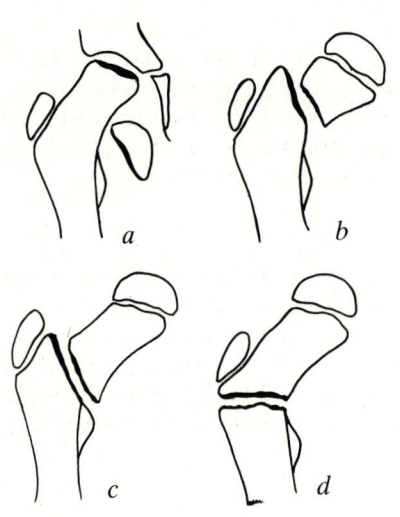

Fig. 7.11. Femoral neck fracture in children. *a*, Traumatic separation of epiphysis. *b*, Transcervical. *c*, Cervicotrochanteric. *d*, Intertrochanteric.

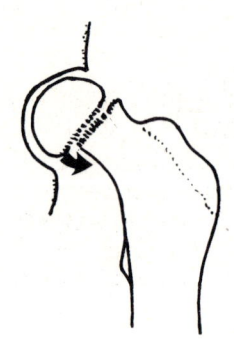

Fig. 7.12. Slipped femoral epiphysis.

7. *Complication of major surgery.* Deep vein thrombosis (15%) and pulmonary embolism (5%) infection (5–10%; worse with posterior incisions), bronchopneumonia, bed-sores, etc.
8. *Dislocations of the prosthesis.* Infrequent after an anterior incision; hip flexion during sitting places the metal head at risk with a posterior approach. Medial migration of the head through the acetabular floor may occur.

Fractures of the Femoral Neck in Children

These account for less than 1% of femoral neck fractures and are usually the result of marked violence such as a road traffic accident or a fall from a tree.

The majority are transverse or midcervical.

True femoral neck fractures are:

Type I (*traumatic separation of the epiphysis*), and

Type II (*a transcervical fracture*) (*Fig.* 7.11*a,b*).

Type I: These can be treated by Buck's traction (2–4 kg attached to the lower limbs through strapping) with the affected limb internally rotated to realign the fragments. This is used for 2–4 weeks. Alternatively, a hip spica can be applied in the same postion.

In *Type II* transcervical fractures the hip is fixed with multiple pins (as for a slipped epiphysis) but the epiphyseal plate is not transgressed or premature closure might result.

(For Types III and IV *see* Trochanteric fractures.)

N.B. Avascular necrosis is variable and may resemble Legg–Perthes disease in the young and requires a non-weight-bearing brace or plaster immobilization (e.g. Petri plasters). Occasionally a rotation osteotomy may have to be performed.

Slipped Femoral Epiphysis
- *In adolescents the upper femoral epiphysis may become acutely displaced at the growth disc, but slipping may occur gradually in 70% of cases.*
- *Although trauma may precipitate a sudden slip (30%) there is always an abnormal weakness of the epiphyseal cartilage, perhaps due to an underlying endocrine disorder. Often the child has a markedly rotund appearance.*

Diagnosis
There is pain in the hip and a limp, but in many cases the pain is *referred to the knee*. With the gradual slip on the earliest X-rays the epiphysis appears wide and 'woolly' and a line drawn along the upper surface of the neck passes above the outer margin of the head, rather than through the lateral third (*Fig. 7.12*). Gradually the downward and posterior slipping of the head becomes obvious. With sudden displacement the shaft is foreshortened and the head obviously displaced postero-inferiorly on the initial films.

Treatment
With *slight displacement* (less than ⅓ of the head diameter) the head is pinned with multiple pins.

With *acute displacement* gentle reduction can be performed under anaesthesia (occasionally open reduction is required). Then the head is fixed with multiple pins.

With a *chronic*, irreducible slipped epiphysis an osteotomy of the femoral neck or upper femur is performed.

Complications
1. *Coxa vara*—when the displacement has not been reduced and the epiphysis has fused. Osteotomy is needed.
2. *Avascular necrosis.*
3. *Osteoarthritis.*
- *Special note: Up to 30% of patients may develop* **bilateral** *slipping within 2 years; these patients must be regularly assessed radiologically.*

Fractures of the Trochanteric Region ('Extracapsular')
(for historical reasons usually included with femoral neck fractures)
Fractures of the *trochanteric* region are:
1. Greater trochanter.
2. Lesser trochanter.
3. Intertrochanteric (may be comminuted).
4. Pertrochanteric.
5. Subtrochanteric.

Fractures of the Greater Trochanter
Usually due to a direct blow and is occasionally displaced by the hip abductors. Such injuries are treated by early mobilization (after 7–10 days) with partial weight-bearing and crutches or a frame (*Fig. 7.13a*). During the period of bed rest Russell traction is used with the limbs in neutral rotation and abduction.

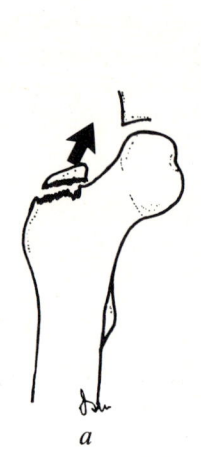

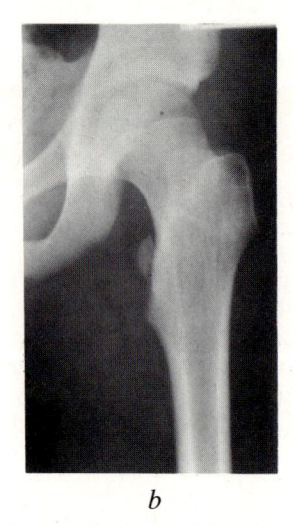

Fig. 7.13. *a*, Fracture of the greater trochanter. *b*, An avulsion fracture of the lesser trochanter in a female runner.

Fractures of the Lesser Trochanter
This structure may be avulsed by the iliopsoas in young sports persons (*Fig.* 7.13*b*) (or a part of a comminuted trochanteric fracture). The patient may rest for 2–3 days, then begin gentle ambulation with crutches for the isolated fracture (*see also*: Comminuted trochanteric fracture).

Intertrochanteric Fractures (extracapsular femoral neck fractures)
Most patients are over 70 years, with women outnumbering men 2:1. These fractures may be *undisplaced* or *displaced; stable* or *unstable* (*Fig.* 7.14).

Type I: *Undisplaced (Stable)*
The fracture line traverses the intertrochanteric region and usually the greater and lesser trochanter are not involved (*Fig.* 7.14*a*). It is often seen in younger (50+) patients after marked trauma (heavy fall, road traffic accident).

Diagnosis
The hip is painful but not rotated nor the limb foreshortened.

Treatment
In the young patient the hip can be maintained in the neutral position by Buck's skin traction for 2 weeks then mobilized non-weight-bearing for 10 weeks.
In the elderly Ender's nail fixation is the method of choice (*Fig.* 7.15*a*).

Type II: *Displaced Fracture* (without medial cortex loss) (sometimes called **pertrochanteric**) (*Fig.* 7.14*b*).
Whereas in subcapital fractures the posterior cortex of the neck was a critical feature for stability in *trochanteric* fractures the *medial femoral cortex* must remain intact for *stability* (*Fig.* 7.15*d*).

153 Fractures of the pelvis, thigh and knee

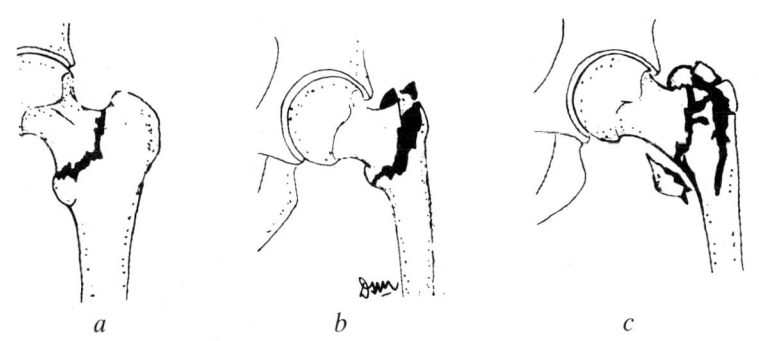

Fig. 7.14. Trochanteric fractures of the femoral neck region. *a,* Intertrochanteric. *b,* Pertrochanteric. *c,* Comminuted.

In this lesion the main fracture line extends along the intertrochanteric region and the upper fragment tilts into varus, while both trochanters are involved.

Diagnosis
The lower limb is externally rotated as well as hip movements being painful.

Treatment
For *younger* patients (65 years or less) a compression screw (*see Fig.* 7.9) (fixed or sliding) attached to a cortical plate can be used; or a fixed-angle nail-plate. A pin-and-plate risks breakage or loosening at the nail-plate junction. These procedures lose 0·5–1 litre of blood, and have all the complications of a major operation.

For *older patients* multiple intramedullary pins (*Fig.* 7.15*b*) inserted by the Ender's method from the medial distal femur is a simple, atraumatic procedure. However, insufficient pins may lead to backward migration, poor control of rotation, with the occasional femoral supracondylar fracture (through the insertion area). However, the blood loss is often as low as 50 ml and infection very rare. Some centres advocate bone cement plus nail-plate fixation to allow early mobilization in the infirm.

Type III: *Displaced Fracture (with medial cortex disruption) (comminuted)*

The damaged medial cortex (*Fig.* 7.14*c*) allows the head to fall into *marked varus,* and the shaft to displace medially behind the neck with the greater trochanter split. The lesser trochanter is also displaced (a key radiological feature).

Diagnosis
As Type II but the limb is shortened and markedly externally rotated (due to the unapposed action of the external rotators on the shaft).

Treatment
The fracture is often difficult to reduce by closed methods and reduction is achieved during internal fixation. However, *for stability* the medial cortex is secured (often after an osteotomy) by a nail-plate (*Fig.* 7.15*c,d*) or compression nail-plate device.

154 An outline of fractures and dislocations

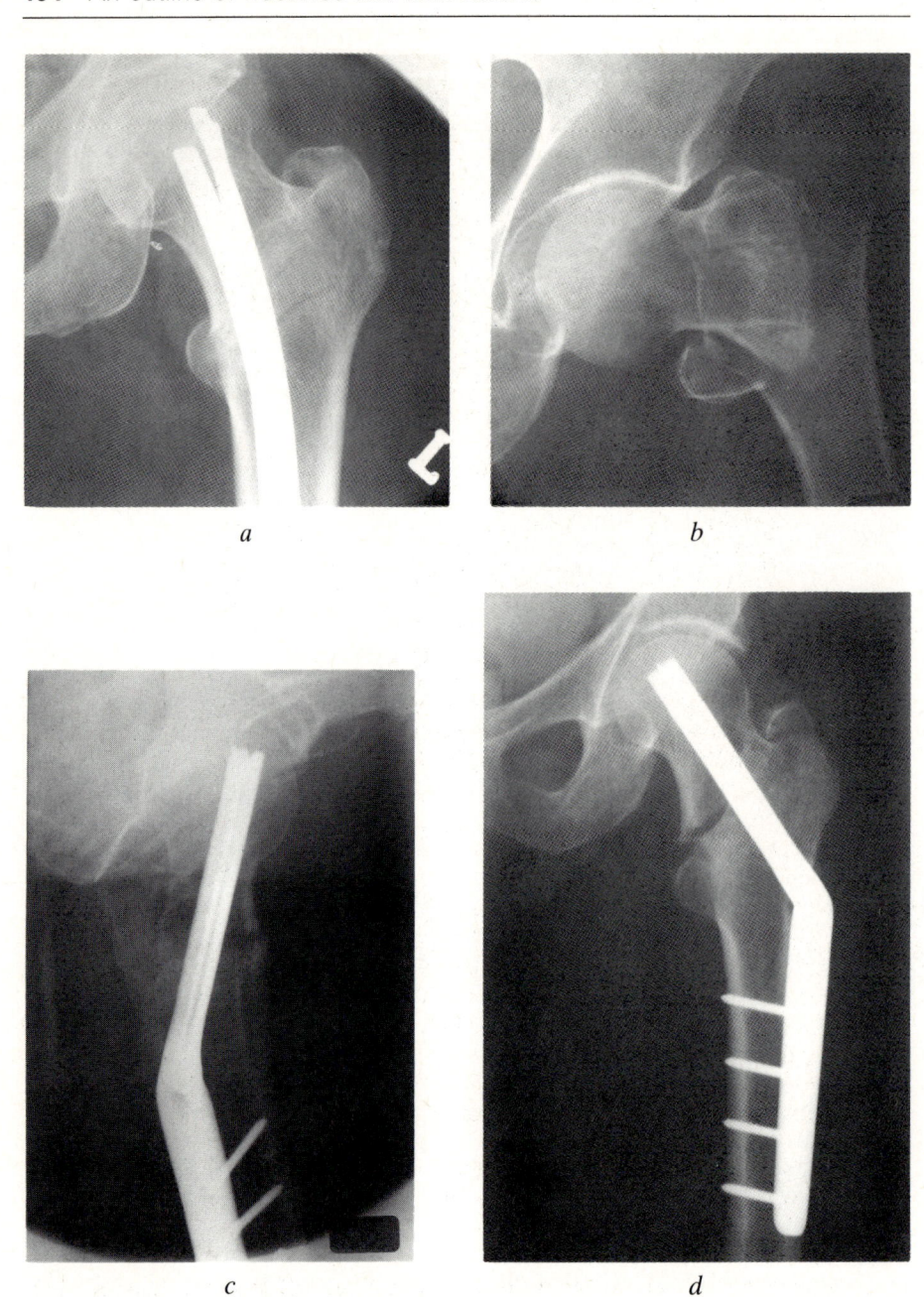

Fig. 7.15. *a*, Ender's nail fixation for a stable trochanteric fracture. *b*, An unstable comminuted fracture. *c*, With excellent cortical apposition (and nail-plated fixation). *d*, Medial cortex stability is important in trochanteric fractures, the slight misalignment in this case caused no loss of fixation.

155 Fractures of the pelvis, thigh and knee

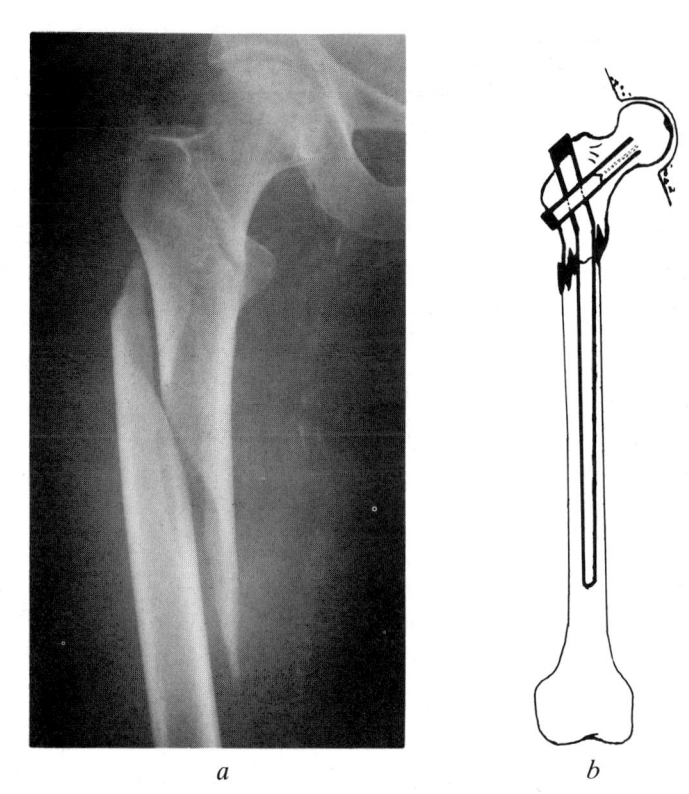

Fig. 7.16. a, Spiral subtrochanteric fracture extending into the intertrochanteric region. *b*, Zickel nail.

Type IV: *Intertrochanteric with Subtrochanteric*

This is rare but extremely unstable (*Fig. 7.16a*). A solid internal fixation device and extended plate is required, often a high-angled (150°) device is needed or, preferably, a Zickel nail technique (*Fig. 7.16b*) (pin in the femoral neck through a nail along the femoral shaft).

(N.B. If the patient is old or very infirm Ender's intramedullary nails can be used to hold the main fragments and to relieve pain. However, there is no stability for mobilization and a de-rotation plaster boot is applied to keep the limb in the neutral position).

With unstable fractures full weight-bearing is delayed for up to 3 months depending on the rate of union; crutches or a walking frame are used.

Complications
1. There is a *mortality rate* of 30% within 1 year of fracture. This is often highest in patients who are subjected to immediate surgery (within 24 hours) without evaluation of their general medical condition and without subsequent correction of blood loss (worse than after subcapital fractures) and electrolytes. During the period of investigation the limb is rested in neutral rotation with Russell traction.
2. The *complications of major surgery* (*see* under subcapital fractures).

3. *Failure of nails, plates, etc.*—either breakage, penetration through head of femur or backing out.
4. *Collapse of fracture* with the head passing into marked varus. This may require a valgus osteotomy.
5. *Fatigue fracture of the femoral neck* (where the nail is too short) or *transverse fracture of the shaft* (where the cortex has been over-drilled during insertion).
6. *External rotation deformity* of the lower limb to malreduction.
7. *Weakness of hip flexion* and consequent difficulty in transferring from bed to chair or getting out of a car due to iliopsoas weakness when the lesser trochanter is displaced.

Intertrochanteric Fractures in Children

Types I and II femoral neck fractures in children were described under subcapital fracture.

Type III (cervicotrochanteric) (*see Fig. 7.11c*) and *Type IV* (intertrochanteric) (*see Fig. 7.11d*) when *undisplaced* are best treated by a plaster spica for 4–6 weeks. *Displaced* fractures need internal fixation with pins in the younger child, but a nail-plate or screw device is used close to puberty and often a plaster spica applied for 3–4 weeks. Complications are as mentioned under 'subcapital children's fracture'—with avascular necrosis occurring in 25% of cases of displaced cervicotrochanteric fractures. The prognosis is better in children under 10 years.

Subtrochanteric Fractures

These fractures (*Fig. 7.17*) are *notorious* for delayed union, non-union and breakage of the fixation device, for the greatest femoral stress during weight-bearing is concentrated on the medial subtrochanteric region. They are best treated by an intramedullary Zickel nail. (N.B. If there is an intertrochanteric component a compression screw plus 12-holed plate can be used). A weight-bearing calliper or cast-brace is employed for 12–14 weeks.

In children a plaster hip spica can be given for 4–6 weeks after reduction, or gallows traction (Bryant's traction) is used when the child is less than 2 years.

• *N.B. With Bryant's traction in older children or those heavier than 15 kg the weights employed or the forces of countertraction can cause skin problems, swollen feet and limb ischaemia, especially if the knee is hyperextended when the popliteal circulation may be affected.*

Stress Fractures of the Femoral Neck

Many elderly patients complain of hip pain without an obvious fracture radiologically; gentle internal rotation may reproduce the discomfort. X-rays taken over 3 weeks at 7–day intervals may reveal the occult stress fracture as bone resorption occurs. Internal fixation may be required to prevent displacement.

In sports people and military recruits a *stress fracture* may occur which can be detected by a bone scan. Activity is curtailed for 3–4 months and spontaneous union occurs.

After *radiotherapy* to the pelvis a fracture may occur in the femoral neck, sometimes with avascular changes in the femoral head. Internal fixation is

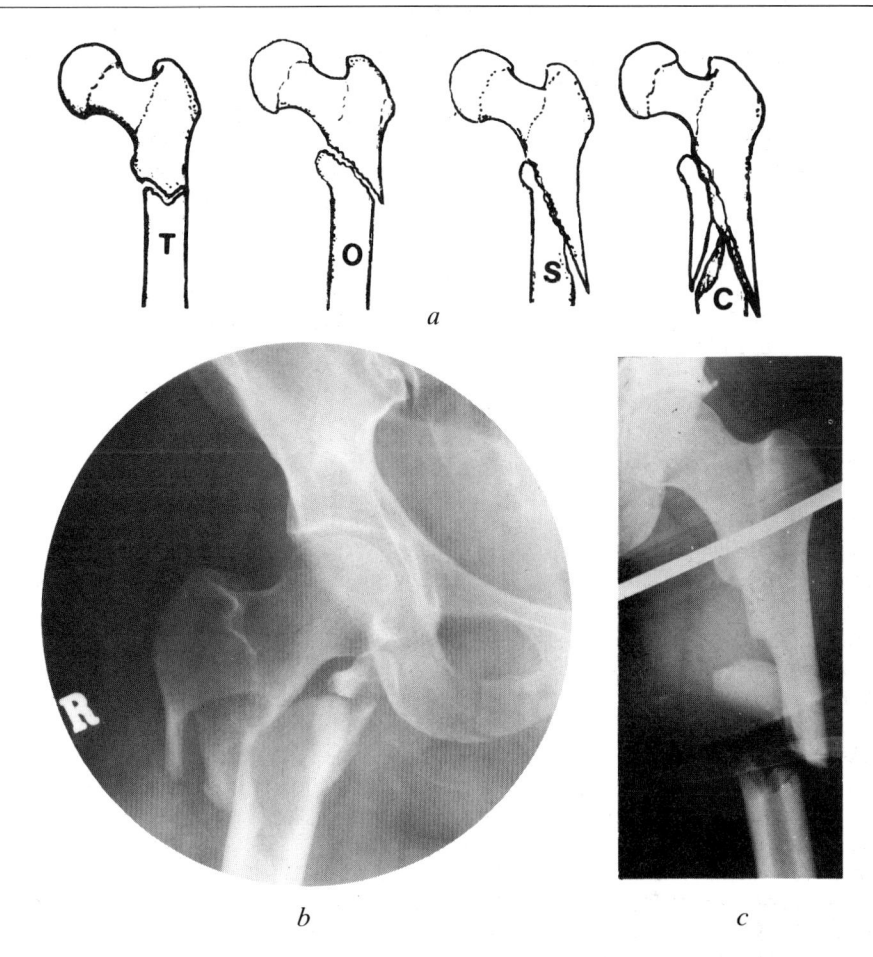

Fig. 7.17. Subtrochanteric fracture classification. *a*, **T** = transverse, **O** = oblique, **S** = spiral, **C** = comminution. *b*, An unusual subtrochanteric fracture with an associated pelvic ramus fracture. *c*, An extremely unstable comminuted fracture following a road traffic accident.

usually required to prevent eventual varus angulation. *Pathological (neoplastic) fractures* are common in the trochanteric region (breast, renal, prostate, lung and blood dyscrasia must be excluded). Usually prosthetic replacement is performed.

- ***Special note: Femoral neck (subcapital) and trochanteric fractures do not demand urgent surgery—a delay of 1 or 2 days is not prejudicial to the final outcome and allows detailed investigation and correction of the impaired medical state (up to 70% are on long-term medication). During this period the limb is rested on a splint or pillow with gentle skin traction (2–5 kg—Russell traction) and the patient is turned regularly for pressure area care, given chest physiotherapy and, if necessary, rehydrated with oral and intravenous solutions.***

- **Fractures of the Femoral Shaft**
    - *These are due to great force and may be associated with 1–2 litres of blood loss, profound shock (if bilateral), other severe injuries (including head, spine, chest, abdomen and pelvis), and later fat embolism.*

They are divided into:
1. Upper third.
2. Middle third.
3. Lower third (including supracondylar) (*see later*)(*Fig.* 7.18).

They may be spiral (usually upper third); transverse or comminuted (middle third); transverse or T- or Y-shaped (lower third).

Diagnosis
This fracture cannot be missed, such is the pain, swelling and deformity.
- *Check circulation in the lower limb—3% have damage to the femoral or popliteal vessels.*
- *Review the patient—one in four (25%) have other major injuries: one in five (20%) are compound.*

Treatment
The injured thigh is supported on a splint during the X-rays. Blood pressure and pulse are assessed and dextrose-saline drip infusion given prior to blood transfusion (usually 1–2 litres depending on estimated loss; more with severe injuries).

Conservative treatment uses the classic Thomas splint (*Fig.* 7.19a) for 12 weeks with traction through the upper tibia (or sometimes lower femur) by a Steinmann pin. Up to 20 kg are used to reduce the fracture slowly over several days, the normal re-aligned curve of the femoral shaft (on the lateral view) being achieved by padding behind the fractured area. A Pearson knee-piece allows knee movements. As an alternative *in the absence of head and other major injuries*, a general anaesthetic is given and the fracture reduced and maintained as above.

If callus is present at 8 weeks and the fracture feels stable a weight-relieving calliper can be used for 6–12 weeks.

However, three months in bed is a very long time, especially for young adults. Thus at 4 weeks (if the fracture feels 'sticky') a cast brace with a flexion knee-hinge can be given and this is worn for 6–8 weeks, the patient being allowed home partial weight-bearing with crutches. This form of treatment is especially useful with comminuted fractures when there is poor stability for internal fixation. Other variants include box-plaster initially and a cast brace at 6 weeks; or a thigh brace at 6 weeks.

Surgical treatment consists of AO plating of the shaft or intramedullary fixation using a stout (e.g. Küntscher) (*Fig.* 7.20a) nail or flexible nails (e.g. Ender) (*Fig.* 7.20b,c).

Open reduction is needed when there is an irreducible fracture due to soft-tissue interposition, with a loose (butterfly) segment (a bone graft can be added, if necessary), and a vessel or nerve injury. Usually a compression plate is applied or a stout intramedullary nail inserted (with spiral fractures cerclage

159 Fractures of the pelvis, thigh and knee

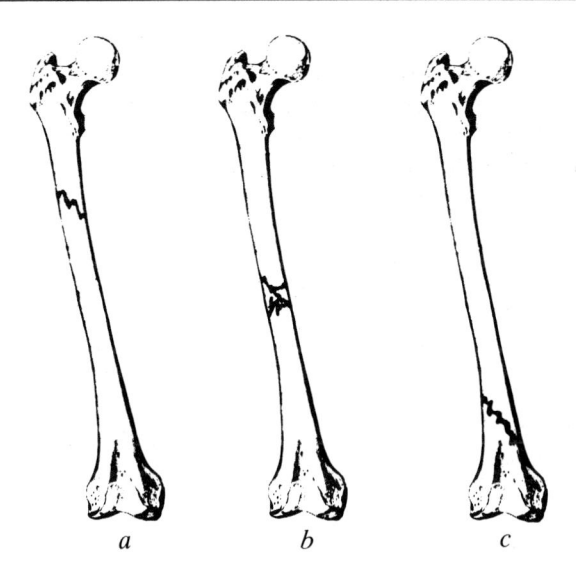

Fig. 7.18. Classification of femoral shaft fracture: *a*, upper, *b*, middle and *c*, lower thirds.

wires can be used in addition). The patient rests for 2 weeks and may be mobilized with limited weight-bearing for 12 weeks.

Closed reduction can be achieved under X-ray control and a stout intramedullary nail inserted from the trochanteric region, or Ender's nails from the medial femoral condyle. The blood loss is minimal with these techniques, less than 100 ml being reported with Ender's method. Patients can mobilize at 10 days and the majority return home at 3 weeks. However, unless the fracture is very stable (e.g. transverse) weight-bearing should not be allowed for 12 weeks. An external fixator gives rapid mobilization within 1 week.

Complications
1. *Shock.*
2. *Other major injuries* (head, spine, thorax, etc.).
3. *Fracture–dislocation* or *dislocation* of the *same hip* (*Note*: if the upper fragment is *adducted* look carefully at the hip X-ray—it should be abducted by the strong hip abductors).
4. *Femoral* or *popliteal* vessel injury.
5. *Sciatic nerve injury.*
6. *Fat embolism.*
7. *Major infection* (20% have compound wound, 1–5% infection after surgical intervention).
8. *Ligamentous* and *meniscal injuries* in the *knee* complicate 10% of cases and account for knee problems 6–9 months later when full weight-bearing and exercises begin in earnest.
9. *Tibial shaft fracture* (the *floating knee*) (*Fig.* 7.21); 14% of patients have an upper tibial fracture which allows the knee to 'float'.
10. *Non-union, delayed union, malunion, malrotation* and *shortening*.

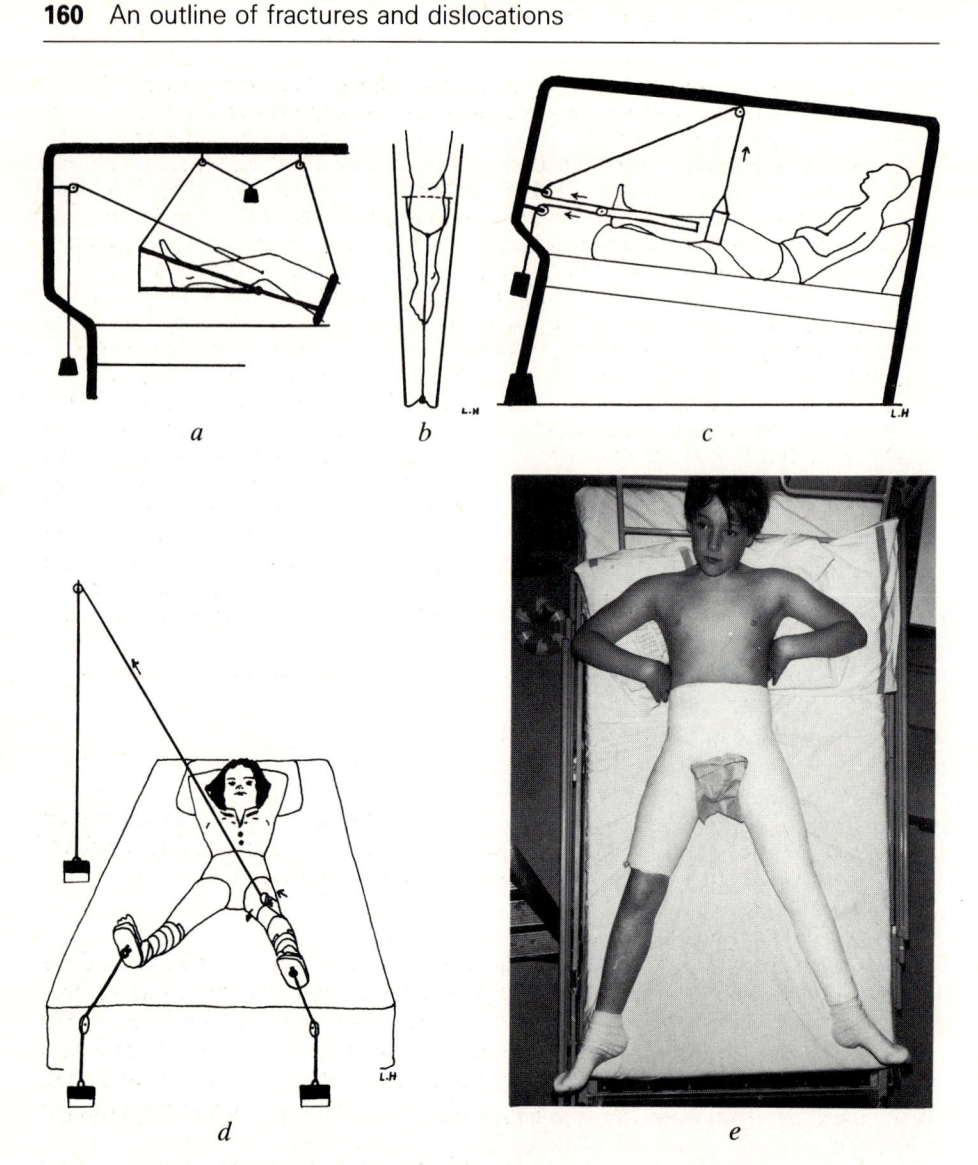

11. *Late osteoarthrosis* hip and knee (from impact) during the violent phase of injury.
12. *Refracture* (may require internal fixation and bone-grafting).
13. *Knee stiffness*. This is more common after conservative treatment with tibial traction (when excessive loading is placed through the knee ligaments). Adhesions between the quadriceps and the fracture site may occur. Thus, in all patients knee mobilization is a priority with either a knee-piece (Pearson's), or a split bed. Intramedullary fixation allows early knee mobilization, although there is often soreness after Ender's nail fixation which persists for 4 weeks, although eventually full flexion is achieved.

Fig. 7.19. *a*, In *sliding* (or suspended or balanced) skeletal *traction* a metal splint (usually Thomas) is used with the thigh resting on padded cotton straps. A pulley system elevates the ring which should be 2·5–5 cm (1–2 in) greater than the thigh girth (at the groin). Both the hip and knee are flexed by 15–20°. Traction (7–10 kg initially, increasing by 1–2 kg to 15 kg) is applied through a tibial pin with the leg resting on a Pearson knee-piece (with foot support) suspended from the end of the splint. The bed may be elevated 30° but counter traction is through the cords that suspend the splint from the beams. The apparatus is supported by weights to allow balance of the limb. N.B. The groin and buttock must be regularly cleaned, powdered and kept free of undue pressure which can cause skin ulceration. Physiotherapy encourages thigh muscle contractions and knee mobility. *b*, In *fixed traction* in an adult the tibial pin cord is tied to the end of the Thomas' splint. (N.B. In children skin traction is used and attached to the splint in the same way. The circulation should be watched in the foot.) The splint is suspended from an overhead beam. *c*, In *Russell's traction* the limb rests on one or two pillows with the knee slightly flexed with a padded canvas sling; 2–3 kg are applied through skin traction using foam rubber strips (adhesive plaster can cause skin blistering). The foot of the bed is elevated for counter traction. This method is good for fractures and problems around the hip but not for femoral shaft fractures because of the lack of support under the broken area. *d*, In *Buck's traction* the limbs rest on the bed and 2–3 kg are applied through skin traction: any rotatory malalignment is corrected by rotation straps. The skin and foot circulation are regularly assessed for blistering and venous engorgement. *e*, A *hip spica*.

If knee flexion is less than 90° at 4–6 months a manipulation can be carried out under general anaesthesia, or reverse dynamic slings applied. Elongation or freeing of the quadriceps may be desired.

Femoral Shaft Fractures in Children

In children under 2 years, or less than 15 kg, gallows traction is used for 2–3 weeks (*see under* Trochanteric fractures, for complications). Some centres routinely use a hip spica immediately rather than risk ischaemic and skin problems. Older children are placed on a Thomas' splint for 2–3 weeks with skin traction (*see Fig.* 7.19*b*) (either to achieve or maintain reduction), and then given a hip spica for 1 month. Always check circulation and skin in the affected limb daily.

Special note: In children non-union is *not a feature*, internal fixation is *not* required, overgrowth of the femur in the injured limb is *not* a problem. Shortening often resolves by 2 years. However, in children over 10 years, shortening, if over 2 cm (due to overlap of fragments), may only slowly alter. Thus with a femoral shaft fracture in this age group (over 10's) traction is used for 4 weeks and the position checked by weekly X-rays.

Fractures of the Lower Femur: Supracondylar

Although the supracondylar fracture (*Fig.* 7.22) does occur within the lower third these fractures demand special consideration because they may involve the knee and often occur in the elderly with porotic bones. It is also worth noting that vascular injuries occur less commonly with fractures of the

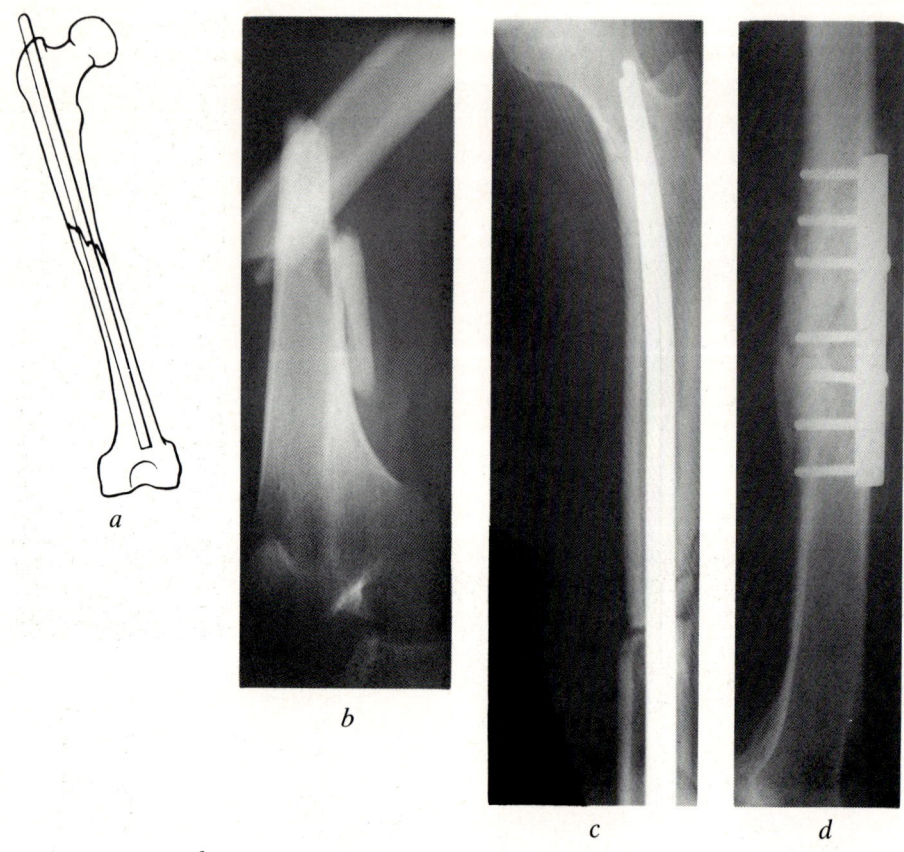

Fig. 7.20. *a*, The internal fixation of a femoral shaft fracture by a Küntscher nail. *b, c*, Ender's nails. *d*, A compression plate (at 6 months).

lower third and that the standard intramedullary nail gives *useless* fixation because of the flared distal femur.

These fractures are:
Undisplaced: Transverse (including epiphyseal) or T-shaped.
　　　　　　Avulsion (from condyles).
　　　　　　Unicondylar (may be lateral or medial).
Displaced: Oblique or transverse or unicondylar.
　　　　　　Comminuted (involving femoral shaft).

Diagnosis
Usually an elderly patient falls on to the flexed knee. There is immediate pain and swelling with effusion. The lower fragment may be tilted backwards by the gastrocnemius.

Treatment
The knee is aspirated and a plaster cylinder applied for 4–6 weeks (a hinge can be used) in *undisplaced* fractures.

163 Fractures of the pelvis, thigh and knee

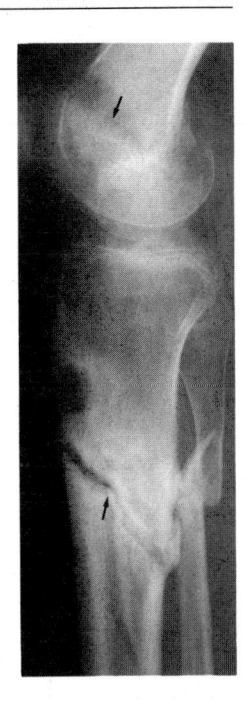

Fig. 7.21. The 'floating knee' in a 20-year-old involved in a road traffic accident, treated conservatively in a plaster for 8 weeks, result at 6 months.

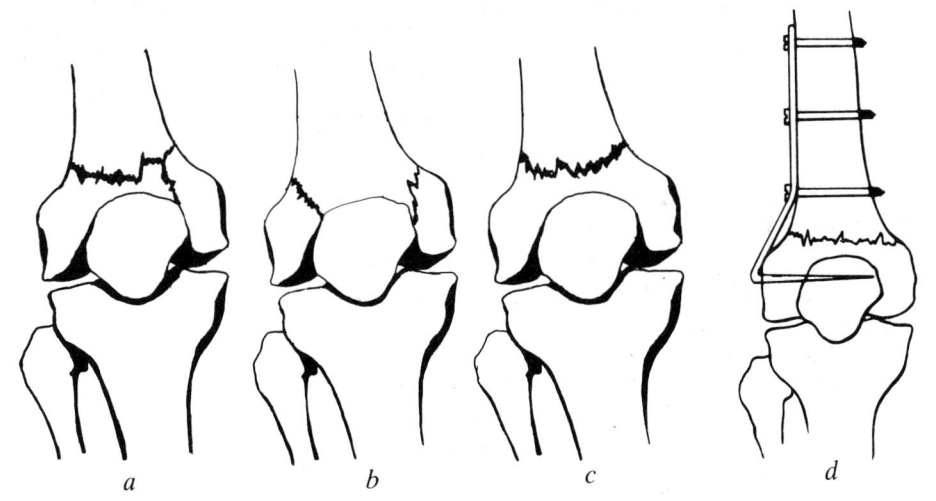

Fig. 7.22. Classification of femoral supracondylar fracture. *a*, T-shaped. *b*, Lateral or medial condyle. *c*, Transverse. *d*, Fixation with a condylar blade-plate.

With *displaced* fractures internal fixation with a supracondylar blade-plate (*Fig.* 7.22d) or screws are required with accurate reduction of the femoral articular surface. A plaster may be used for 2–4 weeks if there is any doubt about stability, otherwise early knee movements are encouraged. *Epiphyseal* injuries need gentle reduction and plaster immobilization for 4 weeks; arrest of growth is fairly infrequent.

With *non-union* (usually comminuted fractures) a blade-plate and bone graft can be used but in very refractory cases an intramedullary nail can be driven through the femur and across the knee and removed when union has occurred at 6–9 months; or early ambulation with a cast-brace is used for 6–8 weeks.

• Fractures of the Patella

These may be *undisplaced* or *displaced* (*Fig.* 7.23) but are almost always intra-articular. They may be caused by direct trauma or a muscle-pull in sport.

They are divided into:
1. Osteochondral fracture.
2. Transverse.
3. Stellate or comminuted.
4. Avulsion of inferior pole (not intra-articular).

Diagnosis
Knee pain and swelling, often with a palpable gap in the patella.

Treatment
Undisplaced fractures need aspiration of haemarthrosis, a plaster cylinder for 1 month then quadriceps exercises and knee mobilization.

Displaced fractures need accurate reduction or osteoarthrosis eventually develops at the patellofemoral joint. With *transverse* fractures a compression screw is used; with *comminution* but only *slight* displacement, a cerclage or tension-band wiring is the method of choice. With a *small, loose fragment* the piece can be excised. However, with *severe comminution* the patella is completely excised.

Quadriceps exercises begin after 24 hours but exercises to regain flexion and hyperextension commence at 2–4 weeks depending on the surgical technique used. The limb is rested in a plaster backslab for 1–2 weeks.

Avulsion of the *inferior pole* may occur in vigorous sport; this is not an intra-articular fracture and does not need open reduction. A plaster or thick crêpe-and-wool (Jones support) is used for 2–3 weeks.

Complications
These include quadriceps weakness after patellectomy, knee stiffness and osteoarthrosis if a step remains in the patella. (N.B. Congenital bipartite patella often occurs in both knees and the edges are smooth. Fractures are rare at the upper lateral corner of the patella where this condition is seen.)

• Dislocation of the Patella (including subluxation)

Lateral dislocation (or subluxation) (*see Fig.* 2.19) is a common knee problem in teenage girls (medial subluxation is rare).

165 Fractures of the pelvis, thigh and knee

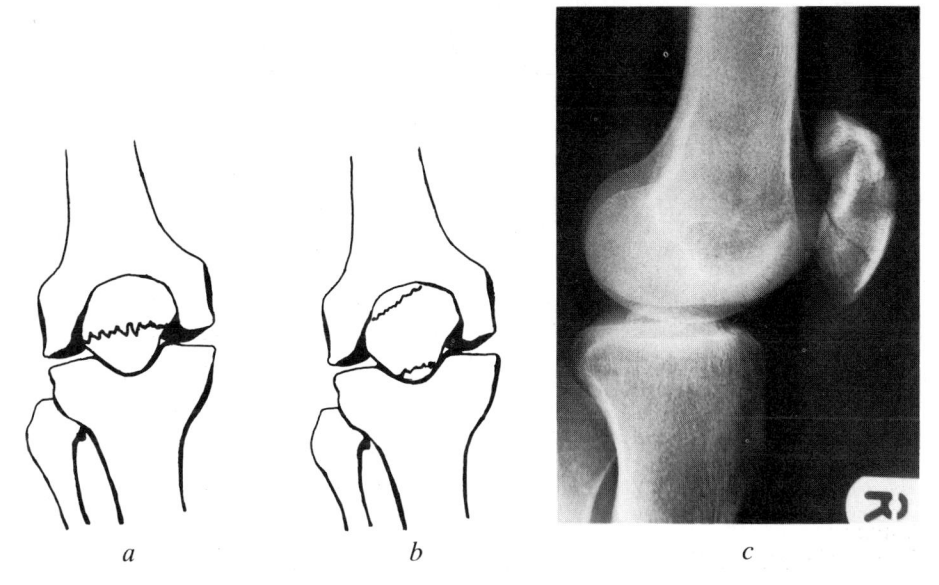

Fig. 7.23. Classification of a patellar fracture. *a*, Transverse. *b*, Upper and lower poles. *c*, Comminuted.

The condition may be associated with capsular laxity or familial joint hypermobility, a high patella (patella alta), a deficient lateral condyle, fibrosis of vastus lateralis, or a valgus knee.

The displacing force is usually a blow on the inner aspect.

The patella may spontaneously reduce or require an anaesthetic—the former is much more frequent.

Diagnosis
The patient points to the area of dislocation (laterally) and recounts how the knee 'gave way' or 'snapped back' into position. Clinical examination reveals instability of the medial supporting structures as the patella is pushed laterally.

Treatment
With the first dislocation the knee may need aspiration and a plaster cylinder applied for 2–3 weeks. With recurrent dislocation the retinaculum on the outer aspect is incised and the medial retinaculum overlapped to affect medial placement.

(A patellar tendon transplant to a lower, medial situation on the tibia risks undue compression of the patella on the femoral condyle and osteoarthrosis). Any osteochondral fragment detached from the patella (or occasionally femoral condyle) needs removal from the knee.

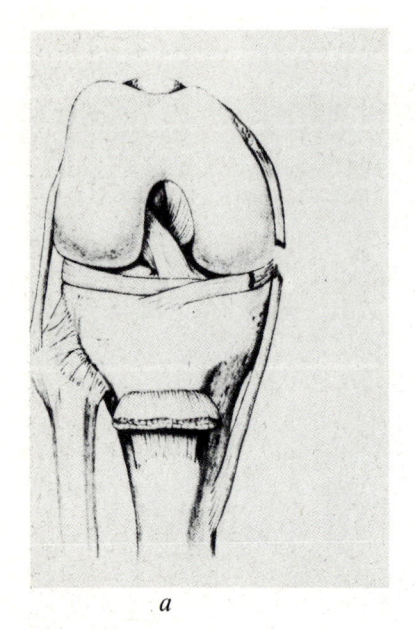

Fig. 7.24. *a*, Medial ligament injury. *b*, Stress film (the air in the joint outlines the medial meniscus).

- **Ligament Injuries in the Knee***
  - *Isolated ligament injuries are uncommon, the intimate proximity of all these structures renders whole groups vulnerable to injury either by direct or indirect forces.*
  - *The importance of the close attachment of the capsule is often forgotten in the search for ligamentous damage; stretching or avulsion of the capsule adds greatly to instability.*
  - *Many muscles blend with the capsule (e.g. semimembranosus into the posterior capsule) and act as dynamic stabilizers. Good muscle tone can, in many respects, compensate for some ligamentous weakness.*
  - *Knee ligaments can be damaged with femoral and tibial shaft fractures, the soft-tissue injury being overshadowed by the fracture.*

With *collateral ligaments* (*medial* and *lateral*) the joint becomes unstable at 30° of flexion when the anterior cruciate is relaxed. *Strains* and *partial* tears are treated with strapping or crêpe support for 2–3 weeks (*see* Chapter 1). Such injuries usually involve the superficial component.

---

* N.B. These injuries have been fully detailed in *Injuries in Sport*, Wright-PSG and only a short synopsis is given here.

167 Fractures of the pelvis, thigh and knee

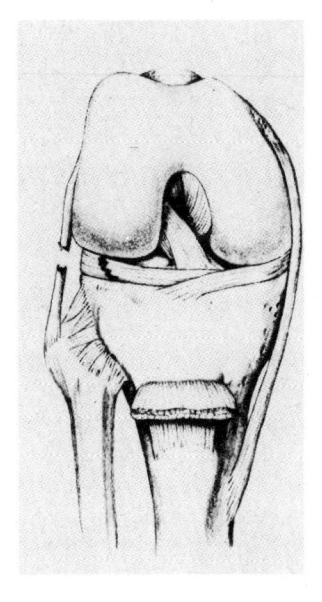

Fig. 7.25. *a*, Lateral ligament injury. *b*, Avulsion of the fibular head by the lateral ligament.

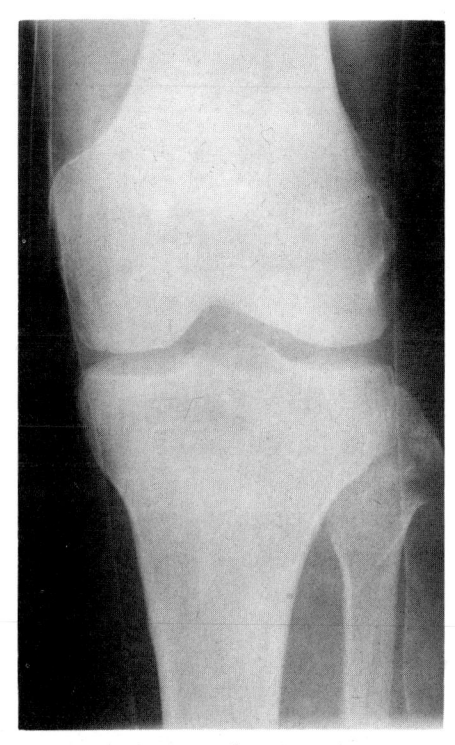

Medial Ligament (*Fig.* 7.24)
Complete tears usually involve both the superficial and deep components; abduction stress at 30° indicates instability. There may be an avulsion fracture from the condyles or a medial meniscus injury. The ligament is repaired. However, if other structures are not involved conservative treatment with a plaster (above knee) for 4–6 weeks gives equally good results in some series as operative treatment.

Lateral Ligament (*Fig.* 7.25)
The adduction stress test at 30° indicates complete tearing and the ligament is repaired with a plaster for 4–6 weeks.

Anterior Cruciate (*Fig.* 7.26)
A blow on the knee causing hyperextension accompanied by a sudden 'pop' may indicate a complete tear (or avulsion of the anterior tibial spine). With the knee flexed to 90° the tibia can be drawn forward. The Lachman test (*Fig.* 7.26e) correlates better with an isolated anterior cruciate tear than does the anterior drawer test. Isolated tears can be repaired or the avulsed spine re-attached. Good thigh muscle tone can compensate for a lax anterior cruciate if the diagnosis has been missed or repair has been inefficient. Synthetic

168 An outline of fractures and dislocations

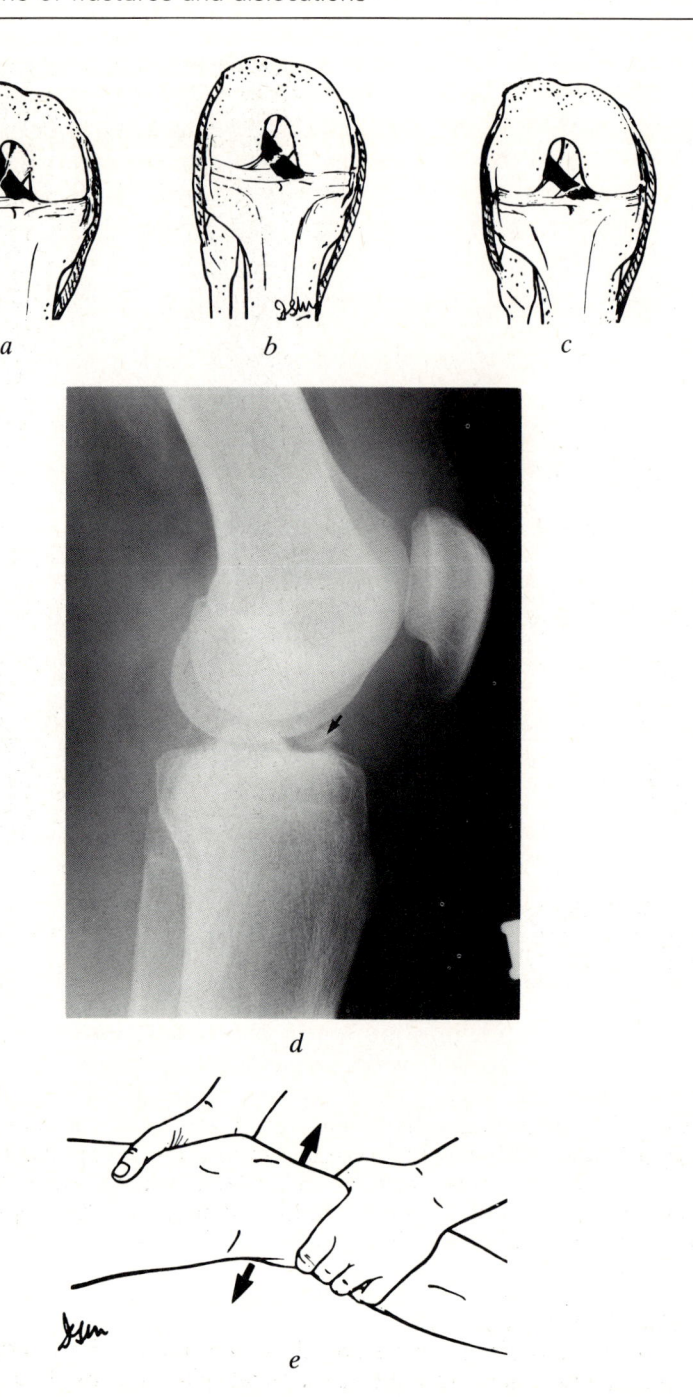

Fig. 7.26. Anterior cruciate tears at upper (*a*); middle (*b*); and lower (*c*), levels; when there may be avulsion of the anterior tibial spine (*d*); *e*, Lachman test showing mobility of the tibia on the steadied thigh.

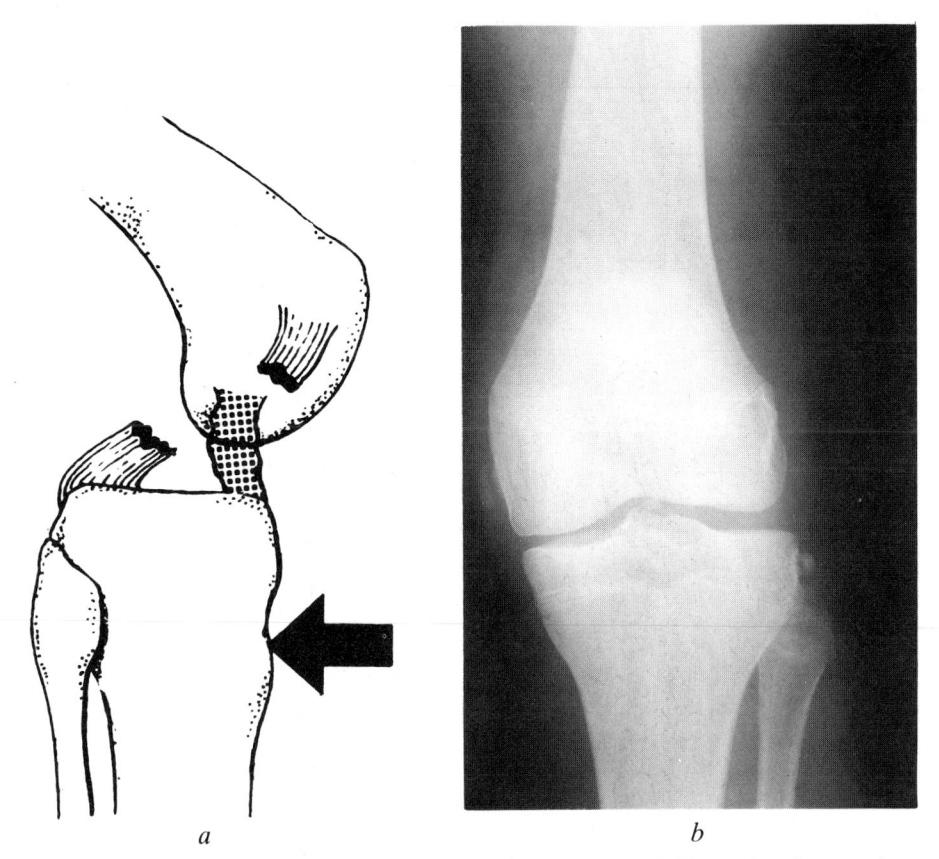

Fig. 7.27. *a,* Posterior cruciate injury. *b,* An unusual X-ray showing previous damage to the medial ligament, lateral ligament and avulsion of the posterior cruciate (posterior spine).

materials (Terylene and carbon fibre, etc.) have been used to replace badly damaged ligaments but their success over the long term has not been fully evaluated. Fascial strips (e.g. patellar retinaculum) and tendons (e.g. semitendinosus) have been used with limited success. After repair a plaster is worn for 4–6 weeks in extension.

Posterior Cruciate (*Fig.* 7.27)
There is a positive drawer test; the tear is often in the mid-portion or from the femoral attachment; sometimes the tibial spine is avulsed. Direct repair can be carried out and a plaster applied in 45° of flexion for 4–6 weeks. Tendon transfers and synthetic materials have been used for chronic posterior cruciate instability with limited success (*see* Anterior cruciate).

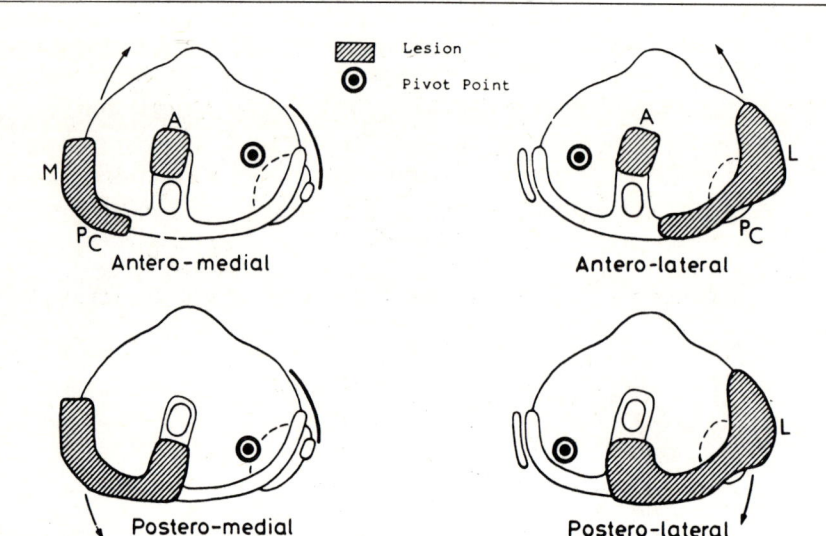

Fig. 7.28. Patterns of rotatory instability.

Rotatory Instability (*Fig.* 7.28)

With an *intact posterior cruciate* the tibia commonly rotates in an *anteromedial* or *anterolateral* direction depending on which ligaments are damaged. With the knee flexed to 90° the foot is rotated and the tibia pulled first forwards and then pushed backwards when any abnormal movements of the tibial condyles can be seen. With anteromedial instability, for example, the medial tibial plateau becomes prominent with external rotation of the foot and anterior pulling. A positive anterior drawer sign in neutral rotation with prominence of the lateral tibial condyle indicates anterolateral instability.

In the 'jerk' test the valgus loaded knee is extended from 90° of flexion and between 30–15° a jerk is experienced as the lateral tibial condyle subluxes anteriorly and then reduces.

For *anteromedial* instability surgical repair of the medial and anterior cruciate ligaments is performed with either partial meniscectomy or preservation of the medial meniscus. Sometimes the damaged medial meniscus has to be excised. With *anterolateral* instability the anterior cruciate and lateral meniscus are resutured (if the meniscus is badly torn it is excised). The lateral ligament and iliotibial tract are also repaired.

After repair the limb is immobilized in a long leg plaster with 30° of flexion for 3 weeks and a hinged cast brace applied for 4 weeks.

Sometimes a combination of anteromedial and anterolateral instability exists and may only be diagnosed with the patient under a general anaesthetic; prior to surgery both instabilities must be tested even if one is apparent clinically.

Posterolateral rotatory instability is less common but early repair of the posterolateral soft tissues (cruciate ligament, lateral ligament, capsule, gastrocnemius and popliteus) gives good results.

oblique tear   transverse tear   anterior horn tear

posterior horn tear   bucket handle tear

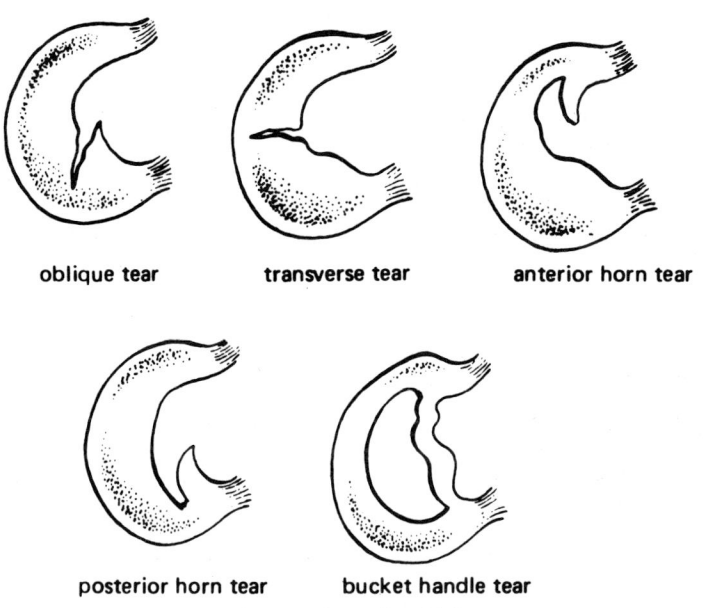

Fig. 7.29. Types of meniscal injury.

- **Meniscal Injuries** (*Fig.* 7.29)
    These are:
1. Subluxation (usually anterior horn).
2. Peripheral tear (usually mid-portion).
3. Partial tear (oblique, bucket-handle).
4. Horizontal tear.

    • *Every effort must be made to preserve the meniscus, especially if there is ligamentous injury. The worst results of any knee ligament injury occur when the meniscus has been removed.*
    • *The meniscus acts as a weight-bearing, load-distributing cruciate in the horizontal situation, preventing lateral or medial subluxation of the femoral condyles on the tibial plateau. They prevent shear forces and fissuring or blistering of the hyaline cartilage, i.e. eventual osteoarthrosis. Removal of the meniscus is equivalent to removal of a cruciate.* (N.B. Thus, if the anterior cruciate is damaged and a medial meniscectomy is performed, two out of three restraining structures are torn; when the medial collateral is injured it is then three out of three and gross disruption!)
    With anterior horn subluxation, a partial tear or a horizontal tear there is instability but generally no locking; with a bucket handle tear or a peripheral detachment there is locking as well. Only when there are numerous tears (footballer's meniscus), transverse tears or major detachment is a total meniscectomy performed: otherwise small tags or the bucket-handle are removed, leaving the intact meniscus behind (*partial* meniscectomy). Small peripheral tears or anterior horn subluxations are repaired and the results are good (*see Injuries in Sport* for a full account).

- **Other Knee Injuries**

Avulsion of the tibial spines (*see Figs.* 7.26d, 7.27b). These are in reality cruciate injuries but easily treated. The anterior tibial spine is reduced in 5° flexion of the knee (*not* full extension); if irreducible it can be fixed with a small pin or screw or pullthrough wire. A plaster is worn for 6 weeks. Rarely is the posterior tibial spine avulsed—it may require internal fixation.

Avulsion of the tibial tubercle or *tibial apophysis* (acute Osgood-Schlatter's syndrome) requires a plaster cylinder for 3–4 weeks in extension to relax the patellar tendon. *Avulsion of the inferior pole of the patella* is similarly treated.

Dislocation of the knee is a rare but *very serious injury* with a 30% incidence of popliteal artery and posterior tibial nerve disruption. The cruciates are completely torn. The femoral condyles may pass anterior, posterior or lateral to the tibial plateaux; or there may be an associated tibial condylar fracture. Reduction is urgently carried out, an aspiration of haemarthrosis performed and a plaster backslab given for 1 week. The knee can be assessed for stability and operative intervention performed to repair torn structures. When there are condylar fractures these are fixed with screws or pins. Often the results with limited repair are surprisingly good.

8

Fractures of the leg, ankle and foot

●Upper Tibial Fractures—Condylar

A fall from a height or a direct blow, e.g. from a car bumper, can cause an upper tibial fracture (*Fig. 8.1a*). The knee ligaments may be torn at the same time (*see* Chapter 1).

Fractures are *undisplaced* or *displaced*:
lateral condyle (60%)
medial condyle (15%)
both (i.e. comminuted) (25%)

Undisplaced fractures are treated by aspiration of the haemarthrosis and a plaster cylinder for 4 weeks. Crutches or a frame are used during this period to prevent compression and displacement.

● **It is often advantageous to use a crêpe-and-wool support after aspiration in the fit adult who can easily manage crutches.** Quadriceps exercises begin as soon as possible. Some centres advocate restricted weight-bearing for 12 weeks to avoid undue compression.

Displaced fractures require accurate reduction and internal fixation (*Fig. 8.1b*). However, the contralateral ligament injuries may require suture. A cast brace or plaster cylinder is worn for 2–3 weeks, then mobilization begins. When there is comminution a bone graft may also be required. The extent of the comminution can be assessed by computerized tomography before surgery, if necessary. Since this fracture is intra-articular the most frequent complication is localized osteoarthrosis. Fractures of the upper fibula may also coexist.

● **Fractures of the Tibial Shaft** (with fibular fractures)
● *The tibia and fibula are commonly broken together* (*Fig. 8.2*), **but because of the tibia's subcutaneous position infection and non-union are more common than in any other long bone fracture.** The tibia (and fibula) can be considered in three areas: upper (excluding condylar), middle and lower thirds (excluding malleoli).

The fibula carries at least one-sixth of the static loading on the leg and the presence of the intact fibula indicates a less severe trauma than when both bones are broken, thus the prognosis for tibial union is better in one respect: however,

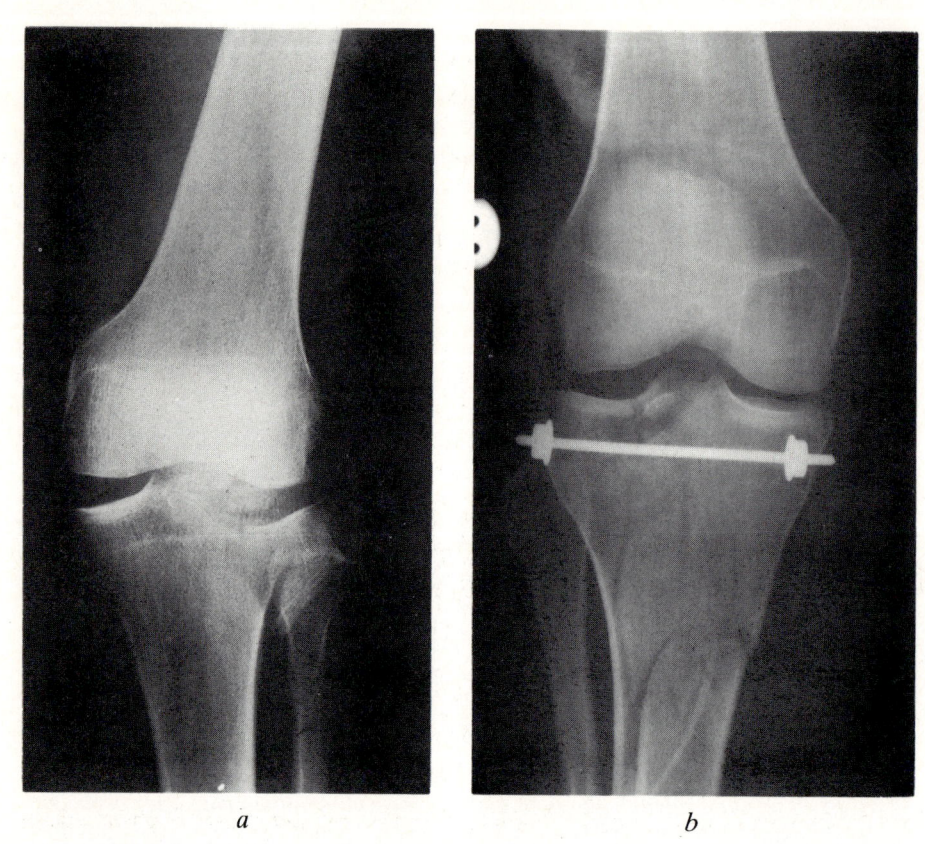

Fig. 8.1. *a*, A fracture of the lateral tibial condyle. *b*, Accurately reduced fracture fixed with a Webb screw.

since the fibula tends to act as a spring the tibial fracture is rotated internally leading to a varus deformity and a maintained gap.
- *Up to 26% of patients with an intact fibula may show delayed or non-union plus angulation.*

Because of the stabilizing effect of the fibula and interosseous membrane there is no more shortening at 1 or 2 weeks than seen on the initial X-ray.

- **Stable Fracture**
1. Stress
2. Greenstick
3. Transverse
4. Short oblique
5. Intact fibula
6. Epiphyseal injuries

Stress Fractures

Stress fractures are found in the tibia and fibula due to bone failure in repeated loading, such as road-running, jogging, etc. There is local bone tenderness and X-rays usually show the crack (with sclerosis), although in the early stages an isotope study may be needed. These fractures respond to rest for 2–3 months.

Greenstick, Transverse and Short Oblique Fractures (*Fig. 8.2a,b,c*)

Common from kicks in soccer and direct impact during a fall.

Diagnosis

There is local bone tenderness, usually in the middle third of the tibia where this fracture is common. The fibula is usually fractured. Many are undisplaced.

Treatment

If there is displacement the fracture is reduced by either allowing the leg to hang vertically with the knee flexed over the plaster table (gravity-assisted) or by gentle traction with the knee slightly flexed over a plaster post. Since the bone is subcutaneous the accuracy of reduction is easily verified. A long leg plaster is applied for 4–6 weeks and gentle weight-bearing can begin at 3–4 weeks; or a cast brace (patella-bearing) can be used for 6–8 weeks. X-rays are taken at weeks 1 and 3.

Complications

These will be discussed at the end of the section.

Tibial Fractures with an Intact Fibula

These are usually easily reduced but the fracture must be observed for rotation and angulation with X-rays at 1 and 3 weeks. A plaster is worn for 6 weeks (as above).

Epiphyseal Injuries

Epiphyseal injuries of the lower tibia (*Fig. 8.2d*) may be displaced and are occasionally confused with an ankle fracture. Reduction is easy and a plaster worn for 3–4 weeks. Injuries to the *upper tibial epiphysis* are rare but occasionally displacement leads to popliteal vessel damage. The treatment is as for lower epiphyseal injuries. Scanograms to estimate leg length are required yearly until fusion.

- **Unstable Fractures**
1. Spiral or sharp oblique (*Fig. 8.2e*)
2. Comminuted (*Fig. 8.2f*)
3. Segmental (*Fig. 8.2g*)
4. Small segment above the ankle (*Fig. 8.2h*)

176 An outline of fractures and dislocations

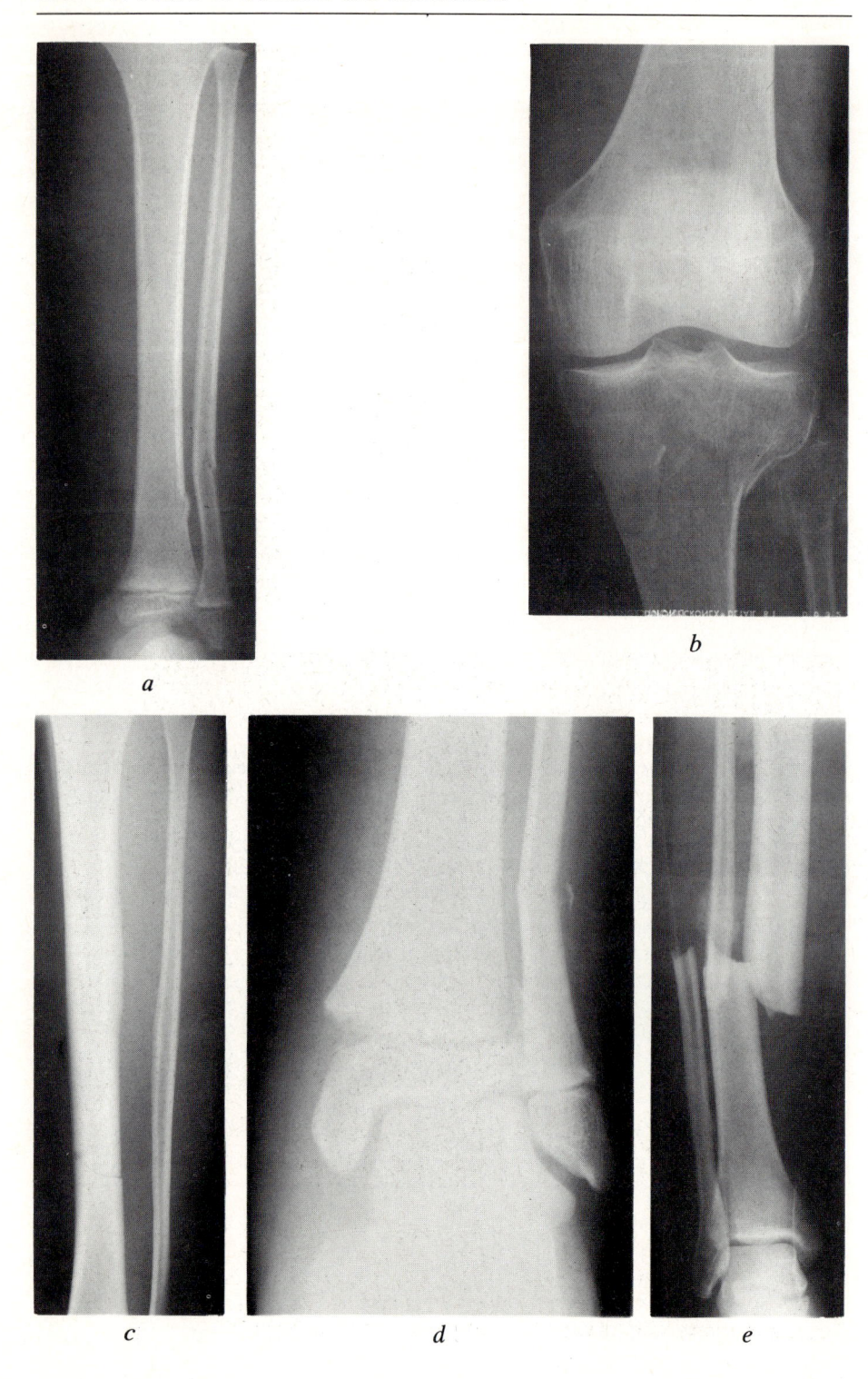

a

b

c *d* *e*

177 Fractures of the leg, ankle and foot

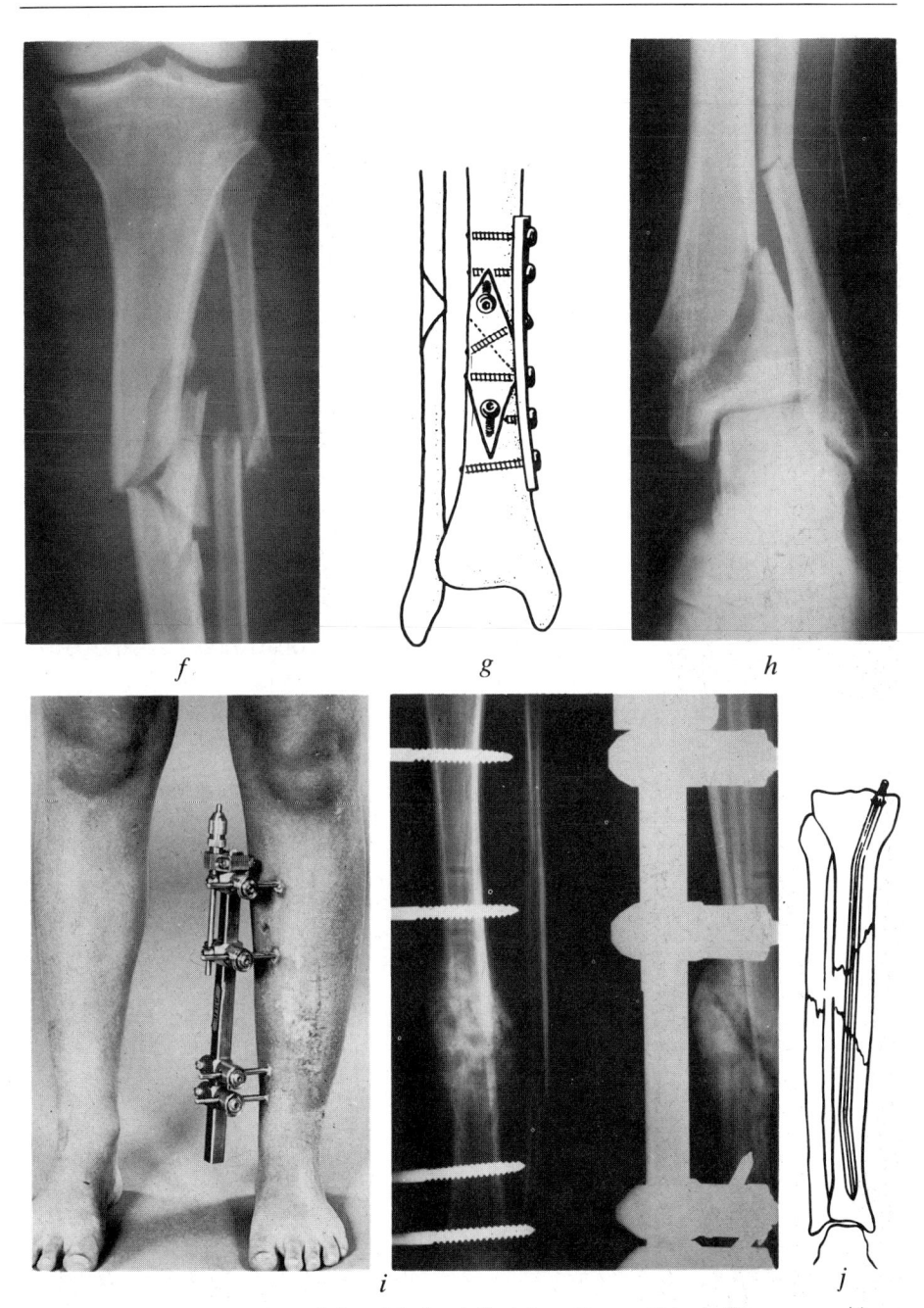

Fig. 8.2. Fractures of the tibia (and fibula). *a*, Greenstick. *b*, Transverse (there may be lateral popliteal nerve damage). *c*, Midshaft tibia (typical soccer injury). *d*, Epiphyseal injury. *e*, Displaced oblique (unstable). *f*, Compound, comminuted (unstable). *g*, Plating (compression). *h*, Lower tibia with valgus angulation (may resemble a Potts fracture clinically). *i*, External fixation device. *j*, Intramedullary nail.

Diagnosis
The swelling and deformity are obvious. These fractures are often compound and the wound dictates surgical treatment. They are generally found in the upper and middle thirds.

Treatment
An attempt is made at closed reduction but if the fracture cannot be aligned a *spiral* or *sharp oblique* fracture (*without a wound*) is usually treated by a screw or compression plate fixation. The patient is mobilized as soon as operative discomfort allows. With *comminuted* or a *segmental fracture* the leg is reduced under general anaesthesia and transfixed with pins above and below the fracture line. These pins are incorporated either in a plaster or in an external fixation device. The latter method is preferable because it allows regular three-dimensional adjustment (*Fig. 8.2i*). It is used for 6–12 weeks depending on union. A segmental fracture can also be treated by an intramedullary nail (*Fig. 8.2j*) inserted close to the tibial tubercle. The method of alignment through a pin in the calcaneus (with traction) has been largely supplanted by the external fixation device.

With a *compound* injury the wound is excised. If it is situated away from the fracture, is small and adequately excised, the fracture can be treated by plating or screw fixation. With a larger wound an intramedullary nail can be inserted from above. Generally, it is wise to avoid metal fixation when there is danger of infection and an external fixation device or cast-brace is used depending upon the relative degree of stability after reduction.

Small segment fractures of the lower tibia should be stable since they are often transverse but slight dorsiflexion of the foot in plaster tilts the fragment backwards; it is corrected by allowing 5–10% of equinus. The plaster is worn for 6 weeks.

Complications
1. *Non-union.* 20% of compound fractures may suffer this complication, usually treated by bone-grafting and compression plating; electromagnetic techniques can be used (Chapter 3). A technique using a vascular pedicle graft of fibula has recently been introduced.
2. *Infection.* Acute infection needs antibiotics, special consideration is given for tetanus and gas gangrene; chronic infections may need excision of sequestrum and long-term antibiotics.
3. *Skin loss.* May require transfer of flaps, or a pedicle graft from the other leg.
4. *Malunion, rotation, angulation, shortening.* These are common in comminuted fractures and where there has been bone loss.
5. *Associated rupture of the knee collateral ligaments* can occur in 10% of cases, especially when there is comminution (*Fig. 8.3*).
6. *Compartmental syndromes.* These are due to extensive soft-tissue swelling in the four leg compartments, the deep posterior compartment being especially vulnerable. Pain and anaesthesia occur usually in the distribution of the posterior tibial nerve. If the pressure is raised when measured directly or if there is a suggestion clinically, the fascia is split, and a skin graft may be required.

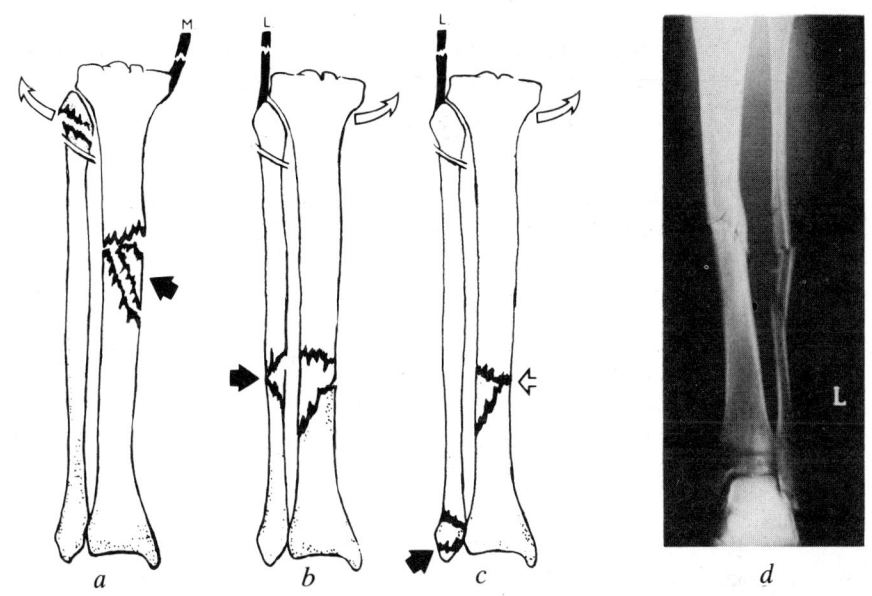

Fig. 8.3. Patterns of knee ligament injury with tibial shaft fractures (*a,b,c* refer to level of fibula fracture). *d*, This 30-year-old man had a lateral ligament injury.

7. *Osteoarthrosis of the ankle.* An alteration in the alignment of the tibia causes undue stress on the ankle joint and eventual osteoarthrosis; in addition, long periods of immobilization in plaster lead to joint changes. The tibial deformity should be corrected by an osteotomy and internal fixation, except in the infirm and elderly, when a calliper can be used.
8. *Associated fractures of the femur* (floating knee) (*see* Chapter 7).
9. *Clawing of the toes, intermuscular adhesions (calf)* may occur from muscle ischaemia or adhesions between the fracture area and the gastrocnemius–soleus complex. These require surgical release or Achilles tendon lengthening.
10. *Persistent valgus deformity* with angulation of a lateral condylar fracture which has compressed under weight-bearing.

● *A special note must be made about infected non-union.* This occurs when the plate has been removed because of infection and the fracture fails to unite or a refracture occurs. The dead bone must be removed and a graft can be applied through an incision (usually posterior) with use of the fibula as a strut.

● **Fractures of the Fibula Shaft Alone**

Fractures of the *shaft* alone (*Fig.* 8.4) are found in soccer and other contact sports. No reduction is required and either a firm strapping or a below-knee walking plaster is used for 3 weeks. With *avulsion* fracture of the head of the fibula the lateral ligament complex is weakened—a plaster cylinder is used for 4 weeks.

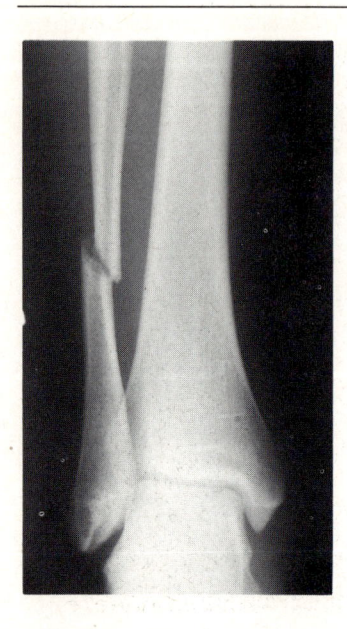

Fig. 8.4. Fibula shaft fracture.

- **Dislocation of the Superior Tibiofibular Joint**
    This is a very uncommon injury (*Fig.* 8.5) due to a fall from a height (parachuting) and described in soccer players, due to a sudden inversion and plantar flexion of the foot pulling the peroneal tendons and extensors of the toes which in turn displace the fibula (anterior). A posterior dislocation occurs with direct violence and a twisting injury to the knee. With the knee flexed the head can usually be replaced by direct pressure under general anaesthesia. A plaster cylinder is used for 2–4 weeks.

- **Fractures and Dislocations of the Ankle**
    - *The ankle is a hinge joint capable of moving in one plane (flexion/extension). This stability has its drawbacks with abnormal force either tearing the related ligaments or fracturing the malleoli (which fit snugly around the talus).*

Sprains and Subluxation of the Ankle
    Such injuries (*Fig.* 8.6) are due to *internal rotation* and *inversion* with a sprain to the lateral ligaments. (N.B. An external rotation and eversion force usually produces fractured malleoli). The weak *anterior talofibular* ligament (anterior slip) tears first; continued inversion leads to disruption of the calcaneofibular (medial slip) and posterior talofibular ligaments (posterior slip). Two out of three ligaments torn leads to gross inversion instability on stress X-rays.

181 Fractures of the leg, ankle and foot

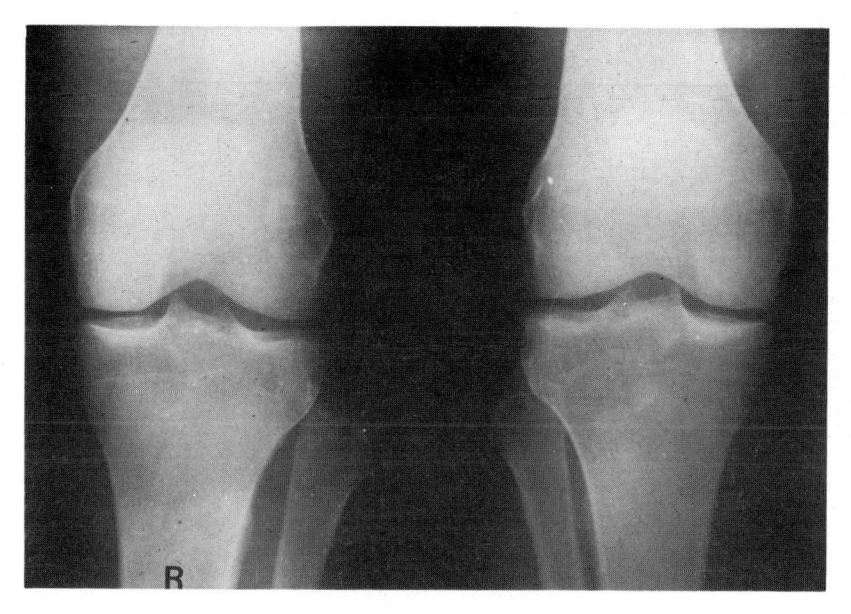

Fig. 8.5. Anterior dislocation of the R superior tibiofibular joint (note prominent fibular head). (Films reversed for comparison.)

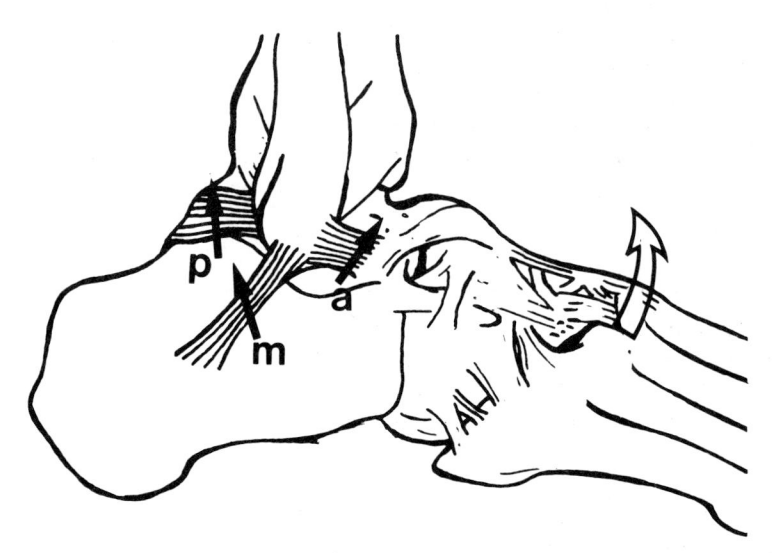

Fig. 8.6. Lateral ligament injuries at the ankle: **a** = anterior slip (anterior talofibular); **m** = middle slip (calcaneofibular); **p** = posterior slip (posterior talofibular).

Forced *plantar flexion* disrupts the anterior slip of both the lateral and medial (deltoid) ligaments and the anterior capsule. This leads to abnormal anterior *subluxation* of the talus in the ankle mortise.

Diagnosis
Tenderness over the affected ligaments with positive stress X-rays or arthrogram in severe cases. With anterior subluxation there may be an abnormal anterior drawer test when the lower tibia is stabilized with one hand and the other grips the heel.

Treatment
Minor strains are treated by U-shaped or figure-of-eight strapping. Partial tears need a below-knee walking plaster for 3–4 weeks. Complete tears require operative repair and plaster immobilization for 4 weeks. Intensive physiotherapy with 'wobble-board' proprioception exercises are needed.

Complications
1. *Acute lateral tears* can become *chronic* with localized pain on inversion and a feeling of instability. Occasionally the ankle 'gives way' (chronic subluxation). Although ultrasonics and ankle exercises often help when there is instability, the torn ligament can be incised and repaired if badly scarred, or a tendon transfer operation used to strengthen the lateral ligament. Usually the peroneus brevis is transferred.
2. *Osteochondral fracture* of the dome of the *talus* (5%).
3. *Fractures of the proximal fibula* (occasionally tibia).
4. *Osteoarthrosis of the ankle*, especially medially where the dome of the talus strikes the lower tibia.
5. *Chronic anterior subluxation* can be treated by the excision of a triangular flap in the anterior capsule which is then sutured to the lower tibia and anterior slip with the foot in dorsiflexion. A plaster is worn for 3–4 weeks.

(N.B. *Tears of the deltoid ligament* are rare on their own but coexist with lateral malleolar fractures; often there is an avulsion injury of talus. They require suture and a below-knee plaster for 4 weeks.)

Fractures of the Ankle
Most ankle fractures are caused by an *external rotation force* (*Fig. 8.7*). In addition there may be supination or pronation. In *supination* injuries the fracture is usually *below* the level of the tibiofibular syndesmosis. With *pronation* injuries the fracture is *above* this level.

With *external rotation* forces involved the following stages can be noted:

I: Tearing of the anterior tibiofibular ligament and anterior capsule.
II: A spiral fracture of the lateral malleolus.
III: A fracture of the posterior tibial margin (up to 25%).
IV: A fracture of the medial malleolus or rupture of the deltoid ligament. The talus may be displaced laterally or posterolaterally.

● *The major concern in ankle fractures is the degree of displacement of the talus*. A mortise view of the ankle is required, with the joint rotated internally 20°. With this anteroposterior view the medial joint space should be approximately the same as the lateral joint space. With displacement of the talus over 1 mm there is a 42% loss of contact in the tibiotalar articulation.

Diagnosis
There is marked swelling and deformity around the ankle and X-rays easily determine the fracture.

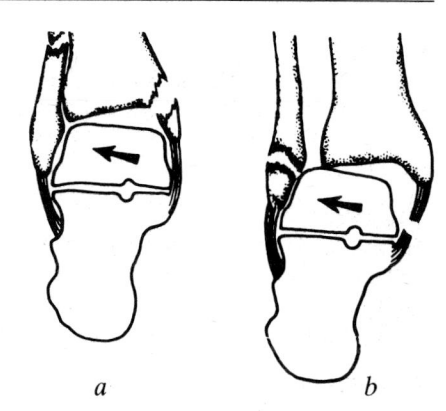

Fig. 8.7. External rotation force causing a fibular fracture: *a*, With pronation. *b*, With supination.

Treatment
Undisplaced Fractures (*Fig. 8.8a,b*)
Undisplaced fractures need a below-knee walking plaster with the foot at a right angle for 4 weeks.

Displaced Fractures (*Figs. 8.8c,d, 8.9*)
These need accurate reduction and closed methods should be performed first. However, because of the marked displacement and swelling it is often difficult to achieve accurate reduction and surgery is regularly required. Soft tissues, especially the tibialis posterior and peroneal tendons, may block reduction. The lateral malleolar fractures can be secured with screws or Rush nails. Medial malleolar fractures need tension band wires or screws; however, too much compression often causes the small fragments to split. It is also important to repair the torn medial or lateral ligament at the same time.

If there is rupture of the syndesmosis and the related interosseous membrane by lateral or posterolateral displacement of the talus (with a fibular fracture above the syndesmosis) the normal length of the fibula must be restored using a semi-tubular 5-holed plate. The syndesmosis and the interosseous membrane can be repaired by direct suture but it is not necessary to transfix the tibia to the fibula with a long screw, for this decreases the rotation in the syndesmosis necessary for normal ankle dorsiflexion. After surgery the limb is placed in a well-padded plaster for 2–4 weeks followed by ankle mobilization exercises. Full weight-bearing is achieved between 6–12 weeks. The circulation must be watched during the first 48 hours after surgery.

Complications
1. *Malalignment* of the talus within the mortise or joint incongruity due to inadequate fixation will lead to *osteoarthrosis* of the ankle.
2. *Malunion* of the fibula may lead to shortening of the malleolus with lateral displacement of the talus. This produces a stiff and painful ankle which eventually becomes osteoarthritic. Osteotomy is required to re-align and lengthen the lateral malleolus.
3. *Non-union* may need freshening of the bone ends and screw fixation, with possible removal of interposing tendon or soft tissues.
4. *Osteoarthrosis of the ankle*.

184 An outline of fractures and dislocations

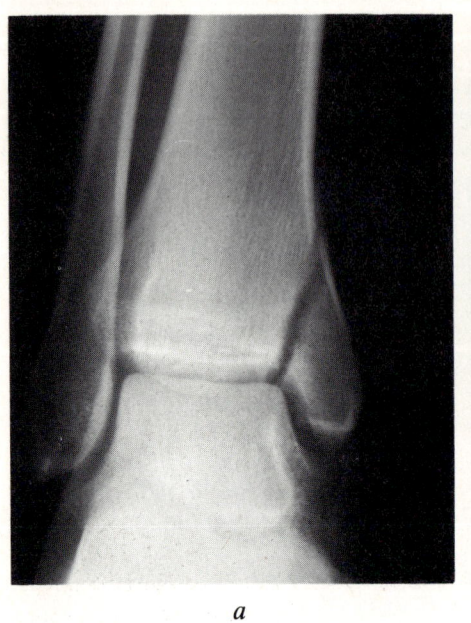

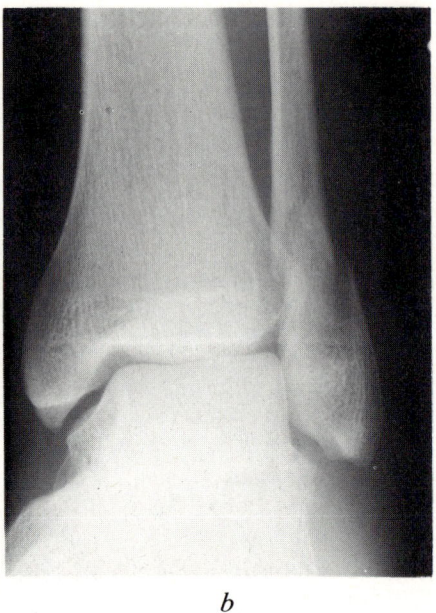

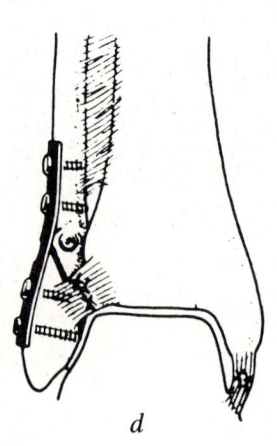

Fig. 8.8. *a*, Undisplaced medial malleolar fracture. *b*, Undisplaced lateral malleolar fracture (there is very slight rotation which needs correction). *c*, Displaced lateral malleolus fracture—note increased joint space medially. *d*, Reduction and fixation with compression plating and ligament repair.

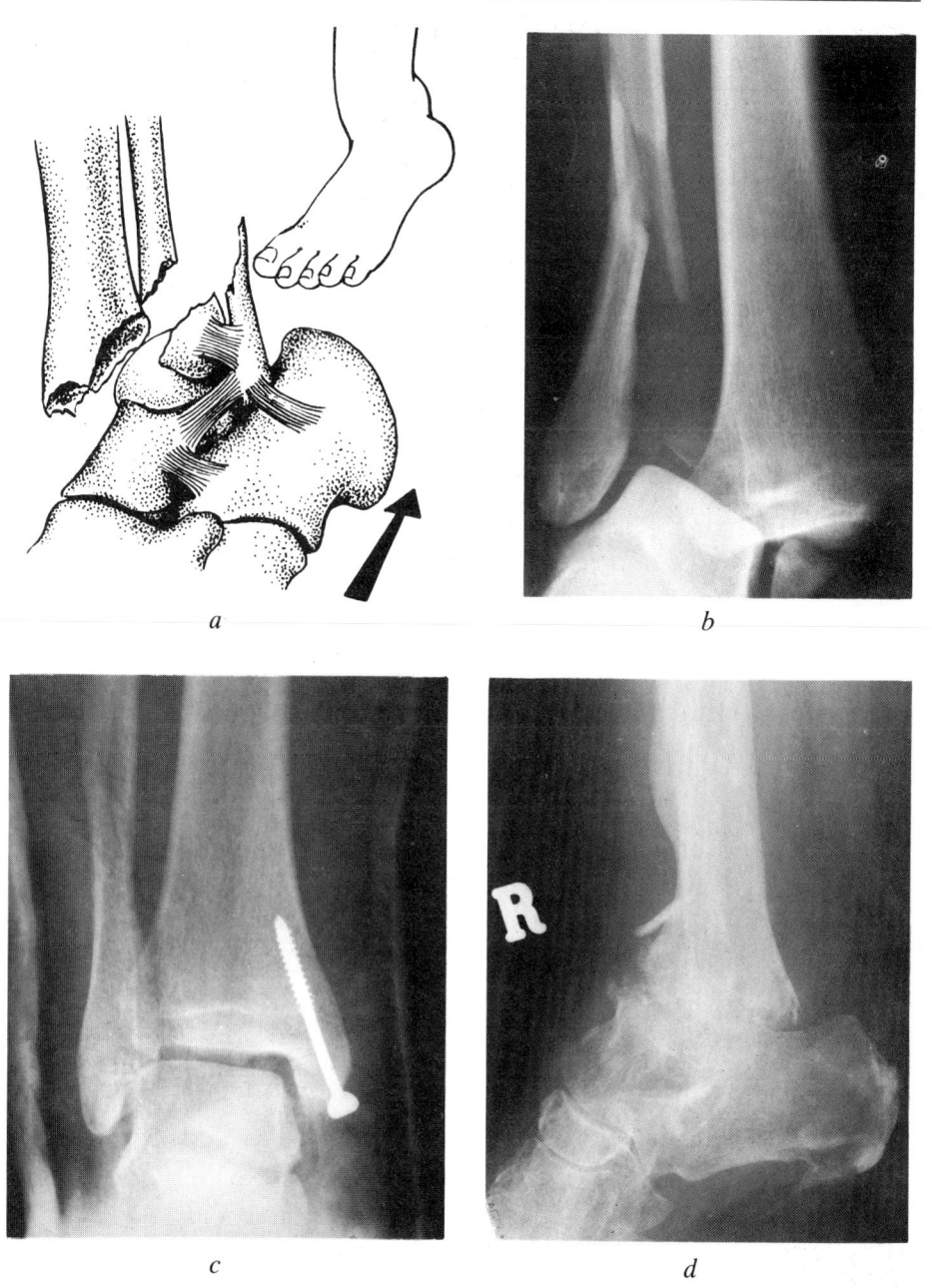

Fig. 8.9. *a*, Fracture-dislocation of the ankle. *b*, Gross disruption with a medial malleolar fracture, lower fibular shaft fracture and displacement of the talus in a 38-year-old man. *c*, Reduction and fixation with a screw (note the fibula is to length, if not a plate would have been applied). Excellent clinical result at 1 year. *d*, A fracture-dislocation 3 years previously in a 40-year-old woman; the talus has undergone avascular necrosis—it was severely displaced initially.

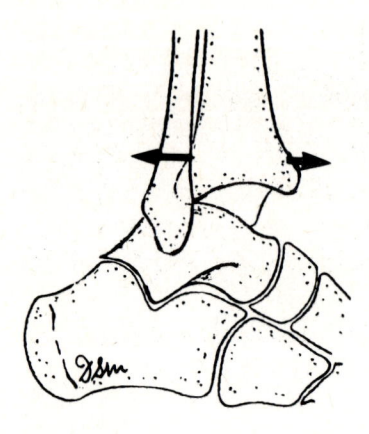

Fig. 8.10. Dislocation of the ankle.

Maisonneuve fracture
Forced external rotation of the foot may cause diastasis of the ankle and a fracture of the fibula just below its neck. The clinician should look carefully for the fibular fracture at this level if there is a deltoid ligament rupture or fracture of the medial malleolus *without* a fracture of the lateral malleolus. Treatment requires plaster for 3–4 weeks with slight displacement, or fixation of the medial malleolus with screws if there is displacement and a light plaster for 4 weeks.

Kerbstone Fracture
This is due to forced plantar flexion producing an avulsion fracture of the posterior tibial margin. It is treated by a below-knee plaster for 3–4 weeks.

Diastasis of the Inferior Tibiofibular Joint
This occurs with an abduction injury, the talus being displaced laterally with the lateral malleolus; the diastasis can be fixed with a transverse screw through the lower fibula into the tibia (*see* Ankle fractures *above*) and removed after 4–6 weeks or a well-moulded plaster used for 4 weeks.

Comminuted Lower Tibial Fractures
These occur with a fall from a height; the calcaneus may also be fractured.

Dislocation of the Ankle Joint (*Fig.* 8.10)
These may be:
Posterior
Anterior
Upward
Lateral

The posterior dislocation is the most common and is due to severe plantar flexion. In all ankle dislocations there may be an associated marginal fracture of the tibia or fibula; with upward dislocation of the talus the fibula usually fractures in its lower third (Dupuytren's fracture) allowing the talus to rest between the tibia and the fibula.

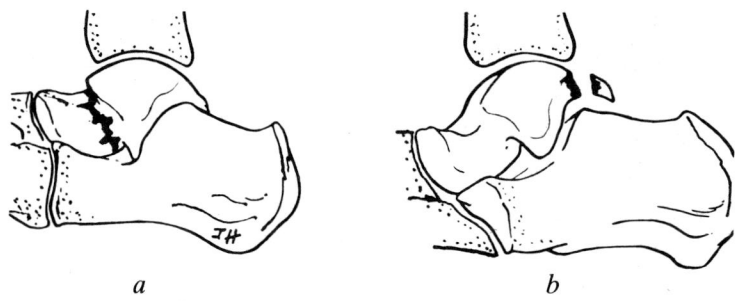

Fig. 8.11. *a*, Fractured neck of talus. *b*, Fractured tubercle of talus.

Diagnosis
There is gross pain and the deformity is obvious.

Treatment
The dislocating force is corrected under general anaesthesia, i.e. with posterior dislocation the foot is dorsiflexed and held in a below-knee plaster for 3–4 weeks in the neutral position. With upward dislocation of the talus the syndesmosis is split and operative intervention is required for replacement. With other forms of dislocation of the ankle joint the fractures may require internal fixation.

Complications
1. The dislocation may be *irreducible*, often due to the displacement of the tibialis posterior tendon or posterior tibial artery and nerve between the medial malleolus and the talus. Operative reduction and internal fixation are required.
2. The fractured *fibula* may become *impacted* behind the tibia and require open reduction (Bosworth fracture).
3. The *dorsalis pedis artery* may become trapped in the extensor retinaculum when there is posterior dislocation of the fibula. Prompt reduction is required to release the damaged vessel. Open reduction and division of the retinaculum is required.
4. *Osteoarthrosis* may develop due to incomplete reduction, irregularity of the fracture line or avascular changes within the talus.

- ### Fractures and Dislocations of the Foot

Fractures and Dislocations of the Talus (*Fig.* 8.11)
The talus may be fractured in the neck, body or tubercle. *Fractures of the neck* are commonly due to road traffic accidents when the brake pedal impacts against the arch of the foot. *Compression fractures* may occur when falling from a height. The tubercle is injured with plantar flexion during sport while jumping or kicking. The posterior tibial margins may also be damaged. The talus may *dislocate* out of the ankle mortise and lie anterior to the lateral malleolus.

188 An outline of fractures and dislocations

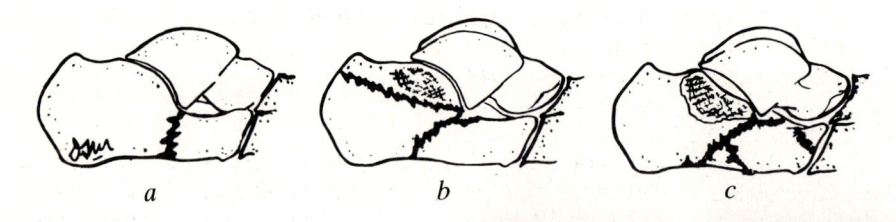

Fig. 8.12. Calcaneal fractures. *a*, Vertical sustenaculum. *b*, Associated with a horizontal fracture to the tuberosity. *c*, Comminuted with anterior process. *d*, Gross comminution with subtalar joint involvement in a 23-year-old scaffold worker who fell 20 feet (also sustaining a fracture of L4).

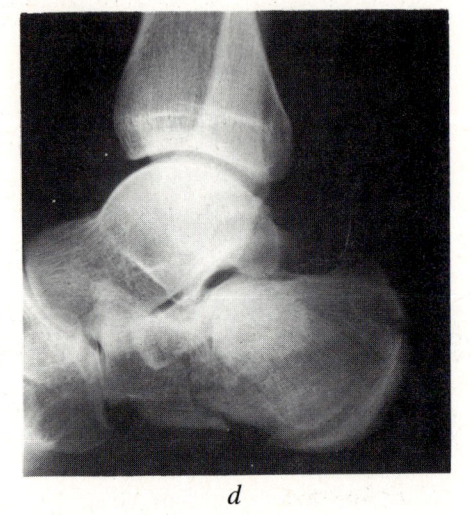

Diagnosis
There is a painful range of ankle movements with associated swelling.

Treatment
With undisplaced fractures closed manipulation can be carried out. However, if there is dislocation and wide separation of the fragments then internal fixation is performed after reduction. A below-knee plaster is used for 4–6 weeks.

Complications
1. *Avascular necrosis.* This occurs when there is a displaced fracture of the talus (*see Fig.* 8.9d).
2. *Non-union and mal-union* may occur after fracture through the neck.
3. *Osteoarthrosis of the subtalar and tibiotalar* joints.
4. *Irreducible dislocation of the talus.* This requires open reduction.
5. *Sheer fractures of the navicular, or avulsion injuries of the metatarsal bones, cuboid and lateral malleolus.*
6. *Formation of loose bodies in the joint from small ostochondral lesions.*

Fractures of the Calcaneus (*Fig.* 8.12)
These are commonly due to a fall from a height and bilateral injuries occur in 20% of cases.
- It is also important to look for associated fractures of the spine, tibia and ankle which occur in 30% of calcaneal fractures. The majority involve the subtalar joint and lead to a permanent degree of stiffness and discomfort.

Fractures of the leg, ankle and foot

Fractures are divided into *displaced* and *undisplaced*:
1. Vertical fracture of the tuberosity.
2. Horizontal fracture of the tuberosity.
3. Fractures of the sustenaculum tali.
4. Fracture of the anterior process.

• *It is important to recognize fractures of the calcaneus with subtalar joint injuries* (*Fig.* 8.12d). There may be a single or several undisplaced cracks into the subtalar joint; or associated with comminution and subtalar joint depression; or with marked spread of the calcaneal fragments.

Diagnosis
The history of a fall from a height with a tender heel requires accurate X-ray evaluation, not only of both heels but also other areas, including the spine.

Treatment
Undisplaced fractures need a below-knee walking plaster for 4 weeks, then partial to full weight-bearing over 6 weeks.

The *displaced* fracture, however, causes many more problems. Closed reduction is often impossible and some centres believe in non-weight-bearing for 6–8 weeks with the limb supported in a crêpe and wool bandage. Other centres believe in open reduction and gentle leverage of the fragments back into position being secured with either screws, stout pins or wires and supplemented by a bone graft.

Complications
1. *Involvement of the subtalar joint* produces pain and stiffness which may require an arthrodesis. Inversion and eversion can be extremely painful.
2. *Painful heel.* Undisplaced fractures may often have localized pain with tenderness over the heel and a diffuse plantar fasciitis.
3. *Stiffness of the foot.* Long immobilization can cause stiffness in the midtarsal region, as well as the subtalar joint.
4. A *chronic stenosing tenosynovitis* of the peroneal tendon below the fibula can cause some foot pain; upward displacement of the tuberosity of the talus can cause relative weakness of the muscles and difficulty in running and jumping.
5. The *sural nerve* may occasionally become stuck behind the ankle and needs freeing.
6. *Osteoarthrosis* may develop and require either a subtalar arthrodesis or a triple arthrodesis. Arthrodesis is best carried out within 6–8 months after the fracture and subtabular arthrodesis by itself may be ineffective in relieving the discomfort. It is often better to carry out arthrodesis of all three joints of the hindfoot.

Fractures of the Navicular (*Fig.* 8.13)

The navicular is the keystone of the medial longitudinal arch. There may be:
1. Stress fracture.
2. An avulsion injury.
3. A fracture of the body.
4. A fracture-dislocation of the body.

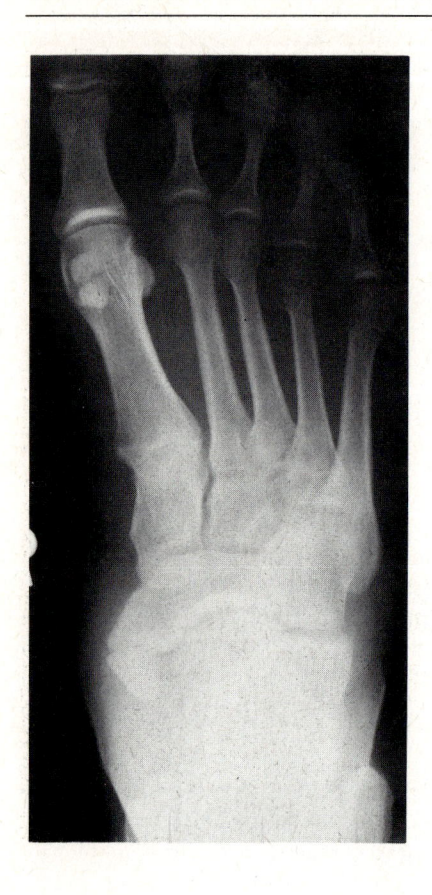

Fig. 8.13. A fracture of the navicular with slight subluxation of the forefoot.

Undisplaced fractures can be treated conservatively with a below-knee plaster for 2–4 weeks; a dislocation may require surgical reduction and fixation with a screw; this is also used if there is bony separation.

Fractures of the Cuboid and Cuneiform Bones
These usually occur as the result of direct violence but there is generally little displacement. Rarely the cuboid or one of the cuneiforms (generally the medial cuneiform) can become dislocated. Open reduction is required with stable fixation with crossed Kirschner wires; a below-knee plaster is used for 4 weeks.

Dislocations and Fracture-dislocations of the Midtarsal Joint
This joint comprises the talonavicular and calcaneocuboid joints. Dislocations are most often medial and generally associated with fractures of the navicular and cuboid. Reduction is usually easily performed and maintained with a below-knee plaster for 4 weeks.

Fracture-dislocations of the Tarsometatarsal Joint (*Fig.* 8.14)
These are often due to a crushing injury which can produce a wide variety

191 Fractures of the leg, ankle and foot

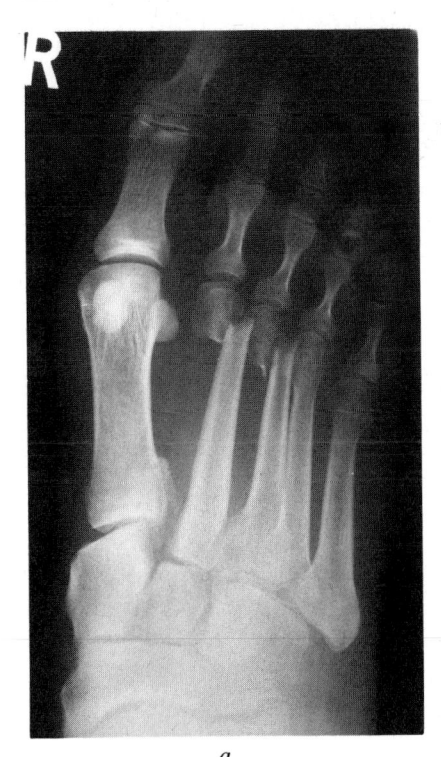

Fig. 8.14. *a*, A fracture-dislocation of the tarsometatarsal joint (with fractures of the 2nd and 3rd metatarsal heads). *b*, Dislocation of the 1st metatarsal.

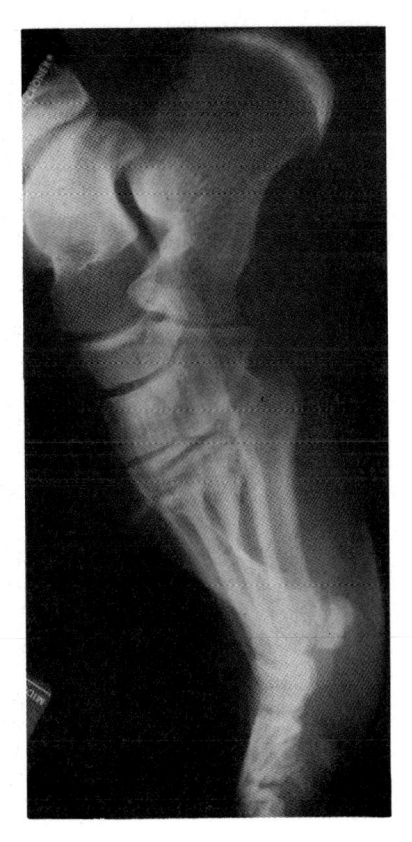

of fractures and dislocations. They were common in the Napoleonic Wars and originally described by Lisfranc. X-rays may show divergent dislocations of the 1st and 2nd metatarsals with the remaining metatarsals moving laterally. There may also be a fracture of the navicular or cuneiform bones. Occasionally there is comminution of the base of the 4th and 5th metatarsals with a fracture of the cuboid.

Diagnosis
There is often marked pain and swelling over the forefoot due to the crushing injury.

Treatment
Manipulation is often successful but the arch of the foot must be restored. If there is interposition of tendons (especially the anterior tibial tendon between the navicular and first cuneiform) open reduction may have to be performed. The fractures can be fixed with plates and screws or by Steinmann pins inserted

192 An outline of fractures and dislocations

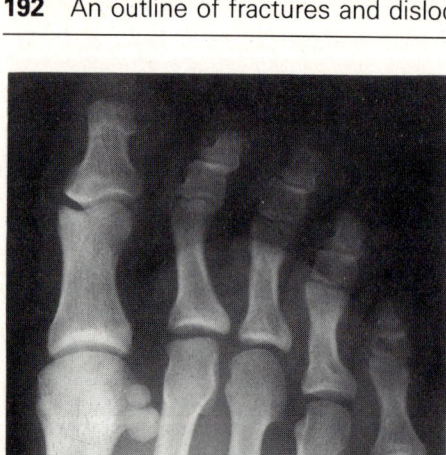

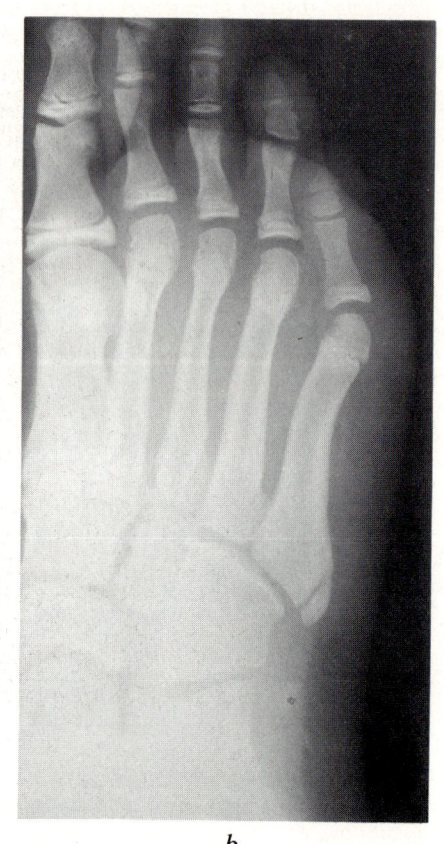

Fig. 8.15. *a*, Transverse fracture 3rd metatarsal. *b*, Avulsion injury base of 5th metatarsal.

through the metatarsals into the tarsal bones. The circulation in the foot must be observed closely for 48 hours, while skin necrosis is not uncommon. No weight-bearing is allowed for 6 weeks, with a plaster (below-knee) being used for 3–4 weeks.

Fractures of the Metatarsals (*Figs.* 8.14, 8.15)

These are commonly displaced and due to direct violence. Occasionally a *stress fracture* occurs in the 2nd or 3rd metatarsal and is known as a march fracture. Fractures without displacement need a below-knee plaster for 3 weeks. However, if displacement occurs the plaster must be moulded to ensure a correct longitudinal and transverse arch. Displacement may require internal fixation with screws or wires.

An *avulsion injury* may occur at the base of the *5th metatarsal* (*Fig.* 8.14*b*). This is due to the pull of the peroneus brevis tendon. Such an injury should be treated with strapping for 2–3 weeks or a below-knee walking plaster, depending on the degree of discomfort.

Fig. 8.16. Dislocation of the terminal phalanx of little toe.

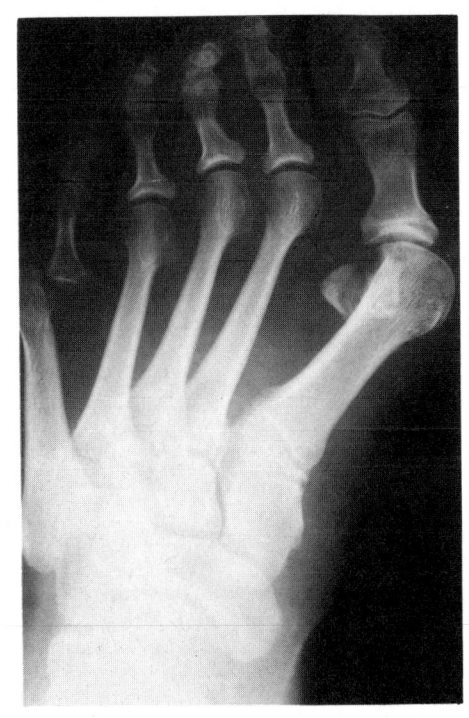

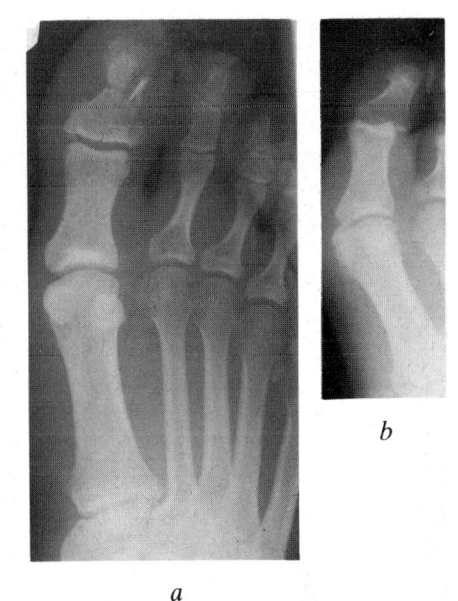

Fig. 8.17. a, Fracture of the terminal phalanx of great toe (often compound). *b*, Dislocation of the terminal phalanx of great toe.

Dislocation of the Metatarsophalangeal Joint
These are uncommon (*Fig.* 8.16) and usually the great toe is involved.

Diagnosis
The deformity is obvious.

Treatment
Closed reduction under general anaesthetic. Occasionally the soft tissues can prevent reduction and surgery is required. A below-knee plaster is used for 3–4 weeks.

Fractures of the Toes
These are usually the result of a crushing injury and the terminal phalanx of the great toe is most often affected (*Fig.* 8.17*a*). As a rule displacement of the fragments is minimal and injuries can be treated by strapping one toe to another for 2–3 weeks.

Dislocation of the Terminal Phalanx
This is easily recognized clinically and on X-rays (*Fig.* 8.17*b*). Reduction is simply achieved under local or general anaesthesia; strapping is used for 1–2 weeks.

Bibliography

Chapter 1

Bennett A. and Harvey W. (1981) Prostaglandins in orthopaedics. *J. Bone Joint Surg.* **63B**, 152.
Dove J. (1980) Complete fractures of the femur in Paget's disease of bone. *J. Bone Joint Surg.* **62B**, 12.
Friedlaender G. E. (1982) Current concepts review: bone-banking. *J. Bone Joint Surg.* **64A**, 307.
Greenfield G. B. (1975) *Radiology of Bone Diseases*, 2nd ed. Philadelphia, Lippincott; Oxford, Blackwell Scientific Publications.
McKibbin B. (1978) The biology of fracture healing in long bones. *J. Bone Joint Surg.* **60B**, 150.
Mickelson M. R. and Bonfiglio M. (1976) Pathological fractures in the proximal part of the femur treated by Zickel-nail fixation. *J. Bone Joint Surg.* **58A**, 1067.
Nordin B. E. C. (ed.) (1976) *Calcium, Phosphate and Magnesium Metabolism*. Edinburgh, Churchill Livingstone.
Osmond-Clarke H. (1950) Half a century of orthopaedic progress in Great Britain. *J. Bone Joint Surg.* **32B**, 620.
Owen R., Goodfellow J. and Bullough P. (ed.) (1980) *Scientific Foundations of Orthopaedics and Traumatology*. London, Heinemann.
Röntgen W. C. (1896) On a new kind of rays. *Nature*, **53**, 274, 377.
Sevitt S. (1981) *Bone Repair and Fracture Healing in Man*. Edinburgh, Churchill Livingstone.
Shanks S. C. and Kerley P. (ed.) (1971) *A Text-book of X-ray Diagnosis*, 4th ed. Vol. VI, Bones, Joints and Soft Tissues. London, Lewis.
Woods C. G. (1972) *Diagnostic Orthopaedic Pathology*. Oxford, Blackwell Scientific Publications.
Wynne-Davies R. and Fairbank T. J. (1976) *Fairbank's Atlas of General Affections of the Skeleton*, 2nd ed. Edinburgh, Churchill Livingstone.

Chapter 2

Adams J. C. (1980) *Standard Orthopaedic Operations*, 2nd ed. Edinburgh, Churchill Livingstone.
Anderson L. D. (1965) Compression plate fixation and the effect of different types of internal fixation on fracture healing. (Instructional Course Lecture, American Academy of Orthopaedic Surgeons.) *J. Bone Joint Surg.* **47A**, 191.
Attenborough C. G. (1953) Remodelling of humerus after supracondylar fractures in childhood. *J. Bone Joint Surg.* **35B**, 386.

Bibliography

Bleck E. E., Duckworth N. and Hunter N. (1974) *Atlas of Plaster Cast Techniques.* London, Lloyd-Luke.

Böhler L. (1929) *The Treatment of Fractures.* Vienna, Maudrich.

Bowker P. et al. (1981) A biomechanical study of cast-brace treatment of femoral shaft fractures. *J. Bone Joint Surg.* **63B**, 7.

Brookes M. (1971) *The Blood Supply of Bone. An Approach to Bone Biology.* London, Butterworth.

Chalmers J., Gray D. H. and Rush J. (1975) Observations on induction of bone in soft tissues. *J. Bone Joint Surg.* **57B**, 36.

Johnson R. M. (ed.) (1980) *Advances in External Fixation.* Chicago, Year Book.

Küntscher G. (1965) Intramedullary surgical technique and its place in orthopaedic surgery. (Instructional Course Lecture, American Academy of Orthopaedic Surgeons.) *J. Bone Joint Surg.* **47A**, 809.

Lister J. (1867) On a new method of treating compound fracture, abscess, etc., with observations on the conditions of suppuration. *Lancet* **1**, 326.

Mattingly S. (ed.) (1981) *Rehabilitation Today.* London, Update.

Müller M. E., Allgöwer M. and Willenegger H. (1979) *Manual of Internal Fixation,* 2nd ed. Berlin-Heidelberg-New York, Springer-Verlag.

Parry C. B. Wynn (1981) *Rehabilitation of the Hand,* 4th ed. London, Butterworth.

Sharrard W. J. W., Sutcliffe M. L., Robson M. J. et al. (1982) The treatment of fibrous non-union of fractures by pulsing electromagnetic stimulation. *J. Bone Joint Surg.* **64B**, 189.

Stewart J. D. M. (1975) *Traction and Orthopaedic Appliances.* Edinburgh, Churchill Livingstone.

Stimson L. A. (1900) An easy method of reducing dislocations of the shoulder and hip. *M. Rec.* **57**, 356.

Uhthoff H. K. (ed.) (1982) *Current Concepts of External Fixation of Fractures.* Berlin, Springer-Verlag.

Williams D. (ed.) (1976) *Biocompatibility of Implant Materials.* London, Sector Publishing Ltd for Pitman Medical.

Chapter 3

Akbarnia B., Torg J. S., Kilpatrick J. et al. (1974) Manifestations of the battered child syndrome. *J. Bone Joint Surg.* **56A**, 1159.

Brighton C. T., Friedenberg Z. B., Zemsky L. M. et al. (1975) Direct current stimulation of non-union and congenital pseudarthroses. *J. Bone Joint Surg.* **57A**, 368.

Brown P. W. (1973) The open fracture. *Clin. Orthop.* **96**, 254.

Central Health Services Council (1970) *The Battered Baby.* London, HMSO.

Eastcott H. H. G. (1973) *Arterial Surgery,* 2nd ed. London, Pitman Medical.

Eisenberg K. S., Sheft D. J. and Murray W. R. (1972) Posterior dislocation of the hip producing lumbosacral nerve-root avulsion. *J. Bone Joint Surg.* **54A**, 1083.

Flint, L. M., Brown A., Richardson J. D. et al. (1979) Definitive control of bleeding from severe pelvic fractures. *Am. Surg.* **189**, 709.

Gossling H. R., Ellison L. H. and Degraff A. C. (1974) Fat embolism: the role of respiratory failure and its treatment. *J. Bone Joint Surg.* **56A**, 1327.

Holden C. E. A. (1979) The pathology and prevention of Volkmann's ischaemic contracture. *J. Bone Joint Surg.* **61B**, 296.

Hood R. W., Bird C. B., Eidemiller L. E. et al. (1978) Ischemia as a cause of non-union of a fracture. *J. Bone Joint Surg.* **60A**, 126.

Medical Research Council (1976) *Aids to the Examination of the Peripheral Nervous System.* London, HMSO.

Mubarak S. J. and Hargens A. R. (1981) *Compartment Syndromes and Volkmann's Contracture.* Philadelphia, Saunders.

Patterson F. P. and Morton K. S. (1973) Neurological complications of fractures and dislocations of the pelvis. *J. Trauma* **12**, 103.
Patzakis M. J., Harvey J. P. and Ivler D. (1974) The role of antibiotics in the management of open fractures. *J. Bone Joint Surg.* **56A**, 532.
Proctor H. and London P. S. (1977) *Principles for First Aid for the Injured*, 3rd ed. London, Butterworth.
Rutherford W. H., Nelson P. G., Weston P. A. M. et al. (1980) *Accident and Emergency Medicine*. Tunbridge Wells, Pitman Medical.
Salter R. B. and Harris W. R. (1963) Injuries involving the epiphyseal plate. *J. Bone Joint Surg.* **45A**, 587.
Sevitt S. and Stoner H. B. (ed.) (1970) *The Pathology of Trauma*. (Supplement 4 of Journal of Clinical Pathology.) London, BMA.
Sunderland S. (1978) *Nerves and Nerve Injuries*, 2nd ed. Edinburgh, Livingstone.
Tachakra S. S. and Sevitt S. (1975) Hypoxaemia after fractures. *J. Bone Joint Surg.* **57B**, 197.
Van Urk H., Perlberger R. R. and Muller H. (1978) Selective arterial embolization for control of traumatic hemorrhage. *Surgery* **83**, 133.

Chapter 4

Allman F. L. (1967) Fractures and ligamentous injuries of the clavicle and its articulation. (Instructional Course Lecture, American Academy of Orthopaedic Surgeons.) *J. Bone Joint Surg.* **49A**, 774.
Arnold J. A., Nasca R. J. and Nelson C. L. (1977) Supracondylar fractures of the humerus. *J. Bone Joint Surg.* **59A**, 589.
Attenborough C. G. (1953) Remodelling of humerus after supracondylar fractures in childhood. *J. Bone Joint Surg.* **35B**, 386.
Baker D. M. and Stryker W. S. (1965) Acute complete acromio-clavicular separation. *JAMA* **192**, 689.
Conner A. N. and Smith M. G. H. (1970) Displaced fractures of the lateral humeral condyle in children. *J. Bone Joint Surg.* **52B**, 460.
Fowles J. V. and Kassab M. T. (1974) Fracture of the capitulum humeri: treatment by excision. *J. Bone Joint Surg.* **56A**, 794.
Hawkins R. J., Koppert G. and Johnston G. (1984) Recurrent posterior instability (subluxation) of the shoulder. *J. Bone Joint Surg.* **66A**, 169.
Holda M. E., Manoli A. and Lamont R. L. (1980) Epiphyseal separation of the distal end of the humerus with medial displacement. *J. Bone Joint Surg.* **62A**, 52.
Holstein A. and Lewis G. B. (1963) Fractures of the humerus with radial-nerve paralysis. *J. Bone Joint Surg.* **45A**, 1382.
Hovelius L. et al. (1983) The coracoid transfer for recurrent dislocation of the shoulder. *J. Bone Joint Surg.* **65A**, 921.
Hume A. C. (1957) Anterior dislocation of the head of the radius associated with undisplaced fracture of the olecranon in children. *J. Bone Joint Surg.* **39B**, 508.
Jefferiss C. D. (1977) Straight lateral traction in selected supracondylar fractures of the humerus in children. *Injury* **8**, 213.
Jones E. R. L. and Esah M. (1971) Displaced fractures of the neck of the radius in children. *J. Bone Joint Surg.* **53B**, 429.
Klenerman L. (1966) Fractures of the shaft of the humerus. *J. Bone Joint Surg.* **48B**, 105.
Leslie J. and Ryan T. (1962) The anterior axillary incision to approach the shoulder joint. *J. Bone Joint Surg.* **44A**, 1193.
Linscheid R. L. and Wheeler D. K. (1965) Elbow dislocations. *JAMA* **194**, 1171.
Loomer R. and Kokan P. (1976) Non-union in fractures of the humeral shaft. *Injury* **7**, 274.

Lunseth P. A., Chapman K. W. and Frankel V. H. (1975) Surgical treatment of chronic dislocation of the sternoclavicular joint. *J. Bone Joint Surg.* **57B**, 193.
McLaughlin H. (1952) Posterior dislocation of the shoulder. *J. Bone Joint Surg.* **34A**, 584.
Mills K. L. G. (1974) Severe injury of the upper end of the humerus. *Injury* **6**, 13.
Neer C. S. (1975) Displaced proximal humeral fractures. *J. Bone Joint Surg.* **52A**, 250.
Osborne G. and Cotterill P. (1966) Recurrent dislocations of the elbow. *J. Bone Joint Surg.* **48B**, 340.
Osmond-Clarke H. (1948) Habitual dislocation of the shoulder. *J. Bone Joint Surg.* **30B**, 19.
Palmer E. E., Niemann K. M., Vesely D. et al. (1978) Supracondylar fracture of the humerus in children. *J. Bone Joint Surg.* **60A**, 653.
Riseborough E. J. and Radin E. L. (1969) Intercondylar T fractures of the humerus in the adult. *J. Bone Joint Surg.* **51A**, 130.
Rowe C. R., Pierce D. S. and Clarke J. G. (1973) Voluntary dislocation of the shoulder. *J. Bone Joint Surg.* **55A**, 445.
Sarmiento A., Kinman P. B., Galvin E. G. et al. (1977) Functional bracing of fractures of the shaft of the humerus. *J. Bone Joint Surg.* **59A**, 596.
Scott J. C. and Orr M. M. (1973) Injuries to the acromio-clavicular joint. *Injury* **5**, 13.
Soltanpur A. (1978) Anterior supracondylar fracture of the humerus (flexion type). *J. Bone Joint Surg.* **60B**, 383.
Wilkins R. M. and Johnston R. M. (1983) Ununited fractures of the clavicle. *J. Bone Joint Surg.* **65A**, 773.

Chapter 5

Aitken A. P. and Nalebuff E. A. (1960) Volar transnavicular perilunar dislocation of the carpus. *J. Bone Joint Surg.* **42A**, 1051.
Anderson L. D., Sisk T. D., Tooms R. E. et al. (1975) Compression-plate fixation in acute diaphyseal fractures of the radius and ulna. *J. Bone Joint Surg.* **57A**, 287.
Borgeskov S., Christiansen B., Kjaer A. et al. (1966) Fractures of the carpal bones. *Acta Orthop. Scand.* **37**, 276.
Bruce H. E., Harvey J. P. and Wilson J. C. (1974) Monteggia fractures. *J. Bone Joint Surg.* **56A**, 1563.
Campbell R. D., Lance E. M. and Yeoh C. B. (1964) Lunate and perilunar dislocations. *J. Bone Joint Surg.* **46B**, 55.
Campbell V. and Waddell J. P. (1980) Surgical treatment of radial head fractures. *J. Bone Joint Surg.* **62B**, 130.
Cooney W. P., Dobyns J. H. and Linscheid R. L. (1980) Fractures of the scaphoid: a rational approach to management. *Clin. Orthop.* **149**, 90.
Coonrad R. W. and Goldner J. L. (1968) A study of the pathological findings and treatment in soft-tissue injury of the thumb metacarpophalangeal joint. *J. Bone Joint Surg.* **50A**, 439.
Dowling J. J. and Blackwell S. jun. (1961) Comminuted Colles' fractures. *J. Bone Joint Surg.* **43A**, 657.
Du Toit F. P. and Gräbe R. P. (1979) Isolated fractures of the shaft of the ulna. *S. Afr. Med. J.* **56**, 21.
Ellis J. (1965) Smith's and Barton's fractures. *J. Bone Joint Surg.* **47B**, 724.
Fernandez D. L. (1982) Correction of post-traumatic wrist deformity in adults by osteotomy, bone-grafting and internal fixation. *J. Bone Joint Surg.* **64A**, 1164.
Fisk G. R. (1984) The wrist. *J. Bone Joint Surg.* **66B**, 396.
Green D. P. and Anderson J. R. (1973) Closed reduction and percutaneous pin fixation of fractured phalanges. *J. Bone Joint Surg.* **55A**, 1651.
Griffiths J. C. (1964) Fractures at the base of the first metacarpal bone. *J. Bone Joint Surg.* **46B**, 712.

Kim W. C. et al. (1983) Failure of treatment of ununited fractures of the carpal scaphoid. *J. Bone Joint Surg.* **65A**, 985.
Linden W. van der and Ericson R. (1981) Colles' fracture. *J. Bone Joint Surg.* **63A**, 1285.
Mikic Z. Dj. (1975) Galeazzi fracture-dislocations. *J. Bone Joint Surg.* **57A**, 1071.
Pollen A. G. (1968) The conservative treatment of Bennett's fracture-subluxation of the thumb metacarpal. *J. Bone Joint Surg.* **50B**, 91.
Samilson R. L. and Prieto V. (1983) Dislocation arthropathy of the shoulder. *J. Bone Joint Surg.* **65A**, 456.
Sarmiento A., Kinman P. B., Murphy R. B. et al. (1976) Treatment of ulnar fractures by functional bracing. *J. Bone Joint Surg.* **58A**, 1104.
Schiller M. G. (1976) Intravenous regional anesthesia for closed treatment of fractures and dislocations of the upper extremities. *Clin. Orthop.* **118**, 25.
Smaill G. B. (1965) Long-term follow-up of Colles' fracture. *J. Bone Joint Surg.* **47B**, 80.
Wright T. A. (1968) Early mobilization in fractures of the metacarpals and phalanges. *Can. J. Surg.* **11**, 491.

Chapter 6

Bedbrook G. M. (1979) Spinal injuries with tetraplegia and paraplegia. *J. Bone Joint Surg.* **61B**, 267.
Bohlman H. H. (1979) Acute fractures and dislocations of the cervical spine. *J. Bone Joint Surg.* **61A**, 1119.
Boshch A., Stauffer E. S. and Nickel V. L. (1977) The risk of neurological damage with fractures of the vertebrae. *J. Trauma* **17**, 126.
Braakman R. and Penning L. (1976) Injuries of the cervical spine. In: *Injuries of the Spine and Spinal Cord*, **26**, 227. New York, Elsevier.
Burke D. C. (1971) Hyperextension injuries of the spine. *J. Bone Joint Surg.* **53B**, 3.
Christensen F. et al. (1978) Computed tomography for a bursting fracture of the lumbar spine. *J. Bone Joint Surg.* **60A,** 1108.
Davies W. E., Morris J. H. and Hill V. (1980) An analysis of conservative (non-surgical) management of thoraco-lumbar fractures and fracture-dislocations with neural damage. *J. Bone Joint Surg.* **62A**, 1324.
De Oliveira J. C. (1978) A new type of fracture-dislocation of the thoracolumbar spine. *J. Bone Joint Surg.* **60A**, 481.
Effendi B. et al. (1981) Fractures of the ring of the axis. *J. Bone Joint Surg.* **63B**, 319.
Fielding J. W. and Hawkins R. J. (1977) Atlanto-axial rotatory fixation. *J. Bone Joint Surg.* **59A**, 37.
Flesch J. R., Leider L. L., Erickson D. L. et al. (1977) Harrington instrumentation and spine fusion for unstable fractures and fracture-dislocations of the thoracic and lumbar spine. *J. Bone Joint Surg.* **59A**, 143.
Handelberg F., Bellemans M. A., Opdecam P. et al. (1981) The use of computerized tomography in the diagnosis of thoracolumbar injury. *J. Bone Joint Surg.* **63B**, 336.
Holdsworth F. W. (1970) Fractures dislocations, and fracture-dislocations of the spine. *J. Bone Joint Surg.* **52A**, 1534.
Prolo D. J., Runnels J. B. and Jameson R. M. (1973) The injured cervical spine. Immediate and long-term immobilization with the halo. *JAMA* **224**, 591.
Ryan M. D. and Taylor T. K. F. (1982) Odontoid fractures. *J. Bone Joint Surg.* **64B**, 416.
Schneider R. C., Livingstone K. E., Cave A. J. E. et al. (1965) 'Hangman's fracture' of the cervical spine. *J. Neurosurg.* **22**, 141.
Smith W. S. and Kaufer H. (1969) Patterns and mechanisms of lumbar injuries associated with lap seat belts. *J. Bone Joint Surg.* **51A**, 239.

Chapter 7

Allen W. C. and Price C. T. (1978) Ligament repair in the knee with preservation of the meniscus. *J. Bone Joint Surg.* **60A**, 61.
Armour P. and Coates R. (1979) The treatment of subcapital femoral fractures by primary total hip replacement. *J. Bone Joint Surg.* **61B**, 386.
Barnes R., Brown J. T., Garden R. S. et al. (1976) Subcapital fractures of the femur. *J. Bone Joint Surg.* **58B**, 2.
Canale S. T. and Manugian A. H. (1979) Irreducible traumatic dislocations of the hip. *J. Bone Joint Surg.* **61A**, 7.
Carnesale P. G., Stewart M. J. and Barnes S. N. (1975) Acetabular disruption and central fracture-dislocation of the hip. *J. Bone Joint Surg.* **57A**, 1054.
Casey M. J. and Chapman M. W. (1979) Ipsilateral concomitant fractures of the hip and femoral shaft. *J. Bone Joint Surg.* **61A**, 503.
Catto M. (1965) A histological study of avascular necrosis of the femoral head after transcervical fracture. *J. Bone Joint Surg.* **47B**, 749.
Cruess R. L., Daoud H. and O'Farrell T. (1982) Quadricepsplasty. *J. Bone Joint Surg.* **63B**, 194.
D'Arcy J. and Devas M. (1976) Treatment of fractures of the femoral neck by replacement with a Thompson prosthesis. *J. Bone Joint Surg.* **58B**, 279.
Dehne E. and Immermann E. W. (1951) Dislocation of the hip combined with fracture of the shaft of the femur on the same side. *J. Bone Joint Surg.* **33A**, 731.
De Lee J. C., Evans J. A. and Thomas J. (1980) Anterior dislocation of the hip and associated femoral head fractures. *J. Bone Joint Surg.* **62A**, 960.
Dunn H. K. and Hess W. E. (1976) Total hip reconstruction in chronically dislocated hips. *J. Bone Joint Surg.* **58A**, 838.
Fountain S. S., Hamilton R. D. and Jameson R. M. (1977) Transverse fractures of the sacrum. *J. Bone Joint Surg.* **59A**, 486.
Garden R. S. (1971) Malreduction and avascular necrosis in subcapital fractures of the femur. *J. Bone Joint Surg.* **53B**, 183.
Hansen S. T. and Winquist R. A. (1978) Closed intramedullary nailing of fracture of the femoral shaft. Part II: Technical considerations. In: Instructional Course Lectures, The American Academy of Orthopaedic Surgeons, **27**, 90.
Holm C. L. (1973) Treatment of pelvic fractures and dislocation. *Clin. Orthop.* **97**, 97.
Hughston J. C., Andrews J. R., Cross M. J. et al. (1976) Classification of knee ligament instabilities. Part I: The medial compartment and cruciate ligaments. *J. Bone Joint Surg.* **58A**, 159.
Hughston J. C., Andrews J. R., Cross M. J. et al. (1976) Classification of knee ligament instabilities. Part II: The lateral compartment. *J. Bone Joint Surg.* **58A**, 173.
Johnson J. T. H. and Crothers O. (1975) Nailing versus prosthesis for femoral neck fractures. *J. Bone Joint Surg.* **57A**, 686.
Jones C. W., Morris J., Shea J. et al. (1977) A comparison of the treatment of trochanteric fractures of the femur by internal fixation with a nail plate and the Ender technique. *Injury* **9**, 35.
Judet R., Judet J. and Letournel E. (1964) Fractures of the acetabulum: classification and surgical approaches for open reduction. *J. Bone Joint Surg.* **46A**, 1615.
Kaufer H., Matthews L. S. and Sonstegard D. (1974) Stable fixation of intertrochanteric fractures. *J. Bone Joint Surg.* **56A**, 899.
McDaniel W. J. and Dameron T. B. (1980) Untreated ruptures of the anterior cruciate ligament. *J. Bone Joint Surg.* **62A**, 696.
Miller C. W. (1978) Survival and ambulation following hip fracture. *J. Bone Joint Surg.* **60A**, 930.
Moore T. M., Meyers M. H. and Harvey J. P. (1976) Collateral ligament laxity of the knee. *J. Bone Joint Surg.* **58A**, 594.

Muckle D. S. (ed.) (1977) *Femoral Neck Fractures*. London, Chapman and Hall.
Muckle D. S. and Miscony Z. (1980) Fractures of the femoral neck in the 'young' elderly. *Injury* **12**, 41.
Muckle D. S. and Siddiqi S. (1982) Ender's nails in femoral shaft fractures. *Injury* **13**, 287.
Neer C. S., Grantham S. A. and Shelton M. L. (1967) Supracondylar fracture of the adult femur. *J. Bone Joint Surg.* **49A**, 591.
Peltier L. F. (1965) Complications associated with fractures of the pelvis. *J. Bone Joint Surg.* **47A**, 1060.
Ratcliff A. H. C. (1974) Fractures of the neck of the femur in children. *Orthop. Clinics N. Am.* **51**, 903.
Rorabeck C. H. and Bobechko W. P. (1976) Acute dislocation of the patella with osteochondral fracture. *J. Bone Joint Surg.* **58B**, 237.
Rothwell A. G. (1982) Closed Küntscher nailing for comminuted femoral shaft fractures. *J. Bone Joint Surg.* **64B**, 12.
Rowe C. R. and Lowell J. D. (1961) Prognosis of fractures of the acetabulum. *J. Bone Joint Surg.* **43A**, 30.
Seinsheimer F. (1978) Subtrochanteric fractures of the femur. *J. Bone Joint Surg.* **60A**, 300.
Sharp I. K. (1973) Plate fixation of disrupted symphysis pubis. *J. Bone Joint Surg.* **55B**, 618.
Swiontkowski M. F., Hansen S. T. and Kellam J. (1984) Ipsilateral fractures of the femoral neck and shaft. *J. Bone Joint Surg.* **66A**, 260.
Tipton W. W., D'Ambrosia R. D. and Ryle G. P. (1975) Non-operative management of central fracture-dislocation of the hip. *J. Bone Joint Surg.* **57A**, 888.
Torg J. S., Conrad W. and Kalen U. (1976) Clinical diagnosis of anterior cruciate ligament instability in the athlete. *Am. J. Sports Med.* **4**, 84.
Trillat A., Dejour H. and Bost J. (1975) Unicondylar fractures of the femur. *Rev. Chir. Orthop.* **61**, 611.
Trueta J. and Harrison M. H. M. (1953) The normal vascular anatomy of the femoral head in adult man. *J. Bone Joint Surg.* **35B**, 442.
Zickel R. E. (1976) An intramedullary fixation device for the proximal part of the femur. *J. Bone Joint Surg.* **58A**, 866.

Chapter 8

Bonnin J. G. (1965) Injury to the ligaments of the ankle. *J. Bone Joint Surg.* **47B**, 609.
Brown P. W. (1974) The early weight-bearing treatment of tibial shaft fractures. *Clin. Orthop.* **105**, 167.
Burwell H. N. and Charnley A. (1965) The treatment of displaced fractures at the ankle by rigid internal fixation and early joint movement. *J. Bone Joint Surg.* **47B**, 34.
Chrisman O. D. and Snook G. A. (1969) Reconstruction of lateral ligament tears of the ankle. *J. Bone Joint Surg.* **51A**, 904.
Clerny G., Jones R. E. and Byrd S. (1981) Complex open tibial fractures managed with external fixation and pedicle muscle flaps. *J. Bone Joint Surg.* **63B**, 630.
Detenbeck L. C. and Kelly P. J. (1969) Total dislocation of the talus. *J. Bone Joint Surg.* **51A**, 283.
Eventov T., Salama R., Goodwin D. R. A. et al. (1978) An evaluation of surgical and conservative treatment of fractures of the ankle in 200 patients. *J. Trauma* **18**, 271.
Joy G., Patzakis M. J. and Harvey J. P. (1974) Precise evaluation of the reduction of severe ankle fractures. *J. Bone Joint Surg.* **56A**, 979.
Keliger B. (1976) Injuries of the talus and its joints. *Clin. Orthop.* **121**, 243.
Kenwright J. and Taylor R. G. (1970) Major injuries of the talus. *J. Bone Joint Surg.* **52B**, 36.

Bibliography

Lambert K. L. (1971) The weight-bearing function of the fibula. *J. Bone Joint Surg.* **53A**, 507.

Lottes J. O., Hill L. J. and Key J. A. (1952) Closed reduction, plate fixation, and medullary nailing of fractures of both bones of the leg. *J. Bone Joint Surg.* **34A**, 861.

Main B. J. and Jowett R. L. (1975) Injuries of the midtarsal joint. *J. Bone Joint Surg.* **57B**, 89.

Muckle D. S. (1981) The unstable knee: a sequel to tibial fractures. *J. Bone Joint Surg.* **63B**, 628.

Muckle D. S. (1982) *Injuries in Sport*. 2nd ed. Bristol, Wright.

Muckle D. S. (1984) Open meniscectomy: enhanced recovery after synovial prostaglandin inhibition. *J. Bone Joint Surg.* **66B**, 193.

Nade S. and Monahan P. R. W. (1973) Fractures of the calcaneum: a study of the long-term prognosis. *Injury* **4**, 201.

Pankovich A. M. (1978) Fracture of the fibula proximal to the distal tibiofibular syndesmosis. *J. Bone Joint Surg.* **60A**, 221.

Pettrone F. A. et al. (1983) Quantitative criteria for prediction of the results after displaced fracture of the ankle. *J. Bone Joint Surg.* **65A**, 667.

Rasmussen P. S. (1973) Tibial condylar fractures. *J. Bone Joint Surg.* **55A**, 1334.

Rowe C. R., Sakellarides H. T., Freeman P. A. et al. (1963) Fracture of the os calcis. *JAMA* **184**, 92.

Sarkisian J. S. and Cody G. W. (1976) Closed treatment of ankle fractures. A new criterion for evaluation—A review of 250 cases. *J. Trauma* **16**, 323.

Sarmiento A. (1974) Functional bracing of tibial fractures. *Clin. Orthop.* **105**, 202.

Staples O. S. (1975) Ruptures of the fibular collateral ligaments of the ankle. *J. Bone Joint Surg.* **57A**, 101.

Trickey E. L. (1975) Treatment of fractures of the calcaneus. *J. Bone Joint Surg.* **57B**, 411.

Wilson D. W. (1972) Injuries of the tarso-metatarsal joints. *J. Bone Joint Surg.* **54B**, 677.

Yablon I. G., Heller F. G. and Shouse L. (1979) The key role of the lateral malleolus in displaced fractures of the ankle. *J. Bone Joint Surg.* **59A**, 169.

Zuchman J. and Maurer P. (1969) Two-level fractures of the tibia. *J. Bone Joint Surg.* **51B**, 686.

Index

Abdominal injury, 65
Acetabulum, fractures, 137, 140, 141
Acromioclavicular dislocation, 74, 76
Adhesions, joint, 59
Ankle, dislocations, 180, 186
    fractures, 180, 182
    sprains, 180
Atlas injuries, 122
Avascular necrosis, 44, 45, 148, 150, 188
Axis injuries, 122

Barton's fracture, 107
Battered baby, 68
Bennett's fracture-dislocation, 116
Bosworth fracture, 187
Boutonnière deformity, 120
Bronchopneumonia, 59
Burns, 65

Calcaneus, fractures, 188
Callus, 14
Capitate subluxation, 114
Carpal, dislocations, 109, 113, 114
Carpal, fractures, 109
Cervical spine, dislocations, 123
    fractures, 122, 124, 127, 128
    fracture-dislocations, 122, 127, 128
Children's fractures, 67
Clavicle, fractures, 70
Coccyx, fractures, 135
Colles fracture, 105
Compartmental syndromes, 178
Compound fractures, 12, 13
Cord damage, 130, 134
Coronoid fracture, 94
Coxa vara, 149

Crush syndrome, 65
Cuboid fracture, 190
Cuneiform fracture, 190

Deep vein thrombosis, 60
Dislocations (*see also under individual joint*), 15, 36
    avulsion injuries, 17
    chronic or missed, 17
    diagnosis, 16
    immobilization, 36
    recurrent, 36
    treatment, 18, 36
    X-rays, 18

Elbow injuries, 89
    dislocations, 91
    recurrent dislocation, 92
Electromagnetic therapy, 43
External fixation, 34, 35, 177

Fat embolism, 62
Forearm fractures, 93, 101
Femur, epiphysis (slipped), 151
    greater trochanter, 151
    head, fractures, 141
    lesser trochanter, 152
    neck, fractures, 143, 145, 151
    neck, fractures (children), 150, 156
    neck, stress fracture, 156
    shaft, fractures, 143, 158, 161
    shaft, fractures (children), 161
    supracondylar, 161
Fibula fractures, 173, 179

204 Index

Foot, dislocations, 187
   fractures, 187
Fractures (*see also under individual bones*)
   AO technique, 31
   around metal, 66
   in children, 67
   complications, 40
   delayed union, 40
   diagnosis, 5
   forces, 1
   functional bracing, 29
   immobilization, 23, 24, 28
   infection, 47
   introduction, 1
   mal-union, 46
   non-union, 40
   open and closed, 12
   open reduction, 30
   pathological, 6
   principles and treatment, 20
   radiological, 3
   rate of union, 14
   reduction, 20, 22, 30
   refracture, 47
   soft tissue injury, 4
   union, 30
Functional bracing, 29

Galeazzi fractures, 99
Gangrene, 49, 52

Hamate, subluxation, 114
Head injury, 64
Hip dislocation, 140, 159
   anterior, 144
   central, 144
   in children, 145
   posterior, 141
Humerus fractures, 83
   condyles, 89
   epicondyles, 89
   epiphyseal, 83, 89
   lower, 86
   shaft, 84
   supracondylar, 86
   upper, 83

Ilium, fractures, 137
Internal fixation, 31
Ischaemic necrosis, 49, 52, 102
Ischium, fractures, 137

Joint injury (*see also* Dislocations), 55

Kerbstone fracture, 186
Knee dislocation, 172
Knee ligament injuries, 4, 159, 166, 172
   anterior cruciate, 167
   medial, 167
   lateral, 167
   posterior cruciate, 169
   rotatory instability, 170
Knee, meniscal injury, 171

Ligament injuries, 4, 19, 159, 166
Lumbar spine, fractures, 131, 134
   fracture-dislocations, 131, 133
Lunate dislocation, 112, 113

Maisonneuve fracture, 186
Meniscal injury, 171
Metacarpal, dislocation, 141
   fractures, 115, 117
Metatarsal, fractures, 192
   fracture-dislocation, 190
Metatarsophalangeal dislocation, 193
Monteggia fracture, 97
Multiple injuries, 64
Muscle ischaemia, 52

Navicular fractures, 189
Nerve damage, 52, 53, 54, 102
Nuclear Magnetic Resonance, 5

Olecranon features, 93
Osgood–Schlatter's (acute), 172
Osteoarthritis, 57

Patella, dislocation, 164
   fractures, 164
   subluxation, 164
Pathological fractures, 6
Pelvis, fractures, 137
   fracture-dislocation, 139
Phalangeal, dislocations, 120
   fractures, 115, 120
Physiotherapy, 38, 39
Plaster-of-Paris, 24
Post-traumatic ossification, 55
Pressure sores, 63
Pseudo-boutonnière deformity, 120
Pubic ramus fractures, 137
Pulmonary embolism, 60, 61
Radius, anterior dislocation, 93, 95, 96, 97
   head fractures, 94

Index

Radius (*cont.*)
    lower (adults), 105
    lower (children), 103
    shaft, 99
    styloid process, 109
    with ulna, 96, 101
Refracture, 47
Respiratory obstruction, 64
Rib fractures, 136
Rotator cuff tears, 82

Sacro-iliac subluxation, 137
Sacrum, fractures, 135
Scaphoid, fractures, 107, 110, 112
Scapula, fractures, 73
Sciatic nerve injury, 143
Seat belt fracture, 134
Severe infections, 65
Shock, 64
Shortening, 57
Shoulder girdle, 70
Shoulder, anterior dislocation, 78
    dislocation, 76, 78
    fracture-dislocation, 80
    posterior dislocation, 79
    recurrent anterior, 81
    recurrent posterior, 81
    subluxation, 76
Shoulder-hand syndrome, 107
Skin problems, 65
Smith's fracture, 107
Soft tissue injuries, 4, 15, 16
Special problems, 65
Spinal injuries, 122
Sprains and strains, 19
Sternoclavicular joint dislocation, 74
Sternal fractures, 136
Subcapital fractures, 145
Subtrochanteric fractures, 155
Sudeck's atrophy, 56
Supracondylar, femur, 161
Supracondylar, humerus fractures, 86

Supraspinatus tears, 82
Swan-neck deformity, 121
Symphysis pubis dislocation, 137

Talus, fracture-dislocation, 187
Tarsometatarsal fracture-dislocation, 191
Tendon injuries, 19, 55
Thoracic spine fracture-dislocation, 130
Thumb, dislocations, 117
    fractures, 116
Tibia, fractures, 159, 173
    condylar, 173
    epiphyseal, 175
    shaft, 173, 175
    spines, 172
    stress fracture, 175
Tibiofibular (inferior) dislocation, 186
Tibiofibular (superior) dislocation, 180
Toes, dislocations, 193
    fractures, 193
Trochanteric fractures, 151

Ulna, dislocation, 93
    fractures, 96
    styloid, 109
    subluxation (lower), 109
    with radius, 96
Unstable joints, 38

Vascular injury, 49
Visceral injury, 58

X-rays, ancillary investigations, 5
    avascular changes, 44
    non-union, 41
    rule of two, 5